Breast Augmentation

Guest Editor

SCOTT L. SPEAR, MD

CLINICS IN PLASTIC SURGERY

www.plasticsurgery.theclinics.com

January 2009 • Volume 36 • Number 1

SAUNDERS an imprint of ELSEVIER, Inc.

W.B. SAUNDERS COMPANY
A Division of Elsevier Inc.

1600 John F. Kennedy Boulevard ● Suite 1800 ● Philadelphia, Pennsylvania 19103-2899

http://www.theclinics.com

CLINICS IN PLASTIC SURGERY Volume 36, Number 1
January 2009 ISSN 0094-1298, ISBN-13: 978-1-4377-0528-7, ISBN-10: 1-4377-0528-6

Editor: Barbara Cohen-Kligerman

Clinics in Plastic Surgery (ISSN 0094-1298) is published quarterly by Elsevier Inc., 360 Park Avenue South, New York, NY 10010-1710. Months of issue are January, April, July, and October. Business and Editorial Offices: 1600 John F. Kennedy Blvd., Suite 1800, Philadelphia, PA 19103-2899. Periodicals postage paid at New York, NY and additional mailing offices. Subscription prices are $352.00 per year for US individuals, $510.00 per year for US institutions, $177.00 per year for US students and residents, $400.00 per year for Canadian individuals, $596.00 per year for Canadian institutions, $454.00 per year for international individuals, $596.00 per year for international institutions, and $224.00 per year for Canadian and foreign students/residents. To receive student/resident rate, orders must be accompanied by name of affiliated institution, date of term, and the *signature* of program/residency coordinator on institution letterhead. Orders will be billed at individual rate until proof of status is received. Foreign air speed delivery is included in all *Clinics* subscription prices. All prices are subject to change without notice. **POSTMASTER:** Send address changes to *Clinics in Plastic Surgery*, Elsevier Periodicals Customer Service, 11830 Westline Industrial Drive, St. Louis, MO 63146. **Customer Service: 1-800-654-2452 (US). From outside the United States, call 1-314-453-7041. Fax: 1-314-453-5170. E-mail: JournalsCustomerService-usa@elsevier.com (for print support) and JournalsOnlineSupport-usa@elsevier.com (for online support).**

Reprints. For copies of 100 or more of articles in this publication, please contact the Commercial Reprints Department, Elsevier Inc., 360 Park Avenue South, New York, New York 10010-1710. Tel.: (+1) 212-633-3812; Fax: (+1) 212-462-1935; E-mail: reprints@elsevier.com.

Clinics in Plastic Surgery is covered in *Current Contents, EMBASE/Excerpta Medica, Science Citation Index, MEDLINE/ PubMed (Index Medicus), ASCA,* and *ISI/BIOMED.*

Printed and bound in the United Kingdom
Transferred to Digital Print 2011

Contributors

GUEST EDITOR

SCOTT L. SPEAR, MD
Professor and Chairman, Department of Plastic
Surgery, Georgetown University Hospital,
Washington, District of Columbia

AUTHORS

WILLIAM P. ADAMS Jr, MD
Associate Clinical Professor, Department
of Plastic Surgery, University of Texas
Southwestern Medical Center, Dallas, Texas

BRADLEY P. BENGTSON, MD
Associate Professor, Department of Plastic
Surgery, Medical Education and Research
Center & Plastic Surgery Associates, Grand
Rapids, Michigan

STEFAN J. CANO, PhD
Lecturer, Neurological Outcome Measures
Unit, Institute of Neurology, National Hospital
for Neurology and Neurosurgery, University
College London, London, England,
United Kingdom

MARK W. CLEMENS, MD
Resident, Department of Plastic Surgery,
Georgetown University Hospital, Washington,
District of Columbia

MARK A. CODNER, MD, FACS
Clinical Assistant Professor, Emory University
School of Medicine; and Paces Plastic Surgery
and Recovery Center, Atlanta, Georgia

JOSEPH H. DAYAN, MD
Chief Resident, Department of Plastic Surgery,
Georgetown University Hospital, Washington,
District of Columbia

ALLEN GABRIEL, MD
Director of Research, Department of Plastic
Surgery, Loma Linda University Medical
Center, Loma Linda, California

JESSE A. GOLDSTEIN, MD
Department of Plastic Surgery, Georgetown
University Hospital, Washington, District
of Columbia

DENNIS C. HAMMOND, MD
Center for Breast and Body Contouring, Grand
Rapids, Michigan

NEAL HANDEL, MD, FACS
Associate Clinical Professor, Division of Plastic
Surgery, The David Geffen School of Medicine,
University of California at Los Angeles,
Los Angeles, California

PER HEDÉN, MD, PhD
Associate Professor in Plastic Surgery,
Akademikliniken, Stockholm, Sweden

MARK JEWELL, MD
Assistant Clinical Professor, Plastic Surgery,
Oregon Health Science University, Eugene,
Oregon

ANNE F. KLASSEN, DPhil
Associate Professor, Department of Pediatrics,
McMaster University, Hamilton, Ontario,
Canada

G. PATRICK MAXWELL, MD
Clinical Professor of Surgery, Department
of Plastic Surgery, Loma Linda University
Medical Center, Loma Linda, California

COLLEEN McCARTHY, MD, MS
Assistant Professor, Department of Plastic
and Reconstructive Surgery, Memorial Sloan-
Kettering Cancer Center, New York, New York

MAURICE Y. NAHABEDIAN, MD, FACS
Associate Professor, Department of Plastic
Surgery, Georgetown University, Washington,
District of Columbia

SALVATORE J. PACELLA, MD, MBA
Attending Surgeon, Division of Plastic Surgery,
Scripps Clinic Medical Group, La Jolla,
California

PRANAY M. PARIKH, MD
Department of Plastic Surgery, Georgetown
University Hospital, Washington, District of
Columbia

KETAN PATEL, MD
Resident, Department of Plastic Surgery,
Georgetown University, Washington, District
of Columbia

ANDREA L. PUSIC, MD, MPH
Assistant Professor, Department of Plastic and
Reconstructive Surgery, Memorial Sloan-
Kettering Cancer Center, New York, New York

PATRICK L. REAVEY, MD
Research Fellow, Department of Plastic
and Reconstructive Surgery, Memorial

Sloan-Kettering Cancer Center, New York,
New York

AMIE SCOTT, BSc
Research Project Coordinator, Department
of Plastic and Reconstructive Surgery,
Memorial Sloan-Kettering Cancer Center,
New York, New York

SCOTT L. SPEAR, MD
Professor and Chairman, Department of
Plastic Surgery, Georgetown University
Hospital, Washington, District of
Columbia

STEVEN TEITELBAUM, MD, FACS
Assistant Clinical Professor of Plastic Surgery,
The David Geffen School of Medicine,
University of California at Los Angeles, Los
Angeles; and Private Practice, Santa Monica,
California

JUSTIN WEST, MD
Resident, Department of Plastic Surgery,
Georgetown University Hospital, Washington,
District of Columbia

Contents

is the accuracy and symmetry of the pocket creation, and the anatomically most critical aspect of this dissection lies at the inframammary fold. The inframammary approach unquestionably offers the greatest visualization of this area and results in the least damage to normal tissue.

The Periareolar Approach to Breast Augmentation   45

Dennis C. Hammond

Incision placement in patients undergoing augmentation mammaplasty is an important element of the overall strategic plan of the procedure. Whatever incision location is chosen, access to the breast must be sufficient to afford accurate dissection of the pocket, to allow easy insertion of the implant, and to provide for precise hemostasis. At the same time, the incision should be placed where the resulting scar will be inconspicuous and well hidden. For many surgeons, the periareolar approach satisfies all of these requirements. This article describes the various advantages associated with the periareolar incision for breast augmentation and provides the technical details to enable best use of the technique.

The Transaxillary Approach to Breast Augmentation   49

Salvatore J. Pacella and Mark A. Codner

The transaxillary approach to breast augmentation provides patients with an option for augmentation that avoids any visible scars on the breast. The versatility of the endoscopic technique allows the surgeon to reliably dissect the submuscular pocket under direct visualization and to control the position of the inframammary fold while still enabling the use of any of a wide variety of both saline and silicone implants. This article addresses issues related to patient selection and preoperative assessment of this technique as well as technical aspects of performing this operation. In addition, the article reviews postoperative management of the endoscopic augmentation patient and describes potential complications associated with this technique.

Transumbilical Breast Augmentation   63

Neal Handel

Transumbilical breast augmentation was first described in the literature more than 15 years ago. Since its introduction, this procedure has been controversial and has never been widely adopted by plastic surgeons. This article reviews the history of transumbilical breast augmentation; describes a simplified, nonendoscopic approach to insertion of saline implants via the umbilicus; and discusses the advantages, disadvantages, and limitations of this technique.

Form-Stable Silicone Gel Breast Implants   75

Mark Jewell

This article addresses the question of what is the optimal shape for a breast implant. It is oriented toward processes, system engineering, and operational excellence versus being a treatise on the author's personal technique.

Mastopexy combined with augmentations is considered to be a technically advanced and difficult procedure; thus, many surgeons recommend doing this procedure in two separate stages to minimize the risk for complications. A one-stage procedure has, however, several advantages. Even if one-stage mastopexy augmentations are more technically demanding to perform and even if a slightly increased risk for healing problems exists, these procedures can be performed safely if the planning and surgical technique are accurate. The planning and surgical technique described in this article have been used by the author for the past 10 years, with moderate modification in the twenty-first century, leading to a predictable outcome with a low degree of reoperations and complications. This article describes in detail the surgical technique and planning.

Primary augmentation/mastopexy is associated with a significantly higher complication rate than primary augmentation alone. Despite this, its popularity has steadily increased. This demand has led to the need for careful preoperative planning and surgical execution to minimize the most frequent complications. This article focuses on the authors' experience with the technical aspects of the procedure.

For more than 40 years capsular contracture has plagued plastic surgery as the most common complication of aesthetic and reconstructive breast surgery. This article reviews the basis for capsular contracture and defines the methods to prevent it and treat it when it occurs. Capsular contracture is most commonly a result of a subclinical colonization of the implant pocket with bacteria. Sound techniques—including precise, atraumatic, bloodless dissection; appropriate triple antibiotic breast pocket irrigation; and minimizing any points of contamination during the procedure—have produced very low capsular contracture rates. Treatment of capsular contracture is most often surgical total capsulectomy with site change when indicated and replacement with a new implant.

The management of common and uncommon problems following breast augmentation can pose a challenge in some situations. The diversity of these problems is remarkable and different principles and concepts should be adhered to for optimal management. This article reviews some of these problems and hopefully provides solutions for prevention and management.

Clinics in Plastic Surgery

THE CLINICS ARE NOW AVAILABLE ONLINE!

Access your subscription at:
www.theclinics.com

Clinics in Plastic Surgery

Preface

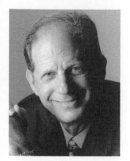

Scott L. Spear, MD
Guest Editor

This issue of the *Clinics in Plastic Surgery* follows by approximately 7 years the last volume on breast augmentation, which was edited by John Tebbetts. During these 7 years, both the surgery and the implants associated with breast augmentation have continued to evolve and improve. Most notably, silicone breast implants were approved by the FDA for sale in November 2006. At this moment, the next generation of silicone breast implants, described as cohesive gel, form stable, or "gummy bear" implants, are under review by the FDA and most likely will be approved by the end of 2008 or early 2009.

Surgical practices are also showing evidence of some change, with growing emphasis on improved patient education, preoperative planning, surgical technique, and algorithms for postoperative care.

It is certainly hoped by now that the implants used are more durable and will last longer. In addition, it is hoped, by better patient evaluation, preoperative planning, and surgical technique that there will be fewer complications and fewer patients who need to undergo revision.

This issue of the *Clinics in Plastic Surgery* on breast augmentation is a combination of technical articles, articles of historical interest, and articles describing overall patient management. Some of the material in the issue is evolutionary, while some is more revolutionary. It is my hope that by reading through the articles that follow, any surgeon involved in breast augmentation will have a stronger grasp of the milieu surrounding breast implants and breast augmentation. I also hope that by becoming familiar with the contents of this issue, the reader will be able to perform the surgery and care for the patient in a more competent fashion.

The process of elective breast implant surgery for breast augmentation has special elements. On the one hand, it has the potential for providing enormous value and benefit to the patient. An implant properly manufactured and designed, appropriately selected and placed in a technically excellent fashion has the potential to provide many years of benefit to the woman who receives it. On the other hand, because it is an implantable device, the surgery needs to be performed with the understanding that this has the potential for being a lifelong addition to the woman's life. The good may last for a long time, but any damage from the surgery or the implant has the potential for also leaving long-term and lasting effects.

The articles in this issue are designed to empower surgeons to take full advantage of this surgical opportunity so that the vast majority of women benefit and the fewest possible number of women are harmed by this well-intended surgery.

I would like to thank all of the contributors and authors to this issue of the *Clinics in Plastic Surgery*. The rewards for writing such manuscripts are few, but the service provided to the readers of this text is enormous.

Scott L. Spear, MD
Department of Plastic Surgery
Georgetown University Hospital
3800 Reservoir Road, NW, 1 PHC
Washington DC 20007

E-mail address:
spears@gunet.georgetown.edu

Clin Plastic Surg 36 (2009) xi
doi:10.1016/j.cps.2008.09.001

The Evolution of Breast Implants

G. Patrick Maxwell, MD, Allen Gabriel, MD*

KEYWORDS

• Breast • Implants • Gel • Augmentation

Female glandular hypomastia is a frequently encountered entity that occurs either developmentally or by postpartum involution. Historically, women have long sought breast enlargement to improve physical proportions, to foster a more feminine appearance, or to enhance self-image.

Following the introduction of the silicone gel prosthesis in 1962,[1] breast augmentation has become one of the most frequently performed operations in plastic surgery.[2] It is estimated that more than 1% of the adult female population in the United States (between 1 and 2 million) has undergone breast augmentation.[3] The women undergoing breast implantation have been scientifically scrutinized since its inception and found to range from outgoing healthy individuals with a desire for aesthetic improvement to women with depression, low self-esteem, negative body image, and sexual inhibitions.[4,5] The popularity of the procedure is thought to be based on the satisfaction of the patients' results.[6] Women in general have enhanced self-image, increased self-assurance, improved sexual functioning, and better interpersonal relationships after augmentation.[7]

Czerny[8] reported the first augmentation mammaplasty, in which he transferred a lipoma to the breast, in 1895. Longacre[9] attempted autogenous "flap" augmentations in the 1950s, and the use of various injectable substances, such as petroleum jelly, beeswax, shellac, and epoxy resin, soon followed.[10] Uchida[11] reported the use of injectable silicone in 1961. Solid materials implanted in the 1950s and early 1960s included polyurethane, Teflon, and polyvinyl alcohol formaldehyde (the Ivalon sponge).[10] Although none of these methods proved satisfactory, the introduction of the silicone

gel breast implant in 1962 by Cronin and Gerow[1] began the modern era of breast augmentation.

The silicone gel implants commercially available in the United States today are a refined and safer device than their predecessors. Silicone development evolved to meet the needs of the aircraft-engineering industry during World War II. Because of its softness and inert nature, it attracted interest from the medical sector and was soon evaluated as an implantable medical device by plastic surgical researchers.[12,13] The Cronin and Gerow mammary implant of the 1960s, which was manufactured by Dow Corning (Midland, Michigan),[1] was composed of a viscous silicone gel contained within a thick silicone shell in the shape of a teardrop. Seams were present at the periphery of the device, and Dacron fixation patches were placed on the posterior surfaces to help ensure proper position (**Fig. 1**). These early devices had such a high incidence of capsular contracture that a new generation of silicone implants was developed by various manufacturers in the mid to late 1970s to produce a more natural result. These implants were round and characterized by a seamless, thin, smooth silicone shell. There were no fixation patches, and the silicone gel was less viscous than in first-generation implants. Whereas the incidence of capsular contracture may have been improved somewhat, the incidence of silicone gel "bleed" and shell rupture was enhanced (especially from manufacturers who made very thin shells).[14] Gel bleed is a phenomenon whereby low-molecular-weight particles of silicone gel diffuse or leak through the silicone elastomer shell, giving a sticky feel to the surface. It has been theorized that silicone bleed could promote capsule

Department of Plastic Surgery, Loma Linda University Medical Center, Loma Linda, CA, USA
* Corresponding author.
E-mail address: gabrielallen@yahoo.com (A. Gabriel).

Clin Plastic Surg 36 (2009) 1–13
doi:10.1016/j.cps.2008.08.001

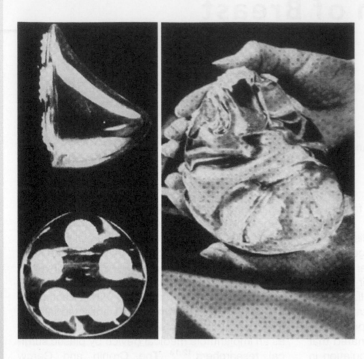

Fig. 1. The original Cronin-Gerow silicone implant introduced in 1962 had an anatomic (teardrop) shape, smooth surface, and posteriorly placed Dacron patches to help maintain the implant's position. (*From* Cronin TD, Gerow FJ. Augmentation mammoplasty: a new natural feel prosthesis. In: Transactions of the Third International Congress of Plastic Surgery, October 13–18, 1963. Amsterdam: Excerpta Medica Foundation; 1963. p. 41–9; with permission.)

contracture.[15,16] Whether it is caused by silicone bleed or other factors, capsule contracture has been the biggest clinical problem with the use of smooth-surfaced silicone gel implants.

The third generation of smooth-surfaced silicone implants, developed in the early to mid-1980s, focused on improving the strength and integrity of the silicone shell and on minimizing the silicone bleed phenomenon.[17,18] This generation of implants was characterized by two layers of high-performance elastomer with a thin fluorosilicone barrier coat in between (produced by McGhan Medical, Heyer-Schulte, Dow Corning, and Cox-Uphoff). There are data to suggest that these improvements enhanced shell life and lessened capsule contracture. Third-generation silicone gel implants with the application of a textured surface can be considered fourth-generation devices, and cohesive silicone gel-filled implants can be considered fifth-generation devices (**Table 1**). These are discussed in the following paragraphs.

SALINE-FILLED IMPLANTS

The inflatable saline-filled implant was first reported by Arion[19] in France in 1965. The impetus for its development was to allow smaller incisions through which a noninflated device could be inserted and then inflated with its liquid filler material. Saline implants were subsequently developed by American manufacturers and underwent clinical evaluation in the early 1970s.[20,21] The

emphasis for the inception of and interest in these devices was focused on their inflatable nature, allowing smaller incisions, not on the character or safety of the liquid filler or an attempt to lessen the rates of capsular contracture.

Although it is generally accepted that the contracture rate with saline implants is relatively low, two qualities of these devices have plagued their clinical use. The foremost was their deflation rate. The original French implant manufactured by Simaplast was found to have a deflation rate near 75% at 3 years and was withdrawn from the market. Heyer-Schulte developed an American saline implant in 1968. Whereas silicone gel implant shells are high-temperature vulcanized platinum cured, the shells for saline-filled implants were made thicker and cured by a room-temperature vulcanized process. This significantly decreased the deflation rate, and all American-made saline implants have since had shells cured by this process.[22]

A second factor found to increase deflation rates was valve failure.[23] The original Heyer-Schulte prosthesis had a retention (leaflet) valve, which was subsequently replaced by a diaphragm valve. Saline implants currently manufactured in the United States by Mentor (which purchased Heyer-Schulte) and Allergan (formerly INAMED and McGhan Medical) have diaphragm valves and room-temperature vulcanized cured shells.

The other characteristic of saline implants that has been a problem relates to the saline itself, which may transmit visible surface wrinkles and

Table 1
Evolution of silicone gel-filled breast implants

First Generation (1962–1970)	Thick, two-piece shell
	Smooth surface with Dacron fixation patches
	Anatomically-shaped (teardrop)
	Viscous silicone gel
Second Generation (1970–1982)	Thin, slightly permeable shell
	Smooth surface (no Dacron patches)
	Round shape
	Less viscous silicone gel
Third Generation (1982–1992)	Thick, strong, low-bleed shell
	Smooth surface
	Round shape
	More viscous silicone gel
Fourth Generation (1993–present)	Thick, strong, low-bleed shell[a]
	Smooth and textured surfaces
	Round and anatomically-shaped
	More viscous (cohesive) silicone gel[a]
Fifth Generation (1993–present)	Thick, strong, low-bleed shell[a]
	Smooth and textured surfaces
	Round and diverse anatomical shapes
	Enhanced cohesive & form-stable silicone gel

[a] In accordance with technical parameters established by the ASTM.

a knuckle-like feel in volumetrically underfilled devices. When the device is overfilled, it may feel and look like a firm ball and transmit a peripheral "scalloping" look. For these reasons, saline implants historically perform better under thicker tissue, and surgeons generally fill implants to the recommended volume or just beyond. Saline implants are also heavier than silicone gel implants on a volumetric basis and may cause more tissue thinning with inferior displacement of the implant over time.

DOUBLE-LUMEN IMPLANTS

The original double-lumen implant was developed by Hartley[24] as a means of countering capsular contracture. It was constructed of an inner silicone gel-filled lumen surrounded by an outer saline inflatable shell. The conceptual of the device is the initial inflation of the outer saline shell to make a larger pocket, with subsequent percutaneous deflation to leave the smaller silicone gel-filled shell within a larger pocket. The device became

popular without going through these machinations as a fixed-volume, two-chamber device or as a drug delivery device, which allowed the addition of steroids or antibiotics to the outer saline-filled chamber.

Cox-Uphoff developed a "reverse double-lumen" implant,[25] which had an outer silicone gel-filled shell surrounding an inner inflatable shell. Today, the only double-lumen device on the United States market is the Mentor Becker, an expander-implant used primarily for reconstruction.[26] This device was originally developed as a saline device but was subsequently converted to a reverse gel and saline double-lumen design to minimize deflation rates.

TEXTURED-SURFACE IMPLANTS

Early attempts at augmentation with polyurethane sponge were not successful, but in 1970, Ashley[27] reported the favorable use of a silicone gel implant covered with a thin layer of polyurethane foam. Although the foam was placed on the implant primarily to maintain its position, clinical use seemed to show a lessened incidence of capsular contracture.[28,29] Throughout the 1980s, increasing numbers of plastic surgeons found polyurethane-covered silicone gel implants to produce aesthetically pleasing results with low capsular contracture rates.[30–32] The polyurethane surface adhered to the surrounding tissues, subsequently delaminated, and created a relatively noncontractible capsule.[33] Unlike smooth-surfaced implants that had to be mobile within their pocket, polyurethane-covered implants could be immobile yet soft. These devices had reached a zenith of popularity by 1990, when questions of the safety of polyurethane foam breakdown products caused Bristol-Myers Squibb,

which owned Surgitek (the company manufacturing the implants), to withdraw from the breast implant market.[34]

The favorable clinical outcomes and commercial success of polyurethane-covered implants (**Fig. 2**) led American implant manufacturers to develop textured silicone surfaces in the hope of achieving similar results. In 1986, McGhan Medical introduced Biocell textured implants and expanders, and Mentor introduced Siltex textured implants. These remain the two textured surfaces available in the United States today. Dow Corning subsequently introduced its MSI "structured surface" in 1990, but the company withdrew from the market in 1992.

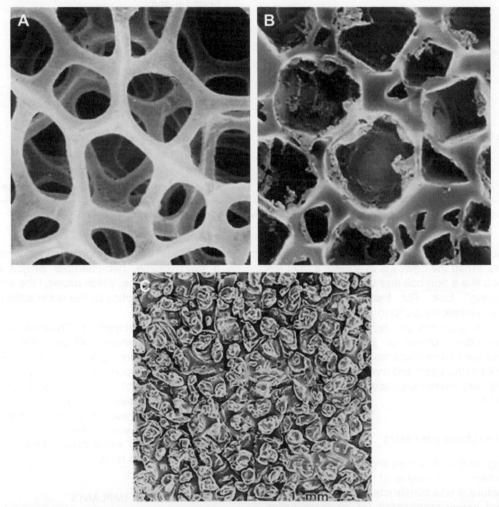

Fig. 2. (*A*) Polyurethane foam gains tissue adherence and delaminates from the implant. No longer available in the United States, this texture fostered the development of textured silicone surfaces. (*B*) Biocell is an aggressive silicone textured surface that adheres to surrounding tissue by an adhesive effect. (*C*) Siltex is a less aggressive silicone textured surface that does not demonstrate any adhesive effect and does not gain tissue adherence. (*From* Maxwell GP, Hammond DC. Breast implants: smooth versus textured. Adv Plast Reconstr Surg 1993;9:209; with permission.)

Biocell is an aggressive open-pore textured silicone surface composed of irregular pores having an average density of 3.1 pores/mm^2 with a mean pore size of 289 μm (range, 37–648 μm). Created by a lost-salt technique, these interconnected pores promote adherence to the surrounding, developing capsule through an adhesive effect.[35–37] This tissue adherence, which is clinically similar to that seen with the polyurethane foam surface, differs in that there is no delamination of the texture as occurs with polyurethane. The adhesive effect and tissue adherence are enhanced in Biocell-covered expanders; these have the added mechanical advantage of expansion pressure, which pushes the textured surface into the developing capsule and imparts its mirror image into the surrounding tissue.[38] Whereas adherence may not occur around the entire device or with all Biocell breast implants, there is a high friction coefficient around these devices, making them relatively immobile. Similar to the polyurethane implants, "immobility with softness" characterizes Biocell-covered implants. Prospective clinical studies have demonstrated that Biocell textured implants have a significantly lower incidence of capsule contracture than do their smooth counterparts, whether they are filled with silicone gel[39] or saline.[40]

Siltex is a less aggressive textured silicone surface created as a negative contact imprint off texturing foam (see **Fig. 2**). It is characterized by a raised, dense pattern of irregular nodules ranging in height[35] from 65 to 150 μm and in width from 60 to 275 μm. Siltex does not adhere to the surrounding tissue and is not characterized by immobility with softness, as are polyurethane and Biocell.[37] Whereas Siltex-covered implants move within their surrounding pocket similar to smooth-walled implants, prospective clinical studies have shown a significantly lower incidence of capsule contracture compared with their smooth counterparts, whether they are filled with silicone gel[41,42] or saline.[43]

Other textured-surface devices that have been available in the past or are currently available outside the United States include the MSI pillar-structured texture previously manufactured by Dow Corning[44] and the polyurethane foam-covered implant manufactured by Silimed in Brazil.[45]

ALTERNATIVE FILLER IMPLANTS

When safety issues with silicone gel implants became a concern, investigators looked for alternative filler substances. Three actually came to market. Polyvinylpyrrolidone is a low-molecular-weight "bio-oncotic" gel thought to be more radiolucent than silicone. It composed the fill material of the Misti Gold implant introduced in 1991 by Bioplasty.[46] NovaMed purchased this company, and the polyvinylpyrrolidone implant is currently still available outside the United States under the name NovaGold. In December 2000, the British Medical Devices Agency issued a device alert regarding this implant and other alternative filler devices, citing the opinion that studies demonstrating the safety of these devices are lacking.[47]

LipoMatrix manufactured triglyceride-filled implants termed "trilucent implants" in 1994. Soybean oil composed the fill material, which was said to be radiolucent. Problems with oil bleed,[48] tissue irritation, and a rancid or foul smell[49] were reported, and the implants were withdrawn from the market in 1999.

Hydrogel implants are filled with an organic polymer, which is a mixture of polysaccharide and water. These implants have been manufactured in France by PIP and Arion. There have been reports of swelling of hydrogel (and polyvinylpyrrolidone) implants after implantation caused by osmotic gradient pressure.[47] The British Medical Devices Agency alert of 2000 also applied to these devices. None of these alternative filler devices is available in the United States.

ENHANCED COHESIVE SILICONE GEL IMPLANTS

All silicone gel implants are cross-linked to maintain a gel consistency, and all silicone gel has cohesive properties. As the cross-linking is increased, the consistency or firmness of the liquid-feeling gel changes to that of a soft cheese. The enhanced cohesive nature of these implants makes them form stable. This refers to the implant's maintaining its shape in all positions (shape maintenance). These implants are designed in various anatomic dimensions in addition to round shapes and are collectively referred to as "cohesive silicone gel implants." These form-stable implants are currently popular worldwide and undergoing Food and Drug Administration (FDA)–approved clinical trials in the United States (**Fig. 3**).[45]

ANATOMIC SHAPED IMPLANTS

The original Cronin and Gerow silicone gel implants had a teardrop shape, as did a number of the early saline- and gel-filled devices. Problems with capsular contracture, however, led manufacturers to design round, smooth-surfaced low-profile implants, which move within their surgical pockets. These round, smooth designs

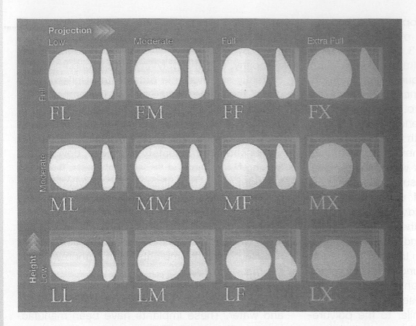

Fig. 3. Style 410 Matrix (IN-AMED) of enhanced cohesive silicone gel implants offers varying heights and projections of shaped devices for breast augmentation and reconstruction. L, low; M, moderate; F, full; X, extra. (*Courtesy of* INAMED Health, Santa Barbara, CA.)

dominated the market for nearly 20 years. Only when the phenomenon of immobility with softness was appreciated was the creation of anatomic devices clinically appropriate.[38–51] The polyurethane Optimum and Replicon devices (no longer available) were early generation anatomic-shaped implants popular in the 1980s.[28,29] The adherence of the polyurethane surface lent itself to the "stacking" of these implants, one on top of another, to produce an anatomic shape with enhanced projection.[51–53]

The tissue adherence observed with tissue expanders that had the Biocell surface led McGhan to develop anatomically shaped expanders and subsequently an internally stacked Style 153 gel anatomic-shaped implant.[35,38,51,54] Favorable clinical experience and advanced product design led to a matrix of variable height-to-width ratio anatomic expanders and implants, the Style 133 expanders and Style 410 Matrix cohesive implants (see **Fig. 3**). The latter enjoy widespread international use in aesthetic surgery[45,55] and have completed their initial FDA clinical Investigative Device Exemption study in the United States, awaiting longer follow-up.

Silimed (Brazil) markets polyurethane-covered cohesive silicone gel implants in anatomic shapes.[34] These devices also enjoy international popularity, but no clinical investigative studies have taken place in the United States.

Mentor introduced a midheight Siltex anatomic-shaped tissue expander in 1997 and other height options in 2003. In the fall of 2002, an Investigative Device Exemption study on a midheight anatomic cohesive gel implant was initiated.

These contour-shaped devices are covered with the Siltex texture. Because tissue adherence does not generally occur, the pocket must be exact and only minimally larger than the footprint of the reduced height device to minimize the possibility of implant rotation.[56,57]

Anatomic-shaped saline inflatable implants are available in the United States manufactured by both Mentor and INAMED (McGhan), and there is debate among plastic surgeons about the merit of each relative to the resultant breast form.[58–62] This debate seems confined to saline-filled implants alone because virtually all tissue expanders marketed for breast reconstruction in the United States are textured and anatomically shaped. It is predicted that once cohesive gel anatomic implants and other gel implants are available in the United States, the issue will be of less concern as evidenced by surgeons' preferences worldwide.

SAFETY AND REGULATORY ISSUES CONCERNING BREAST IMPLANTS

In 1976, the US Congress passed a Medical Device Amendment to the Food, Drug, and Cosmetic Act that gave the FDA authority over medical devices. Implants on the market at the time or those considered "substantially equivalent" to those marketed before 1976 were grandfathered in and allowed to remain in use until the FDA could formally review their safety and efficacy. In 1988, the FDA called for the manufacturers of silicone gel-filled implants to submit their Premarket Approval Applications containing data adequate to substantiate the safety and efficacy of the devices they were marketing. In November 1991, the FDA convened an advisory panel of experts to hold public hearings and evaluate the manufacturers' data. The panel concluded that more research was necessary (to establish safety and efficacy) but recommended continued availability of implants while that research was performed. In January 1992, however, the FDA Commissioner went against the recommendation of the advisory panel and called for a voluntary moratorium on the use of silicone gel implants. After further evaluation of the situation by the advisory panel (who thought there was a public need for the devices), the FDA Commissioner, in April 1992, ruled that although silicone breast implants were not necessarily unsafe, the law required more data to substantiate safety and efficacy than the manufacturers had supplied.[62,63] The use of silicone gel implants was restricted to clinical trials until the data were produced. This was interpreted by the media and the public at large that silicone gel implants were "banned" because they were not safe. This effectively took silicone gel implants off the market for breast augmentation in the United States for the next 12 years.

The media frenzy surrounding this issue was further heightened by several lay jury court decisions that found silicone implants to be responsible for women's pathologic conditions. This led to the filing of thousands of product liability lawsuits against the implant manufacturers. This culminated in a class action lawsuit involving more than 400,000 women.[22] Unable to withstand the financial pressure to defend this massive number of cases, Dow Corning filed for Chapter 11 and Bristol-Myers Squibb withdrew from the market. Ultimately, a settlement of approximately $4 billion was reached, and Mentor and McGhan were left as the only two American manufacturers of saline and silicone breast implants.

Concerns relating to the safety of foreign materials implanted in the female breast began in Japan in 1964 when the term "human adjuvant disease" was suggested on speculation of an association between paraffin breast injections and connective tissue disease-like symptoms in several women.[64] In the 1980s, several reports questioned a link between silicone gel breast implants and various collagen vascular diseases.[65–67] Questions were raised as to whether silicone leaked into the body and caused pathologic conditions. Whereas increased levels of silicone were found within the surrounding tissue capsule[68,69] and axillary lymph nodes, no correlation with symptoms or any disease could be established. Likewise, no specific antibodies to silicone could be found.[70,71]

Amid this background of lawsuits, public concerns, and implant restrictions, the scientific data began to prevail, demonstrating the safety of silicone gel and the lack of its correlation with any disease or pathologic condition. By the late 1990s, approximately 20 epidemiologic studies and other important scientific investigations found no increased risk for development of connective tissue disorders in women with breast implants.[22] In addition, respected independent scientific groups including the Independent Review Group in England,[72] the Institute of Medicine,[10] and the National Science Panel[73] (appointed by the judge of the class action litigation), after carefully reviewing all scientific data available, found no relationship between silicone gel implants and connective tissue disease.

The other health issue that clouded the breast implant arena in the early 1990s was the possibility of a polyurethane foam breakdown product being carcinogenic. Specifically cited was a National Cancer Institute study in which mice fed extremely high doses of 2,4-toluenediamine showed an increased incidence of breast cancer.[74] Because the foam used to cover the Surgitek implant was produced by a mixture of 2,4- and 2,6-toluenediisocyanate, the FDA questioned whether the polyurethane itself or one of its biodegradation products could be carcinogenic in patients after breast implantation. Scientific scrutiny of patients in whom these devices had been implanted found minimal exposure to 2,4-toluenediamine,[75] and the FDA ultimately concluded that it was unlikely any woman with polyurethane-covered implants was at increased risk for development of cancer.[76] Before these scientific findings of safety, however, Bristol-Myers Squibb failed to make premarket approval for the FDA in April of 1991 and withdrew these devices from the market.

Despite this decade of turbulence, the future of silicone gel implants looks bright. No fill material has been found to be as safe and as functional as silicone. Saline clinical inadequacies (in certain situations) are well appreciated by American plastic surgeons. Manufacturing practices of silicone gel implants have been improved and brought into compliance to ensure better-quality products.

CURRENT STATUS OF SILICONE GEL IMPLANTS

The Premarket Approval Application for silicone gel breast implants submitted by INAMED in December 2001 was heard by the FDA expert advising panel in October 2003. After intense scrutiny of the data submitted, and public testimony, the panel recommended approval of the application "with conditions," setting the stage for the return to market of silicone gel implants in the United States. The panel found no evidence to support that silicone gel implants cause disease. They did, however, question the adequacy of the length of follow-up on the studies.

In January 2004, the Commissioner of the FDA went against the panel's recommendation and asked for additional data with longer follow-up from all manufacturers on silicone gel implants. In addition, more information was requested on life expectancy of implants, causes and effects of shell failure, and clinical evaluation of possible "silent rupture" of implants.

On November 17, 2006 the FDA approved the premarket application data. In connection with the approval, the FDA has asked for conduction of postapproval studies, to track the devices. It is crucial for plastic surgeons to support this initiative and comply with the postapproval studies provided by both manufacturers (Allergan and Mentor).

CAPSULAR CONTRACTURE

Capsular contracture results from an exaggerated scar response to a foreign prosthetic material. All surgical implants undergo some degree of encapsulation, but clinical problems arise when this scar formation becomes excessive, much in the same way as hypertrophic and keloid scars represent the unchecked proliferation of the normal healing process. Baker[77] proposed a clinical classification

system in 1975 that remains the most commonly used reporting system.

Capsular contracture remains the most common complication of breast augmentation, with rates reported between 0.5% and 30%. As such, the evolution of breast augmentation mammaplasty has been driven by the need to prevent the development of capsular contracture. The first Dow Corning teardrop-shaped smooth-surfaced silicone implants were found to have an unacceptably high rate of capsular contracture. These implants were placed in a retroglandular position and fixed in place by a Dacron patch on the posterior aspect of the device. The first advancement in prosthetic design was the removal of the Dacron patch with the belief that the Dacron was initiating an inflammatory response resulting in formation of a capsule around the implant. When this failed sufficiently to lower the rate of capsule formation, smooth round devices with thinner shells and less viscous silicone gel were developed. Displacement exercises and implant massage were advocated. Although the rate of capsular contracture was improved, these implants were complicated by high rates of rupture and bleed.

The double-lumen implant was developed with the idea that capsule formation was inevitable. With a larger outer saline-filled lumen, the capsule could be allowed to form and the outer lumen drained, leaving a large pocket for a soft gel implant.[24]

Table 2
Saline-filled breast implants

Model	Surface	Shape	Projection
INAMED Style 68LP	smooth	round	low
INAMED Style 68MP	smooth	round	moderate
INAMED Style 68HP	smooth	round	high
INAMED Style 168 BIOCELL	textured	round	moderate
INAMED Style 468 BIOCELL BioCurve	textured	anatomic	moderate
INAMED Style 163 BIOCELL BioCurve	textured	anatomic	moderate[a]
INAMED Style 363LF BIOCELL BioCurve	textured	anatomic	full[b]
Mentor Smooth Round Moderate Profile	smooth	round	moderate
Mentor Smooth Round High Profile	smooth	round	full
Mentor Siltex Round Moderate Profile	textured	round	moderate
Mentor Siltex Contour Profile Moderate	textured	anatomic	moderate
Mentor Siltex Contour Profile High	textured	anatomic	fill

[a] Style 163 implants are designed with moderate projection and full height.
[b] Style 363LF implants are designed with full projection and low height.

In the late 1970s, the thinking began to shift away from the prosthetic device to the surgical technique. Implant placement moved from the subglandular position to the subpectoral position. This was done in the belief that the active contraction of the pectoralis major muscle would provide internal massage of the implant, maintaining its pocket and ensuring its softness. Subsequent research has confirmed a significant decrease in capsular contracture by this surgical approach.[78–81] With the devices available at the time, the key to maintaining implant softness was to allow implant mobility within the breast pocket. This remained true until the advent of textured surface implants.

In 1970, Ashley[27] introduced the polyurethane-coated silicone breast implant, the use of which became popular in the United States in the 1980s. A dramatic decrease in capsular contracture to less than 3% was noted in multiple studies.[82–84] The polyurethane was found to delaminate from the surface of the implant during the course of the first few months and favorably affect the collagen orientation in the developing periprosthetic space.[85] This allowed the implant to remain soft in a pocket that does not undergo any significant degree of contracture. It was possible to have an immobile implant that remained soft in a fixed pocket. A large study demonstrated that there was no statistical significance between the rates of capsular contracture whether the prosthesis was placed in a subpectoral or a subglandular plane.[32] This type of implant became popular with many plastic surgeons until it was removed from the United States market in early 1991 because of concerns about the potential toxicity of polyurethane breakdown products.

Multiple studies have confirmed that textured surfaces significantly decrease or delay the occurrence of capsular contracture for silicone gel implants placed in a retroglandular position.[39,41,86–88] The data are less clear with retroglandular saline-filled devices.[40,43,89,90]

With the restriction of silicone gel implants in 1992, the implant manufacturers made the rapid transition to enhanced production of various saline-filled implants. The silicone implant data were extrapolated to the saline device, and textured saline implants were initially popular. One observed benefit of the saline-filled devices was a significant decrease in rates of capsular contracture;[91–94] however, problems were seen with widespread use of these devices, including palpable shell folding or "knuckling," visible rippling, and palpability. Many of these problems could be minimized by subpectoral implant placement. This

Table 3
Silicone gel-filled breast implants

Model	Surface	Shape	Projection
INAMED Style 10	smooth	round	moderate
INAMED Style 15	smooth	round	intermediate
INAMED Style 20	smooth	round	full
INAMED Style 110 BIOCELL	textured	round	moderate
INAMED Style 115 BIOCELL	textured	round	intermediate
INAMED Style 120 BIOCELL	textured	round	full
INAMED Style 153 BIOCELL dual-lumen	textured	anatomic	full
INAMED Style 410 BioDIMENSIONAL	textured	anatomic	matrix[a]
Mentor Smooth Round Moderate Profile	smooth	round	moderate
Mentor Smooth Round Moderate Plus Profile	smooth	round	intermediate
Mentor Smooth Round High Profile	smooth	round	full
Mentor Siltex Round Moderate Profile	textured	round	moderate
Mentor Siltex Round Moderate Plus Profile	textured	round	intermediate
Mentor Siltex Round High Profile	textured	round	full

[a] Style 410 implants are available in 12 different combinations of low, moderate, and full height, and low, moderate, full and extra projection.

resulted in the preferred use by most American surgeons of round, smooth-walled, saline-filled implants placed in a subpectoral pocket (**Tables 2 and 3**). Whereas capsular contracture rates were minimized, so was the surgeon's ability to control shape and form.

NOW AND THE FUTURE

Recently, both manufactures reported their long-term follow-up data. The results were very strong and supportive. Mentor's Core MemoryGel 10-year study included 1007 women at 3-years follow-up with 8.1% capsular contracture,[95] whereas Allergan's 10-year core study included 940 women at 6-years follow-up with 14.8% capsular contracture for augmentation mammaplasty.[96]

Both manufacturers had less capsular contractures with the highly cohesive gel implants. The Mentor CPG gel study at 2-year follow-up showed a 0.8% capsular contracture in augmentation mammaplasty.[97] Allergan's style 410 highly cohesive breast implant core study at 3 years showed a 1.9% capsular contracture rate.[98]

The data provided by both manufacturers demonstrate safety and efficacy of these medical devices. The journey is not yet over, because clinicians have to strive to provide continuous data and science followed by extensive education and improvement of surgical techniques for improved clinical outcomes in the future.

REFERENCES

1. Cronin TD, Gerow FJ. Augmentation mammoplasty: a new natural feel prosthesis. Transactions of the Third International Congress of Plastic Surgery, October 13–18, 1963. Amsterdam: Excerpta Medica Foundation; 1963. p. 41–9.
2. National Clearing House of Plastic Surgery Statistics, 2001 Data. Arlington Heights, Ill, American Society of Plastic Surgeons.
3. Terry MD, Skovron ML, Garbers S, et al. The estimated frequency of cosmetic breast augmentation among U.S. women 1963 through 1988. Am J Public Health 1995;85:1122.
4. Baker JL Jr, Kolin IS, Bartlett ES. Psychosexual dynamics of patients undergoing mammary augmentation. Plast Reconstr Surg 1974;53:652.
5. Shipley RH, O'Donnell JM, Bader KF. Personality characteristics of women seeking breast augmentation, comparison to small-busted and average-busted controls. Plast Reconstr Surg 1997;60:369.
6. Hetter GP. Satisfaction and dissatisfaction of patients with augmentation mammaplasty. Plast Reconstr Surg 1979;64:151.
7. Druss R. Changes in body image following augmentation breast surgery. Int J Psychoanal Psychother 1973;2:248.
8. Czerny V. Plastic replacement of the breast with a lipoma. Chir Kong Verhandl 1895;2:216.
9. Longacre JJ. Correction of the hypoplastic breast with special reference to reconstruction of the nipple type breast with local dermofat pedicle flaps. Plast Reconstr Surg 1954;14:431.
10. Bondurant S, Ernster V, Herdman R, editors. Safety of silicone breast implants. Washington, DC: National Academy Press; 2000.
11. Uchida J. Clinical application of crosslinked dimethylpolysiloxane, restoration of breast, cheeks, atrophy of infantile paralysis, funnel-shaped chest, etc. Japanese Journal of Plastic and Reconstructive Surgery 1961;4:303.
12. Brown JB, Fryer MP, Randall P, et al. Silicones in plastic surgery: laboratory and clinical investigations, a preliminary report. Plast Reconstr Surg 1953;12:374.
13. Marzoni FA, Upchurch SE, Lambert CJ. An experimental study of silicone as a soft tissue substitute. Plast Reconstr Surg 1959;24:600.
14. Feng LJ, Amini SB. Analysis of risk factors associated with rupture of silicone-gel breast implants. Plast Reconstr Surg 1999;104:955.
15. Barker DE, Retsky MI, Schultz S. Bleeding of silicone from bag-gel breast implants, and its clinical relation to fibrous capsule reaction. Plast Reconstr Surg 1978;61:836.
16. Caffee HH. The influence of silicone bleed on capsule contracture. Ann Plast Surg 1986;17:284.
17. Price JE Jr, Barker DE. Initial clinical experience with low bleed breast implants. Aesthetic Plast Surg 1983;7:255.
18. Barker DE, Retsky MI, Searles SL. New low bleed implant: Silastic II. Aesthetic Plast Surg 1985;9:39.
19. Arion HG. Retromammary prosthesis. C R Soc Fr Gynecol 1965;5.
20. Regnault P, Baker TJ, Gleason MC, et al. Clinical trial and evaluation of a proposed new inflatable mammary prosthesis. Plast Reconstr Surg 1972;50:220.
21. Rees TD, Guy CL, Coburn RJ. The use of inflatable breast implants. Plast Reconstr Surg 1973;52:609.
22. Young VL, Watson ME. Breast implant research. Clin Plast Surg 2001;28:451.
23. Lavine DM. Saline inflatable prostheses: 14 years experience. Aesthetic Plast Surg 1993;17:325.
24. Hartley JH Jr. Specific applications of the double-lumen prosthesis. Clin Plast Surg 1976;3:247.
25. Colon GA. The reverse double-lumen prosthesis: a preliminary report. Ann Plast Surg 1982;4:293.
26. Becker H. The expander mammary implant. Plast Reconstr Surg 1987;76:631.
27. Ashley FL. A new type of breast prosthesis: preliminary report. Plast Reconstr Surg 1970;45:421.

28. Ashley FL. Further studies on the natural-Y breast prosthesis. Plast Reconstr Surg 1972;49:414.

29. Capozzi A, Pennisi VR. Clinical experience with polyurethane-covered gel-filled mammary prostheses. Plast Reconstr Surg 1981;68:512.

30. Herman S. The Meme implant. Plast Reconstr Surg 1984;73:411.

31. Melmed EP. Polyurethane implants: a 6-year review of 416 patients. Plast Reconstr Surg 1988;82:285.

32. Hester TR Jr, Nahai F, Bostwick J, et al. A 5-year experience with polyurethane-covered mammary prostheses for treatment of capsule contracture, primary augmentation mammoplasty, and breast reconstruction. Clin Plast Surg 1988;15:569.

33. Sinclair TM, Kerrigan CL, Bantic R. Biodegradation of the polyurethane foam covering of breast implants. Plast Reconstr Surg 1993;92:1003.

34. Hester TR Jr, Tebbetts JB, Maxwell GP. The polyurethane-covered mammary prosthesis: facts and fiction. Clin Plast Surg 2001;28:579.

35. Barone FE, Perry L, Maxwell GP, et al. The biomechanical and histopathologic effects of surface texturizing with silicone and polyurethane in tissue implantation and expansion. Plast Reconstr Surg 1992;90:77.

36. Maxwell GP, Hammond DC. Breast implants: smooth versus textured. Advances in Plastic and Reconstructive Surgery 1993;9:209.

37. Danino AM, Basmacioglu P, Saito S, et al. Comparison of the capsular response to the Biocell RTV and Mentor 1600 Siltex breast implant surface texturing: a scanning electron microscopic study. Plast Reconstr Surg 2001;108:2047.

38. Maxwell GP, Falcone PA. Eighty-four consecutive breast reconstructions using a textured silicone tissue expander. Plast Reconstr Surg 1992;89:1022.

39. Hakelius L, Ohlsen L. Tendency to capsule contracture around smooth and textured gel-filled silicone mammary implants: a 5-year followup. Plast Reconstr Surg 1997;100:1566.

40. Burkhardt B, Eades E. The effect of Biocell texturizing and povidone-iodine irrigation on capsule contracture around saline-inflatable breast implants. Plast Reconstr Surg 1995;96:1317.

41. Coleman DJ, Foo IT, Sharpe DT. Textured or smooth implants for breast augmentation? A prospective controlled trial. Br J Plast Surg 1991;44:444.

42. Malata CM, Felderg L, Coleman DJ, et al. Textured or smooth implants for breast augmentation? Three year followup of a prospective randomized controlled trial. Br J Plast Surg 1997;50:99.

43. Burkhardt BR, Demas CP. The effect of Siltex texturing and povidone-iodine irrigation on capsule contracture around saline inflatable breast implants. Plast Reconstr Surg 1994;93:123.

44. Batra M, Bernard S, Picha G. Histologic comparison of breast implant shells with smooth foam and pillar microstructuring in a rat model. Plast Reconstr Surg 1995;95:354.

45. Heden P, Jernbeck J, Hober M. Breast augmentation with anatomical cohesive-gel implants. Clin Plast Surg 2001;28:531.

46. Ersek RA, Salisbury AV. Textured surface, non-silicone-gel breast implants: four years clinical outcome. Plast Reconstr Surg 1997;100:1729.

47. Spear SL, Mardini S. Alternative filler materials and new implant designs. Clin Plast Surg 2001;28:435.

48. Choudhary S, Cadier MAM. Local tissue reactions to oil-based breast implant bleed. Br J Plast Surg 2000;53:317.

49. Papanastasiou S, Odili J, Newman P, et al. Are triglyceride breast implants really biocompatible? Ann Plast Surg 2000;45:172.

50. Rohrich RJ, Beran SJ, Ingram AE Jr, et al. Development of alternative breast implant filler material: criteria and horizons. Plast Reconstr Surg 1996;98: 455.

51. Hester TR, Cukic J. Use of stacked polyurethane-covered mammary implants in aesthetic and reconstructive breast surgery. Plast Reconstr Surg 1990; 10:503.

52. Hammond DC, Perry LC, Maxwell GP, et al. Morphologic analysis of tissue expander shape using a biomechanical model. Plast Reconstr Surg 1993;92:255.

53. Maxwell GP. Breast reconstruction utilizing subcutaneous tissue expansion followed by polyurethane-covered silicone implants. [discussion]. Plast Reconstr Surg 1991;88:640.

54. Maxwell GP, Spear SL. Two-stage breast reconstruction using biodimensional system. Santa Barbara (CA): McGhan Medical Corporation; 1995.

55. Bronz G. A comparison of naturally shaped and round implants. Aesthetic Surgery Journal 2002;22: 238.

56. Baeke JL. Breast deformity caused by anatomical or teardrop implant rotation. Plast Reconstr Surg 2002; 109:2555.

57. Hamas RS. The postoperative shape of round and teardrop saline-filled breast implants. Aesthetic Surg J 1999;19:369.

58. Hamas RS. The comparative dimensions of round and anatomical saline-filled breast implants. Aesthetic Surg J 2000;20:281.

59. Hobar PC, Gutowski K. Experience with anatomic breast implants. Clin Plast Surg 2001;28:553.

60. Tebbetts JB. Breast augmentation with full-height anatomic saline implants: the pros and cons. Clin Plast Surg 2001;28:567.

61. Tebbetts JB, Tebbetts TB. The best breast: the ultimate discriminating woman's guide to breast augmentation. Dallas (TX): CosmetXpertise; 1999.

62. Kessler DA, Merkatz RB, Schapiro RA. A call for higher standards for breast implants. JAMA 1993; 270:2607.

63. Kessler DA. The basis of the FDA's decision based on breast implants. N Engl J Med 1992;326:1713.

64. Miyoshi K, Miyamura T, Kobayashi Y, et al. Hyper-gammaglobulinemia by prolonged adjuvanticity in men: disorders developed after augmentation mammoplasty. Jpn Med J 1964;2122:9.

65. Van Nunen SA, Gatenby PA, Basten A. Post-mammoplasty connective tissue disease. Arthritis Rheum 1982;25:694.

66. Spiera H. Scleroderma after silicone augmentation mammoplasty. JAMA 1988;260:236.

67. Endo LP, Edwards NL, Longley S, et al. Silicone and rheumatic diseases. Semin Arthritis Rheum 1987;17:112.

68. Peters W, Smith D, Lugowski S, et al. Analysis of silicon levels in capsules of gel and saline breast implants and of penile prostheses. Ann Plast Surg 1995;34:578.

69. Schnur PL, Weinzweig J, Harris JB, et al. Silicon analysis of breast and periprosthetic capsular tissue from patients with saline- or silicone-gel implants. Plast Reconstr Surg 1996;98:798.

70. Barnard JJ, Todd EL, Wilson WG, et al. Distribution of organosilicon polymers in augmentation mammoplasties at autopsy. Plast Reconstr Surg 1997;100:197.

71. Rohrich RJ, Hollier LH, Robinson JB Jr. Determining the safety of the silicone envelope: in search of a silicone antibody. Plast Reconstr Surg 1996;98:455.

72. Independent Review Group. Silicone-gel breast implants: the report of the Independent Review Group. Available at: www.silicone-review.gov.uk.

73. Diamond BA, Hulka BS, Kerkvliet NI, et al. Silicone breast implants in relation to connective tissue diseases and immunologic dysfunction: a report by a National Science Panel to the Hon. Sam C. Pointer, Jr. (coordinating judge for the Federal Breast Implant Multidistrict Litigation). Birmingham (AL): Federal Judicial Center; 1998. Available at: http://www.fjc.gov/BREIMLIT/SCIENCE/report.htm.

74. National Cancer Institute Report. Bioassay of 2,4-diaminotoluene for possible carcinogenicity. Bethesda (MD): National Institutes of Health; 1979. DHEW publication NIH-79-1718.

75. Hester TR, Ford NF, Gale J, et al. Measurement of 2,4-toluenediamine in urine and serum samples from women with Meme and Replicon breast implants. Plast Reconstr Surg 1997;100:1291.

76. MDDI Reports. Polyurethane foam-covered breast implant cancer risk negligible. The Gray Sheet July 3, 1995.

77. Baker Jr. JL. Classification of spherical contractures. Presented at the Aesthetic Breast Symposium. Scottsdale, Arizona; August 1975.

78. Biggs TM, Yarish RS. Augmentation mammaplasty: retropectoral versus retromammary implantation. Clin Plast Surg 1988;15:549.

79. Gutowski KA, Mesnafx1 GT, Cunningham BL. Saline-filled breast implants: a Plastic Surgery Educational Foundation multicenter outcomes study. Plast Reconstr Surg 1997;100:1019.

80. Puckett CL, Croll GH, Reichel CA, et al. A critical look at capsule contracture in subglandular versus subpectoral mammary augmentation. Aesthetic Plast Surg 1987;11:23.

81. Woods JE, Irons GB, Arnold PG. The case for submuscular implantation of prostheses in reconstructive breast surgery. Ann Plast Surg 1980;5:115.

82. Handel N, Silverstein MJ, Jensen JA, et al. Comparative experience with smooth and polyurethane breast implants using the Kaplan-Meier method of survival analysis. Plast Reconstr Surg 1991;88:475.

83. Gasperoni C, Salgarello M, Gargani G. Polyurethane-covered mammary implants: a 12-year experience. Ann Plast Surg 1992;29:303.

84. Penisi VR. Long-term use of polyurethane breast prostheses: a 14-year experience. Plast Reconstr Surg 1990;86:368.

85. Smahel J. Tissue reactions to breast implants coated with polyurethane. Plast Reconstr Surg 1978;61:80.

86. Embrey M, Adams EE, Cunningham B, et al. A review of the literature on the etiology of capsular contracture and a pilot study to determine the outcome of capsular contracture interventions. Aesthetic Plast Surg 1999;23:197.

87. Ersek RA. Molecular impact surface textured implants (MISTI) alter beneficially breast capsule formation at 36 months. J Long Term Eff Med Implants 1991;1:155.

88. Pollack H. Breast capsular contracture: a retrospective study of textured versus smooth silicone implants. Plast Reconstr Surg 1993;92:404.

89. Tarpila E, Ghassemifor R, Fagrell D, et al. Capsular contracture with textured versus smooth saline-filled implants for breast augmentation: a prospective clinical study. Plast Reconstr Surg 1997;99:1934.

90. Fagrell D, Berggren A, Tarpila E. Capsular contracture around saline-filled fine textured and smooth mammary implants: a prospective 7.5-year follow-up. Plast Reconstr Surg 2001;108:2108.

91. Cairns TS, de Villiers W. Capsular contracture after breast augmentation: a comparison between gel- and saline-filled prosthesis. S Afr Med J 1980;57:951.

92. Gylbert L, Asplund O, Jurell G. Capsular contracture after breast reconstruction with silicone-gel and saline-filled implants: a 6-year follow-up. Plast Reconstr Surg 1990;85:373.

93. McKinney P, Tresley G. Long-term comparison of patients with gel and saline mammary implants. Plast Reconstr Surg 1983;72:27.

94. Reiffel RS, Rees TD, Guy CL, et al. A comparison of capsule formation following breast augmentation by saline-filled or gel-filled implants. Aesthetic Plast Surg 1983;7:113.

95. Cunningham B. The Mentor core study on silicone MemoryGel breast implants. Plast Reconstr Surg 2007;120:19S.

96. Spear SL, Murphy DK, Slicton A, et al. Inamed silicone breast implant core study results at 6 years. Plast Reconstr Surg 2007;120:8S.

97. Cunningham B. The Mentor Study on contour profile gel silicone MemoryGel breast implants. Plast Reconstr Surg 2007;120:33S.

98. Bengtson BP, Van Natta BW, Murphy DK, et al. Style 410 highly cohesive silicone breast implant core study results at 3 years. Plast Reconstr Surg 2007;120:40S.

History of Breast Implants and the Food and Drug Administration

Scott L. Spear, MD*, Pranay M. Parikh, MD,
Jesse A. Goldstein, MD

KEYWORDS

- Breast implants • Breast augmentation
- Silicone gel • FDA • Regulation

"Those who cannot remember the past are condemned to repeat it."
—George Santayana

The Food and Drug Administration's (FDA) re-approval of silicone breast implants on November 17, 2006, marked a significant moment in the history of plastic surgery. In addition to preserving choice for women undergoing aesthetic and reconstructive breast surgery, this decision represented the culmination of more than 2 decades of effort by government, industry, and the medical community to respond to public scrutiny over the safety and efficacy of silicone breast implants by obtaining data and finding facts to empower women to make informed decisions. Perhaps most importantly, the lessons learned from the events leading up to the 1992 moratorium on silicone implants and the ensuing pursuit of re-approval transcend the issue of implants. In fact, these lessons may serve as guiding principles for plastic surgeons: innovation is central to our specialty, and the influence of industry is an ever-present force.

The history of silicone breast implants and their federal regulation is a complex tale, whose chief players are the device manufacturers and the FDA. Supporting players in the story include lawyers, the media, Wall Street, public interest groups, Congress, and of course, plastic surgeons. In reviewing the timeline of this story (**Box 1**), six periods emerge: Prologue (1962–1988), Crisis (1988–1992), The Dark Years (1993–1995), Quiet Before the Dawn (1996–2000), Age of Enlightenment (2000–2005), and Promise of the Future (2006–present).

PROLOGUE: 1962–1988

Since the first recorded description by Czerny in 1895 of breast augmentation with an autologous lipoma,[1–3] numerous techniques have been attempted to address women's desires for breast augmentation and reconstruction. Injections of paraffin wax[4–10] and free liquid silicone[11–13] in the early twentieth century led to problems with migration, embolization, and granuloma formation resulting in attempts to better contain such materials. Implantation of sponges made from a variety of plastic polymers was abandoned because of problems with infection, contracture, and tissue ingrowth, which often precluded complete explantation.[14–25] In 1962, Cronin and Gerow[26] (in conjunction with the Dow Corning Center for Aid to Medical Research) first implanted a device containing silicone gel confined within a separate silicone elastomer shell into a patient. This precursor to the modern breast implant was manufactured commercially by Dow Corning starting in 1963,[27] and was exempt from FDA regulations, as it was considered a "medical device" rather than a drug.

With the passage of the Medical Device Amendments Act by the US Congress in 1976,

Dr. Spear is a paid consultant to Allergan, Lifecell, and Ethicon corporations.
Department of Plastic Surgery, Georgetown University Hospital, 1st Floor PHC Building, Washington, DC 20007, USA
* Corresponding author.
E-mail address: spears@gunet.georgetown.edu (S.L. Spear).

Clin Plastic Surg 36 (2009) 15–21
doi:10.1016/j.cps.2008.07.007

Box 1
Regulation timeline

May 1976

Medical Device Amendments Act: Authorizes FDA to regulate medical devices.

June 1988

FDA classifies Silicone implants as class III devices insufficient evidence exists to assure safety and efficacy. Requires premarket approval (PMA).

April 1991

FDA issues a final rule calling for submission of PMAs for silicone gel-filled breast implants.

November 1991

1st FDA General & Plastic Surgery Devices Panel meeting on silicone breast implant. Panel recommends devices stay on market with limited access pending accrual of additional safety data.

November 1991

Hopkins versus Dow Corning case results in 7.3 million dollar award to plaintiff on grounds that Dow withheld information on potential dangers of silicone implants and is guilty of fraud.

January 1992

FDA commissioner David Kessler issues voluntary moratorium issued requesting that industry cease marketing of silicone-gel filled breast implants while FDA reviews new safety and effectiveness information that had been submitted.

February 1992

2nd FDA General & Plastic Surgery Devices Panel meeting on silicone breast implant panel classifies silicone-gel filled breast implants as investigational devices and restricted to participants in clinical trials and adjunct studies for reconstruction and revision purposes only. No longer available for cosmetic breast augmentation.

March 1992

Dow Corning withdraws from silicone-gel implant market.

April 1992

FDA approves Mentor Corporation's adjunct study protocol for its silicone gel-filled breast implants for reconstruction and revision patients only.

July 1997

The Department of Health and Human Services (DHHS) commissions the Institute of Medicine (IOM) to review all past and current scientific research regarding the safety of silicone-gel breast implants.

March 1998

FDA approves Allergan's (formerly Inamed) adjunct study protocol for its silicone gel-filled breast implants for reconstruction and revision patients only.

June 1998

FDA approves Allergan's investigational device exemption (IDE) study for its silicone gel-filled breast implants for a limited number of augmentation, reconstruction, and revision patients.

June 1999

IOM publishes report *"Safety of Silicone Breast Implants."* Distinguishes clearly between local and systemic complications of silicone-gel breast implants and determines that there is insufficient evidence linking silicone-gel implants to systemic health effects.

August 2000

FDA approves Mentor's IDE study for its silicone gel-filled breast implants for a limited number of augmentation, reconstruction, and revision.

October 2003

> 3rd FDA General & Plastic Surgery Devices Panel meeting on silicone breast implants. Guidelines for approvability set forth.

April 2005

> 4th FDA General & Plastic Surgery Devices Panel meeting on silicone breast implants. Panel recommends Inamed devices not be approvable due to issues with double lumen 153 device. Panel recommends Mentor devices approvable.

November 2006

> FDA issues letters to Mentor and Allergan approving their PMAs for silicone gel–filled breast implants.

breast implants were no longer exempt from FDA regulation. Although breast implants were initially "grandfathered" into approval, along with all other devices that predated this legislation, they became subject to FDA regulation and scrutiny. Despite an initial recommendation that year by the FDA's Plastic Surgery Device Advisory panel that breast implants be regarded Class II devices, "subject to general controls and performance standards," no official action was taken until 1982, when the FDA proposed to classify them as Class III devices, "subject to demonstration of safety and efficacy" to remain on the market.

At the same time, clinicians and patients were beginning to discover the long-term results of breast augmentation with early generation breast implants. Experience with capsular contractures led to reoperations that revealed an unexpectedly high rate of ruptured implants. Patient dissatisfaction with device failure and the need for reoperation manifested as legal cases, starting with a little-publicized case in 1977 in which a Cleveland patient with ruptured implants won $170,000 for pain and suffering caused by reoperation for device removal. A subsequent case, Stern v Dow Corning in 1984, resulted in an award of $1.7 million to the patient on the basis of misrepresentation of data from internal studies by the Dow corporation, and drew media attention to the issue of implant safety. Meanwhile, surgeon dissatisfaction with gel bleed and device failure resulted in increased cooperation with manufacturers to improve implant design, and create low-bleed devices with more durable shells that would decrease rupture rates.

In June 1988, 12 years after the FDA assumed the responsibility of regulating medical devices, the FDA finally classified breast implants as Class III devices. This event set into motion a sequence of events that for the first time gave the FDA authority to demand information from manufacturers about the safety and efficacy of their breast implants, and marks the transition to the period of crisis.

CRISIS: 1988–1992

The challenge of producing and providing the information required by the FDA, and demanded by an increasingly concerned and anxious patient population, was a significant one. Initial efforts to address this challenge were limited by manufacturers' sluggish response to the new FDA classification, and their reluctance to accept that the availability of silicone implants could now be restricted. This task was made all the more difficult by an often sensationalistic media coverage of the silicone breast implant issue, which unilaterally presented the concerns of patients with ruptured implants and ignored input from physicians and manufacturers. Ironically, in their presentation of the issue, the media lacked the very scientific rigor and unbiased honesty for which they faulted device manufacturers and surgeons.[28]

On April 10, 1991 the FDA, released the final rule, which stated that all manufacturers of silicone breast implants had 90 days to submit premarket approval applications (PMAs) demonstrating safety and efficacy of their silicone implants to be able to continue to manufacture and distribute these devices. Some manufacturers such as McGhan & Mentor, who had anticipated the need for such data and had begun their studies a year before the final rule, scrambled to complete their reports by the July 11, 1991, deadline. Other manufacturers such as Bristol-Myers, realized that it was too late to complete their PMAs, and withdrew from the silicone implant market altogether. During the subsequent FDA review of the PMAs that had been submitted in August 1991, several companies including Surgitek and Bioplasty were informed that they lacked sufficient data to even be considered for review, while others such as McGhan were informed that "the PMA lacks information needed to show that there is reasonable assurance that the device is safe and effective for its intended use."[29]

In preparation for the FDA General & Plastic Surgery Devices Panel meeting scheduled for

November 1991, which would review the available data, and recommend a course of action regarding silicone breast implants to the FDA, the American Society of Reconstructive and Plastic Surgeons (ASRPS) formed a task force on silicone breast implants. The goal of this group was to independently review the evidence for and against silicone breast implants, and use these data to more effectively educate the public and advocate at the panel meeting. As this group reviewed the findings of the studies available at the time, it began to be clear that the problems associated with silicone implants were predominantly local musculoskeletal concerns, associated with rupture and capsular contracture, and that there were no data to support an association between silicone implants and systemic disease. When the FDA advisory panel met from November 12 to 14, 1991, their review of the data was consistent with that of the ASRPS task force, and the panel voted *unanimously* to recommend that implants remain on the market for the public health of women undergoing breast reconstruction, while the manufacturers collected additional data.

However, while device manufacturers and organized plastic surgery celebrated this decision, implants continued to suffer major blows in the court of public opinion. At the same time as the panel meeting in November 1991, the San Francisco case of Hopkins v Dow-Corning resulted in an award of 7.3 million dollars to the plaintiff on the grounds that Dow had hidden information from an animal study in which one study animal with an implanted silicone implant had died, and for this reason was guilty of fraud. Despite the panel's findings and recommendation that implants should be left available for public health benefit, the result of this trial was seized by the media, fueling additional outcries from anti-implant activists about the dangers of implants and their need for immediate removal from the market.

To address this tension and stem the tide of class action lawsuits that was rising in response to the Hopkins decision, on January 6, 1992, the FDA announced a voluntary moratorium on silicone breast implants pending another panel meeting in February. At this meeting, the panel reinforced the lack of evidence to support a causal link between ruptured silicone implants and systemic issues such as autoimmune disease. However, the use of silicone implants would be restricted to reconstructive patients, and only in the context of registered core and adjunct studies to more thoroughly evaluate the safety and efficacy of these devices. The moratorium was lifted, but silicone breast implants were severely limited.

THE DARK YEARS: 1993–1995

If the years of crisis starting in 1988 are characterized by mounting legal battles founded on immature science, the period following the April 1992 lifting of the moratorium on silicone breast implants was characterized by extreme litigiousness and a scientific adolescence. Silicone-gel breast implants were no longer FDA approved for cosmetic indications and were limited to reconstruction only in the context of scientific protocols. Media coverage of high profile cases such as Stern v Dow-Corning and Hopkins v Dow-Corning had convinced the public of a connection between systemic connective tissue diseases (CTDs) and silicone implants. And despite a lack of scientific evidence to support these claims, there was also a lack of published studies to refute them.

This period was also marked by larger struggle: the disparity between a demand for scientific rigor from device manufacturers and surgeons and the liberal use of associative evidence by the media and legal community. As protocols were being designed and implemented to identify outcomes with silicone breast implants, court battles were being waged and won by lawyers and patients linking systemic CTDs and silicone-gel implants through anecdote and conjecture alone. Indeed, by May of 1995, when Dow-Corning (the largest implant manufacturer at the time) declared Chapter 11 bankruptcy, they were facing over 20,000 lawsuits from women suffering from various chronic and ill-defined conditions.[30,31]

A year prior in April of 1994, the largest class-action settlement in history was announced, and as part of the global settlement, Dow-Corning was joined by Mentor, Baxter, Bristol-Meyers Squibb, and 3M in paying pay close to $4.25 billion, with Dow-Corning the largest contributor. Any women with silicone implants manufactured by these companies were eligible for compensation based solely on their symptom profile. No proof of causation was required. Not unexpectedly, within a year, over 440,000 women had registered for the class, and 70,000 immediately qualified for compensation.[32]

During the same period, the scientific data began an anemic emergence into the literature. A few studies refuting the correlation between systemic CTDs and silicone-gel implants were published during this period[33–36] but went neglected outside the plastic surgery community. But a few discerning minds began taking notice.

THE QUIET YEARS: 1996–2000

The transition to the next issue of this story is marked by several landmark legal decisions. As silicone implant related trials continued throughout the United States, judges began to see a need for strong, objective data on which they could base their rulings. In April 1996, two federal judges in New York appointed an independent expert panel, impartial to either side of the debate, to review the available literature on breast implants and their medical effects. In addition to helping judges resolve implant-related cases in New York, this decision established the important precedent that medical evidence to be used in the courtroom should be objective and validated. In October 1996, while presiding over breast implant cases in Oregon, Federal Judge Robert E. Jones ruled, after reviewing the conclusions of his own independent panel of scientists, that plaintiffs' lawyers could not present evidence linking silicone implants with systemic disease, as the evidence was not scientifically valid. Around the same time, the California appellate court dismissed 1800 breast-implant related lawsuits on similar grounds of lack of valid evidence that implants were associated with systemic diseases.

In June 1999 when the Institute of Medicine of the National Academy of Sciences published its 400-page report on silicone breast implants in response to a congressional request for a conclusive review of the literature, and found no link between implants and connective tissue diseases, cancer causation, neurologic disease, diseases in children, or interference with cancer treatment, the media began to take notice. In a 1999 *Washington Post* editorial, "Study Again Clears Silicone; Breast Implants Said to Cause No Major Disease"[37] the editors alleged that lawyers had recklessly overshot provable science, but had focused attention on the manufacturers' failure to adequately test their devices. As the tide of litigation began to quiet, the community was ready for the data.

THE AGE OF ENLIGHTENMENT: 2000–PRESENT

The period after 2000 was the beginning of the enlightenment. Inamed (formerly McGhan) and Mentor received approval of their saline implant PMAs on May 10, 2000. As the body of international literature on implants continued to grow, it became clear that problems with implants were not systemic, but rather local, and consisted chiefly of capsular contracture, rupture, and reoperations. In 2003, the FDA announced another Advisory Panel for Silicone Breast Implants, 11 years after the prior panel resulted in implant moratorium. Amidst another emotionally charged audience, Inamed presented their data on silicone devices. Despite concern about rupture rates, gel

bleed, and a reoperation rate of 20%, testimony regarding ongoing work to address these concerns and a proactive approach to addressing proposed approval conditions resulted in a 9 to 6 decision in favor of Inamed's PMA for silicone gel breast implants.

In January 2004, the FDA again rejected the panel's recommendation and released a set of proposed standards for safety and efficacy of silicone gel implants. Additionally, they announced a fourth panel to take place in April 2005 to reconsider the issue. The climate of this meeting was marked by a strong presence by organized plastic surgery, with the public testimony evenly divided between anti-implant activists relaying negative patient experiences, and plastic surgeons relaying positive patient experiences. Inamed's presentation of their PMA was rejected 5 to 4, largely because of ongoing concerns with the style 153 double lumen device, and a disproportionately high rupture rate on MRI studies. In contrast, Mentor's PMA presentation dazzled the panel, and earned a 7 to 2 recommendation for approval.

In the discussion between the FDA and the manufacturers that followed the panel meeting, the decision was made to offer preliminary approvals for both Mentor and Inamed's silicone gel implants, under the condition that Inamed's 153 device would specifically be excluded from the approval. Conditions for this approval included a 10-year core study following patients with silicone devices, appropriate patient education and informed consent, a retrieval process to continue tracking device failure, continuing physician education, recommendations on how to manage long-term issues such as device rupture, and the institution of postmarket surveillance and registry.

THE PROMISE OF THE FUTURE: 2006 AND BEYOND

Fourteen years after the moratorium, on November 17, 2006, the FDA approved Allergan (formerly Inamed) and Mentor to resume the manufacture and sale of silicone gel breast implants for general use in the United States, including reconstructive and aesthetic indications. As a result of the vigorous research that resulted in this approval, the informed consent process, the implants themselves, surgical techniques, and methods to ensure longitudinal follow-up matured substantially. With this maturation, and a single-minded commitment to identifying and disseminating the truth, the public's faith in plastic surgery has, for now, been restored. Perhaps one indicator of the restoration of this trust is the continued growth of procedures with breast implants. In 2007, breast augmentation remained the most popular aesthetic surgery procedure performed in the United States, up 6% from 2006 and up 64% from 2000.[38]

Protecting and reinforcing this trust will remain a constant challenge to the plastic surgery community. As the deteriorating economic climate of medicine continues to push other specialties toward performing aesthetic procedures to remain viable, an ever-increasing number of clinicians will seek to incorporate breast surgery into their practices. To retain the confidence of the public it will be critical to ensure that plastic surgeons are equipped with accurate information to counsel patients effectively, the resolve to practice ethically, the foresight to collect data, and the humility to critically assess our own results to continuously improve patient outcomes and safety.

REFERENCES

1. Czerny V. Plastischer ersatz der brustdrüse durch ein lipom. Zentralbl Chir 1895;22:72.
2. Czerny V. Drei plastische operationen. Ver Deutsch Gesell Chir 1895;24:211–7.
3. Czerny V. Drei plastische operationen. Arch F Klin Chir Berl 1895;26:544–50.
4. Gersuny R [Uber eine subcutane prothese]. Zeitschrift Heilkunde Wien u Leipzig 1900;21:199. This was translated as. "Concerning a subcutaneous prosthesis". Euerle R Plast Reconstr Surg 1980;65: 525–7.
5. Thorek M. Amastia, hypomastia, and inequality of the breasts. In: Plastic surgery of the breast and abdominal wall. Springfield (IL): Thomas; 1942. p. 369–86.
6. Harris HI. Research in plastic implants: their use in augmentation for amastia or hypomastia. J Int Coll Surg 1961;35:630–43.
7. Rees TD. Plastic surgery of the breast. In: Converse JM, editor. Reconstructive plastic surgery. Philadelphia: Saunders; 1964. p. 1903–38.
8. Stephenson KL. A history of mammaplasty. In: Masters FW, Lewis JR, editors. Symposium on aesthetic surgery of the face, eyelid, and breast. St Louis (MO): Mosby; 1972. p. 115–29.
9. Lalardrie J, Mouly R. History of augmentation mammaplasty. Aesthetic Plastic Surgery 1978;2: 167–76.
10. Schalk DN. The history of augmentation mammaplasty. Plast Surg Nurs 1988;8:88–95.
11. Sperber PA. Silicone augmentation. In: Treatment of the aging skin and dermal defects. Springfield (IL): Thomas; 1965. p. 73–101.
12. Kagan HD. Sakurai injectable silicone formula. Arch Otolaryngol 1963;78:663–8.
13. Helal B. Toxicology of silicones. Br Med J 1968;3: 184–5.
14. Rubin LR. Polyethylene: a three year study. Plast Reconstr Surg 1951;7:131–42.
15. Naso A. Mastectomia e ricostruzione estetica della regione mammaria con spugna di polietilene. Riforma Med 1953;67:662–4.
16. Giacomelli V. Protesi sostitutiva con spugna di polystan dopo mastectomia. Minerva Chir 1953;8: 584–5.
17. Pangman WJ II, Wallace RM. The use of plastic prosthesis in breast plastic and other soft tissue surgery: clinical experience using Ivalon (polyvinyl) sponge in surgery. West J Surg Obstet Gynecol 1955;63:503–12.
18. Edgerton MT. Augmentation mammaplasty: psychiatric implications and surgical indications. Plast Reconstr Surg 1958;21:279–305.
19. Edgerton MT, Meyer E, Jacobson WE. Augmentation mammaplasty. II. Further surgical and psychiatric evaluation. Plast Reconstr Surg 1961;27: 279–302.
20. Demergian P. Experiences with the newer subcutaneous implant materials. Surg Clin North Am 1963; 32:1313–21.
21. Speirs AC, Blocksma R. New implantable silicone rubbers: an experimental evaluation of tissue response. Plast Reconstr Surg 1963;31:166–75.
22. Regnault P. One hundred cases of retromammary implantation of Etheron followed up for 30 months. Transactions of the Third International Congress Of Plastic Surgery. Amsterdam, The Netherlands: Excerpta Medica Foundation, 1964;74.
23. Calnan JS. Assessment of biological properties of implants before their clinical use. Proc R Soc Med 1970;63:1115–8.
24. Smahêl J, Schneider K, Donski P. Bizarre implants for augmentation mammaplasty: long term reaction to polyethylene strips. Br J Plast Surg 1977;30: 287–90.
25. Rees TD, Höhler H. Plastic surgery of the breast. In: Converse JM, editor. Reconstructive plastic surgery. 2nd edition. Philadelphia: Saunders; 1977. p. 3661–726.
26. Cronin TD, Gerow FJ. Augmentation mammoplasty: a new "natural feel" prosthesis. Transactions of the Third International Congress of Plastic Surgery. Amsterdam, The Netherlands: Excerpta Medica Foundation, 1964;41–9.
27. Braley SA. The use of silicones in plastic surgery. Plast Reconstr Surg 1973;50:280–8.
28. Connie Chung Show, ABC Television; Dec 10, 1990.
29. Letter from FDA to Jan Varner, McGhan (Press Release; Sept 13, 1991).
30. Hazleton RA, Former CEO dow corning. Press release. May 15, 1995. Available at: http://www.sec info.com/dt6y.a3.htm. Accessed June 3, 2008.

31. Renwick SB. Silicone breast implants: implications for society and surgeons. Med J Aust 1996;165:338–41.
32. Spear SL. The breast implant story. Ann Plast Surg 2006;56(5):573–83.
33. Perkins LL, Clark BD, Klein PJ, et al. A meta-analysis of breast implants and connective tissue disease. Ann Plast Surg 1995;35(6):561–70.
34. Sanchez-Guerrero J, Colditz GA, Karlson EW, et al. Silicone breast implants and the risk of connective-tissue diseases and symptoms. N Engl J Med 1995;332(25):1666–70.
35. Peters W, Keystone E, Snow K, et al. Is there a relationship between autoantibodies and silicone-gel implants? Ann Plast Surg 1994;32(1):1–5 [discussion: 5–7].
36. Gabriel SE, O'Fallon WM, Kurland LT, et al. Risk of connective-tissue diseases and other disorders after breast implantation. N Engl J Med 1994;330(24): 1697–702.
37. The Washington Post. Study again clears silicone; breast implants said to cause no major disease. The Washington Post; June 22, 1999, A.02.
38. 2000/2006/2007 National Reconstructive and Cosmetic Plastic Surgery Statistics, American Society of Plastic Surgeons. Available at: http://www.plasticsurgery.org/media/statistics/index.cfm.

Measuring Patient Outcomes in Breast Augmentation: Introducing the BREAST-Q© Augmentation Module

Andrea L. Pusic, MD, MPH[a],*, Patrick L. Reavey, MD[a],
Anne F. Klassen, DPhil[b], Amie Scott, BSc[a],
Colleen McCarthy, MD, MS[a], Stefan J. Cano, PhD[c]

KEYWORDS

- Augmentation mammaplasty • Outcomes • Questionnaire
- Patient satisfaction • Quality of life

Breast augmentation is the most common cosmetic surgery procedure performed in the United States. Approximately 350,000 cosmetic breast augmentation procedures were performed in 2007, a 64% increase since 2000.[1] During this same period, increased surgical experience has led to a wide range of techniques for this procedure.[2,3] In addition, the technology of breast implants has evolved significantly and surgeons now have an array of implants from which to choose.[4–7] With such a rapid expansion in treatment options, it is important to establish a strong evidence base as a guide in making surgical decisions. Surgeons need data to determine whether newer techniques and devices, some of which may carry additional surgical risk and cost, are in fact superior to older ones. Patients as well increasingly demand meaningful data to help them better understand expected outcomes and to play a more active role in making medical decisions.

Traditionally, the discussion of surgical outcomes with patients centered on information about morbidity (eg, surgical scars) and complications. While such data remain important, they are insufficient. Achieving an optimal aesthetic result is a primary focus of breast augmentation. Various methods to measure aesthetic outcome following augmentation have been used in the literature. These include both objective clinician rating of the outcome through photo scoring and, more recently, quantitative analysis of breast volume, contour, projection, and symmetry through the use of sophisticated three-dimensional photography and photo-scoring software.[8] These data provide important information to researchers and clinicians. However, they are not sufficient to complete the outcomes discussion because they fail to take into account the patient's viewpoint, which may differ significantly from that of the clinician evaluator.

A different and increasingly used approach to outcome assessment—an approach that includes the patient's viewpoint—involves the use of patient-reported outcome measures (PROMs). These measures are essentially patient-completed

a Department of Plastic and Reconstructive Surgery, Memorial Sloan-Kettering Cancer Center, 1275 York Avenue, NY 10021, USA
b Department of Pediatrics, McMaster University, 3A-1200 Main Street West, Hamilton, Ontario, Canada
c Neurological Outcome Measures Unit, Institute of Neurology, National Hospital for Neurology and Neurosurgery, University College London, Queen Square, London, England WC1N3BG, UK
* Corresponding author.
E-mail address: pusica@mskcc.org (A.L. Pusic).

Clin Plastic Surg 36 (2009) 23–32
doi:10.1016/j.cps.2008.07.005

plasticsurgery.theclinics.com

questionnaires designed to assess a broader range of health-related outcomes, including patient symptoms, satisfaction, and quality of life. Such measures are based on the view that health is a multidimensional construct and that it is subjective and therefore should be evaluated by asking a person directly. An appropriate PROM is able to measure a wide variety of health-related issues, such as satisfaction with aesthetic appearance, body image, and sexual well-being.

In 2002, the Scientific Advisory Committee of the Medical Outcomes Trust (MOT) published an international consensus of appropriate methods for the development and validation of new PROMs.[9] These guidelines can be simplified to a rigorous three-stage system that includes step-by-step procedures for questionnaire item generation, item reduction, and psychometric evaluation.[10] In 2006, the Food and Drug Administration (FDA) released its Guidance to Industry, which similarly delineated the steps needed to develop a PROM.[11] Both the MOT consensus document and the FDA guidance emphasize the importance of patient involvement in the item-generation phase of questionnaire development. Involving patients ensures that issues most important to them are well represented in the conceptual framework and in the final measure. In addition, input from patients helps researchers identify the specific words and phrases used by patients. Use of exact patient vocabulary aids in ensuring that questionnaire items will be understood and will resonate with patients.

SYSTEMATIC LITERATURE REVIEW

Before development of the BREAST-Q©, we performed a systematic literature review to identify available PROMs for use in breast surgery patients.[12] Our literature search identified 224 articles, which contained a total of 227 instruments. After elimination of ad hoc questionnaires and generic instruments, we identified seven PROMs that measured satisfaction, breast-related quality of life, or both and that had undergone development and validation in a cosmetic or reconstructive breast surgery population. Four of these instruments were specific to breast augmentation.

All four instruments were developed by industry. The McGhan Medical Corporation developed an instrument for its Saline-Filled Mammary Implant Augmentation Clinical Study,[13] and LipoMatrix, Inc. developed a questionnaire for its Breast Implant Replacement Study to evaluate the use of Trilucent breast implants. Dow Corning developed a questionnaire that measures patient satisfaction, psychosocial outcomes, concerns, and benefits-to-risks appraisals in women who had received bilateral breast augmentation with Dow Corning silicone implants.[14] Finally, Mentor developed the Breast Evaluation Questionnaire, which was designed to assess patient satisfaction with aesthetic outcomes among breast augmentation patients.[15] The development and validation process for each of these instruments was evaluated using the criteria established by the MOT. In our systematic review, we found that none of these instruments met accepted development and validation criteria for use in a breast augmentation population.

THE IMPORTANCE OF PATIENT-REPORTED OUTCOME MEASUREMENT

Although breast augmentation is a common procedure for which patient satisfaction and improved quality of life are key outcomes, no adequate outcome measures are available to guide research and clinical care. It is this void that the BREAST-Q© was designed to fill.

A well-developed PROM allows physicians to understand the benefits that breast augmentation may have to a woman's overall quality of life, body image, and psychologic and sexual functioning. In addition, such an instrument may aid researchers in measuring patient satisfaction with surgery-specific issues (eg, breast shape, implant rippling, implant "feel," scar locations). The ability to reliably quantify and compare subjective data could provide a wealth of information that could be used to improve surgical techniques and implant technology. As researchers nationally and internationally begin to use a common metric, we will increasingly be able to compare study results in a meaningful fashion. Furthermore, as we seek to support evidence-based practice and to work more closely with patients in making medical decisions, PROM data will provide valuable direction for surgeons and patients.

In addition to providing data that could lead to improvements in surgical techniques and implant technology, PROM data may aid individual plastic surgeons in their clinical practice. Using newer psychometric methods, a well-developed PROM provides valid assessment of individual patients over time. Thus, clinicians will be able to follow improvement in health outcomes, or to detect concern, among individual patients in their care. Assessment of variables, such as patient satisfaction with care (eg, satisfaction with nurses, office staff), may also provide helpful data that could be used to improve service delivery and thereby the experience for patients. Overall, PROM data will help plastic surgeons provide better care for their patients, but also, from a business standpoint, will assist individual surgeons as they seek to improve customer satisfaction.

DEVELOPMENT OF THE BREAST-Q©

The BREAST-Q© was developed following international guidelines for instrument development.[9–11,16] This process can be divided into a multiphased approach that includes (1) the development of a conceptual framework and item generation, (2) the reduction of items and formation of a scale, and (3) psychometric evaluation of the new measure. In the following sections, we provide a brief overview of the development process for the BREAST-Q© focusing specifically on the Augmentation module. A summary diagram for the development process can be seen in **Fig. 1**.

Development of the Conceptual Framework

After obtaining local institutional ethics review board approval for our study, we conducted a series of in-depth, semistructured interviews with breast surgery patients (augmentation, reduction, reconstruction). A detailed discussion of the findings from our qualitative interview study and the development of the conceptual framework is described elsewhere.[17] Interviews explored issues to do with patient satisfaction and breast surgery–related quality of life. Patients were chosen to ensure that a full spectrum of age, ethnicity, reasons for surgery, and surgery type were represented. Patient interviews were audiotaped and transcribed. Data collection and analysis occurred concurrently to ensure that ideas emerging from our data could be reconfirmed in new data that we collected. Interviews continued within each group until subsequent interviews did not provide any new theoretic insights. Based on these interviews, it was clear that specific issues varied in importance by surgical group. To account for patient differences, we developed separate questionnaires, or modules, for each of three breast surgery groups:

- BREAST-Q© Augmentation module
- BREAST-Q© Reconstruction module
- BREAST-Q© Reduction module

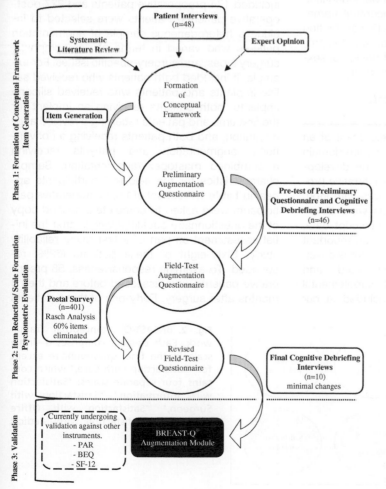

Fig. 1. BREAST-Q© development flowchart. BEQ, Breast Evaluation Questionnaire; PAR, Physician Achievement Review; SF-12, Short-Form-12.

Within the breast augmentation group, a number of common themes were identified. Women described satisfaction, or lack thereof, with reference to breast size, shape, symmetry, cleavage, and how their breasts fit in proportion to the rest of their body. After breast augmentation, women often described feeling more attractive, feminine, and socially confident. Surgery was also seen as a way to bring the body into line with what they perceived to be more "normal" for a woman's body.[18] Finally, women also often expressed concern with aspects of the physician–patient relationship, interactions with office staff, and receipt of preoperative information.

Findings from the patient interviews were combined with issues identified during the systematic literature review (discussed above), and with expert opinion from a panel of plastic surgeons and other health care professionals, to form a conceptual framework of quality of life and patient satisfaction in breast augmentation patients (**Fig. 2**). This model mirrored the main themes discussed by patients, with each identified theme becoming a separate domain. Six key themes were identified that formed the basis of the conceptual framework: (1) satisfaction with breasts, (2) satisfaction with overall outcome, (3) satisfaction with the process of care, (4) psychosocial well-being, (5) sexual well-being, and (6) physical well-being.

Item Generation, Preliminary Scale Formation, and Pretesting

The next phase involved the development of an exhaustive list of potential items for each domain within our conceptual framework. The development of questionnaire items was an iterative process led by the team of investigators with input from expert panel members. Items were developed directly from the interview transcript data, ensuring that all six themes identified as important to women were included and that the items developed retained the patients' own words and phrases. We also incorporated supplemental items from the seven PROMs included in our

systematic review when they covered issues not captured through the interviews.

The preliminary questionnaire was then pretested in a group of breast surgery patients. All 46 participants in this pilot study received the questionnaire by mail and participated in a follow-up cognitive debriefing phone interview. Patients were asked to identify any relevant issues that had been missed, to discuss their understanding of the items, and to identify any ambiguities in the wording of items. They were also asked to comment on the response options and recall period. Based on patient feedback, field-test versions of the questionnaire modules were modified and finalized.

Field Testing and Final Scale Development

The BREAST-Q© Augmentation module was mailed to 551 breast augmentation patients recruited from two centers, one in Cottonwood, Utah, and the other in Vancouver, British Columbia, Canada. The response rate was 72%, yielding a total of 401 field-test participants. This sample included 174 preoperative patients and 227 postoperative patients. Patients were selected to include a heterogeneous sample of augmentation patients who varied in terms of demographics, surgery types, and surgery-specific issues. For example, it included both patients who received saline implants and patients who received silicone implants, both patients receiving an implant for the first time and patients receiving a revised augmentation, and both patients receiving a conventional augmentation and patients receiving a combined mastopexy/augmentation. Sample characteristics for the field-test participants appear in **Table 1**. A subset of 110 postoperative participants were asked to complete a second copy of the questionnaire booklet 2 weeks after the initial assessment as part of a test-retest reliability study. Sixty-eight of these patients (62%) responded. To examine responsiveness, 58 preoperative patients were assessed before and then 3 months after surgery. Forty-one of these patients

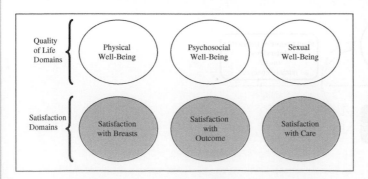

Fig. 2. BREAST-Q© conceptual framework. Each domain comprises a single scale in the final questionnaire except for "Satisfaction with Care," which contains four separate scales: "Satisfaction with Information," "Satisfaction with Surgeon," "Satisfaction with Office Staff," and "Satisfaction with Medical Team."

Table 1		
Sample characteristics of postoperative augmentation field-test patients (227 patients; mean age, 37 years; age range, 18 to 73 years)		
Characteristic	Number	Percentage
Surgery type		
Primary augmentation	187	83
Revision augmentation	23	10
Mastopexy/ augmentation	17	7
Implant type		
Saline	111	49
Silicone	76	33
Not known	40	18
Ethnicity		
White	178	78
Other	38	17
No Response	11	5
Income		
<$39,999	39	17
$40,000–$99,999	109	48
>$100,000	69	30
Relationship		
Partnered	161	70

(71%) responded. For all groups, nonresponding patients did not differ significantly from the study population in terms of age or surgery-specific characteristics.

Rasch[19,20] measurement methods were used to guide scale construction and item reduction. This method of analysis has a number of advantages over traditional psychometric methods based on classical test theory (the current predominant paradigm) and is increasingly used in PROM development as a means to increase the clinical utility of new questionnaires for individual patients. Scale and item scoring with Rasch analyses[21,22] improve the accuracy with which clinical change can be measured. Rasch methods provide estimates for patients (and items) that are independent of the sampling distribution of items (and patients). Among other benefits, using Rasch methods to develop a scale allows for accurate measurement of outcomes for individual patients as well as for larger patient groups. This approach to assessment can help to directly inform patient monitoring, management, and treatment. Other advantages include the potential to bank items, equate scales, administer computerized scales,

and handle missing data.[23–25] We used Rasch analyses for the item reduction process, making final decisions on which items to include or exclude. Approximately 40% of items were retained, while 60% were eliminated because of poor functioning or redundancy. The complete details of the Rasch analysis are published elsewhere.[26]

Final Cognitive Debriefing Interviews

As a final confirmation of the acceptability of the questionnaire, a small sample of postoperative augmentation patients were mailed the item-reduced BREAST-Q© Augmentation module and participated in a cognitive debriefing interview by phone. Just as in phase 1 with the field-test questionnaire, participants were asked to discuss their understanding of the items and to identify ambiguities. Completion time was also examined. This additional feedback led us to make minor changes to the questionnaire.

THE BREAST-Q© AUGMENTATION MODULE
Questionnaire Structure: Scales and Items

The BREAST-Q© Augmentation module has both pre- and postoperative versions. The postoperative questionnaire contains all of the items of the preoperative questionnaire with the addition of postsurgery items and additional scales to measure satisfaction with treatment and process-of-care issues. **Table 2** shows the scale structure with item numbers for both versions.

Each of the scales for both the pre- and postoperative questionnaires can be used independently allowing significant flexibility for use in both clinical research and individual practice. For example, if a researcher is interested in a patient's satisfaction with a new type of implant, he or she may administer only the "Satisfaction with Breasts" scale. Additionally, a private practice surgeon wanting to improve overall patient perceptions of their practice may choose to administer only the "Process of Care" scales.

Completion of the preoperative questionnaire takes approximately 3 to 5 minutes, while the postoperative questionnaire takes about 8 to 10 minutes to complete.

Scale Scoring

Each of the scales for the BREAST-Q© Augmentation module is scored separately and reported on a 0-to-100 scale. A scale of this range makes understanding and comparison of scores easy for patients and clinicians. However, as patients are answering questions on a 1- to 5-value Likert scale, transformation of scores is required to

Table 2
Scale structure of the BREAST-Q© Augmentation module

Preoperative Questionnaire		Postoperative Questionnaire	
Scale	Items	Scale	Items
Satisfaction with Breasts	6	Satisfaction with Breasts	16[a]
Psychosocial Well-being	9	Psychosocial Well-being	9
Sexual Well-being	5	Sexual Well-being	5
Physical Well-being	5	Physical Well-being	7[a]
		Satisfaction with Outcome	8
		Satisfaction with Care	
		Satisfaction with Information	16
		Satisfaction with Surgeon	12
		Satisfaction with Medical Team	7
		Satisfaction with Office Staff	7

[a] These scales include additional items to measure postoperative issues such as scarring.

obtain the 0-to-100 value. Currently, this is achieved by summing the responses within each questionnaire scale and using a conversion table (available with the questionnaire) to obtain the 0-to-100 score. Scoring software is being developed to facilitate calculation of final scale scores and will be available shortly.

PSYCHOMETRIC PROPERTIES OF THE BREAST-Q© AUGMENTATION MODULE

In addition to Rasch analyses, the final scales underwent supplementary psychometric analyses using traditional psychometric methods to provide data that could be compared with existing measures and against current PROM recommendation criteria.[9–11] Each of the scale item responses was summed without weighting or standardization to generate scores. Four traditional psychometric measurement properties were examined: acceptability, reliability, validity, and responsiveness (**Table 3**). The psychometric properties of the BREAST-Q© Augmentation module are presented in **Table 4**.

Internal Consistency Reliability

Internal consistency reliability for the questionnaire was assessed using data from the entire breast augmentation patient sample. The Cronbach's α coefficients for all of the scales ranged from 0.81 to 0.94 and item total correlations ranged from 0.55 to 0.82. These values are well above the recommended criteria of 0.7 and 0.3,[27] respectively, indicating excellent internal consistency reliability.

Test-Retest Reliability

For assessment of test-retest reliability, 68 patients completed the questionnaire twice (response rate 62%) separated by 2 weeks. For five of the scales, the test-retest intraclass correlations were well above the recommended 0.7 criteria[28] (range 0.85–0.94), demonstrating excellent stability.

Responsiveness

Forty-one patients completed the questionnaire before and after surgery to allow for examination of scale responsiveness. Patients had significant improvement in their "Satisfaction with Breasts Scale" scores following breast augmentation (preoperative mean 26 versus postoperative mean 76, $P < .001$). In addition, the calculated effect sizes for the "Satisfaction with Breasts," "Psychosocial Well-Being," and "Sexual Well-Being" scales were all large (effect sizes >0.8) indicating sensitivity of the scales to change (**Table 5**).[29,30]

Face, Content, and Construct Validity

Face and content validity of the BREAST-Q© were established in the development process through patient interviews, cognitive debriefing, and expert review. Construct validity of the BREAST-Q© has been demonstrated with hypothesis testing using data from field test patients. For example, we hypothesized and confirmed that scores on the "Satisfaction with Breasts" scale of the BREAST-Q© Augmentation Module were lower among patients who required a secondary procedure because of complication (eg. capsulotomy) in comparison to patients having the procedure for the first time

Table 3
Description of psychometric properties

Psychometric Property	Definition/Criteria for Acceptability
Acceptability	Quality of data; assessed by completeness of data and score distributions; missing data <5%; maximum endorsement frequencies <80%
Responsiveness	Ability of an instrument's ability to detect change over time or following intervention/surgery; consider effect size or minimal important difference
Reliability	
Internal consistency reliability	The precision of the questionnaire or scale based on the homogeneity (intercorrelations) of the scale's items at one point in time; Cronbach's α >0.7 and item-total correlations >0.3
Interrater reliability	Reproducibility of results between different patients at one point in time
Test-retest reliability	The stability of a scale; assessed on the basis of correlations between repeat administrations of the scale on two occasions; intraclass correlations >0.7 between test and re-test scores
Validity	
Validity within scale	Evidence that the scale measures a single construct and that items can be combined to form a summary score; assessed on basis of internal consistency reliability
Validity comparison with other measures	Comparing scores of questionnaire scales to other accepted related instruments (ie, comparing quality-of-life scale score to score from Short-Form-36)
Validity hypothesis testing	Demonstrate ability to measure expected differences between groups within patient population (eg, satisfaction among patients who had complications compared with those who did not)

Data from Cano SJ, Browne JP, Lamping DL, et al. The patient outcomes of surgery-hand/arm (POS-hand/arm): a new patient-based outcome measure. J Hand Surg [Br] 2004;29(5):477–85; and Scientific Advisory Committee of the Medical Outcomes Trust. Assessing health status and quality-of-life instruments: attributes and review criteria. Qual Life Res 2002;11:193–204.

and patients having a secondary procedure for reasons unrelated to complications. We also hypothesized and confirmed that satisfaction diminished with increasing time since surgery.

Convergent and discriminant validity of the BREAST-Q© Augmentation module relative to other questionnaires is currently being assessed in a sample of 400 postoperative patients in Vancouver. In this study, patients receive the BREAST-Q© Augmentation module by mail along with several other measures that examine similar constructs. These include the Breast Evaluation

Table 4
Psychometric properties of the BREAST-Q© Augmentation module

Scale	Cronbach's α	Item-Total Correlations	Test-Retest Reliability (Intraclass Correlations)
Satisfaction with Breasts	0.91	0.61 (0.45–0.74)	0.85 [0.75, 0.91]
Satisfaction with Outcome	0.92	0.73 (0.58–0.85)	0.88 [0.80, 0.93]
Satisfaction with Information	0.94	0.70 (0.51–0.77)	0.89 [0.82, 0.94]
Psychosocial Well-Being	0.94	0.78 (0.67–0.82)	0.94 [0.89, 0.96]
Sexual Well-Being	0.93	0.82 (0.77–0.87)	0.87 [0.79, 0.92]
Physical Well-Being	0.81	0.55 (0.46–0.61)	0.93 [0.88, 0.96]

Table 5
Effect size in pre- to postoperative patients (n = 41)

	Satisfaction with Breasts	Psychosocial Well-being	Sexual Well-being
Effect size (Cohen's $d = \triangle /SD_{t1}$)	4.0	2.2	3.2

Cohen's d scale: 0.8 "large"; 0.5 "medium"; 0.2"small".[30]

Questionnaire,[15] the Short-Form-12,[31] and the Physician Achievement Review.[32] Discriminant and convergent validity of the BREAST-Q© Augmentation scales will be examined relative to these other measures (ie, quality-of-life scales will be considered relative to the Short-Form-12 scales).

Linguistic Validation

The BREAST-Q© was developed and has been validated in a North American patient population. However, the utility of this instrument will extend beyond this geographic area. As such, the BREAST-Q© is currently undergoing translation and linguistic validation in United States Spanish, in French, and in German.

FUTURE USE AND IMPACT OF THE BREAST-Q© AUGMENTATION MODULE

The BREAST-Q© Augmentation module provides accurate measurement of patient satisfaction and quality-of-life outcomes following breast augmentation. Use of the BREAST-Q© Augmentation module will provide a wealth of essential data to clinicians and researchers that may be used to improve the field of breast augmentation from the perspectives of both surgeons and patients. Among the benefits of this module are its potential contributions to evidence-based practice, device research and development, patient advocacy, and customer satisfaction.

As the field of medicine advances and treatment options increase, greater emphasis is being placed upon evidence-based practice and the use of outcomes data for individual patients in making decisions. As the most important outcomes in plastic surgery are patient satisfaction and quality of life, reliable PROM data are essential to evaluate the benefits of newly developed surgical techniques. Consistent use of the questionnaire will provide a common metric that surgeons can use to compare the results of their technique to those of others. Collecting data of this nature will allow a comprehensive outcomes discussion to determine if advanced and more expensive techniques for augmentation have any additional benefit from a patient perspective.

Implementation of the BREAST-Q© Augmentation module as a common metric will also be useful for industry. Significant research time and funding are directed toward development of new and better breast implants. Some of this effort seeks out improvements that decrease complications. Other effort is involved in improving the shape and feel of the augmented breast. These factors are best assessed from a patient's perspective and can be accurately measured using the BREAST-Q© Augmentation module. As an example, industry studies on new implants may use scores on the satisfaction scales to measure patient perceptions and compare these scores to those of other implant types. In addition to improving implant technology from a patient's perspective, PROM data from the BREAST-Q© Augmentation module will support regulatory efforts by the FDA and industry. The FDA recognizes the importance of PROM data and is moving toward of the assessment of product claims based on such studies. It is clearly anticipated that the FDA will weigh the quality-of-life data in such studies based on the validity and psychometric performance of the PROM being used. The FDA Guidance document has concisely established these expectations for rigorous PROM development and validation.[9–11] The BREAST-Q© Augmentation module has been designed to satisfy these criteria and as such will be useful for pre- and postmarket device evaluation studies.

Patient advocacy is another specific area in which the BREAST-Q© Augmentation module will be useful. The controversy surrounding access to silicone breast implants in the United States illustrates the need for data both to accurately measure the safety of breast surgical procedures and to quantify their benefits to patients. According to data obtained with the BREAST-Q© Augmentation module, breast augmentation patients benefit in terms of their overall satisfaction with their breasts, their psychosocial well-being, and their sexual well-being. Similarly, satisfaction data obtained in breast reconstruction patients using the BREAST-Q© Reconstruction module demonstrate that patients with silicone implants have significantly higher satisfaction than patients with saline implants.[33] Studies evaluating differences in patient satisfaction between different implants may thus provide plastic surgeons with additional data to help women choose among implant types.

Finally, private clinicians will benefit from the use of this questionnaire in their individual practices. As patients are becoming increasingly involved in their own medical care, they are demanding meaningful data to help them better understand expected outcomes. When advising new patients, plastic surgeons who use the BREAST-Q© Augmentation module in their practices will be able to provide tangible evidence of satisfaction from prior patients. This can improve communication with patients, allowing the physician to be more effective in addressing their specific concerns. Furthermore, as increasing data from use of the BREAST-Q© Augmentation module become available, professional societies will be able to provide "benchmarks" for patient satisfaction and quality-of-life outcomes. In addition, breast augmentation patients place substantial importance on the process of care involved in their surgery, including, for example, the preoperative information provided by their surgeon and the way they are treated by their surgeon, his or her nurses, and office staff.[17,34] We developed a number of "Process of Care" scales as part of the BREAST-Q© Augmentation module so clinicians might receive feedback from patients about the entire treatment experience. Surgeons, using their patient information, may then be able to tailor and improve specific aspects of their practice to improve customer satisfaction.

The BREAST-Q© Augmentation module is currently the only questionnaire for use in breast augmentation patients that has been developed using new psychometric methods and validated with strict adherence to the guidelines described by the MOT and the FDA.[9,11] The questionnaire measures the effect of breast augmentation on multiple spheres of patients' lives as well as satisfaction with their surgery and the process of care. The BREAST-Q© Augmentation module has been demonstrated to have excellent psychometric properties, and is currently undergoing additional validation. The use of this questionnaire will provide a wealth of important data to both researchers and clinicians to improve the field of breast augmentation and individual surgeon practices.

REFERENCES

1. American Society of Plastic Surgeons. 2000/2006/2007 National plastic surgery statistics: cosmetic and reconstructive procedure trends. American Society of Plastic Surgeons Web site. 2006. Available at: http://www.plasticsurgery.org/media/statistics/. Accessed May 15, 2008.

2. Goes JCS, Landecker A. Optimizing outcomes in breast augmentation: seven years of experience with the subfascial plane. Aesthetic Plast Surg 2003;27(3):178–84.

3. Hendricks H. Complete submuscular breast augmentation: 650 cases managed using an alternative surgical technique. Aesthetic Plast Surg 2007;31(2):147–53.

4. Gutowski KA, Mesna GT, Cunningham BL. Saline-filled breast implants: a plastic surgery educational foundation multicenter outcomes study. Plast Reconstr Surg 1997;100(4):1019–27.

5. Handel N, Jensen JA, Black Q, et al. The fate of breast implants: a critical analysis of complications and outcomes. Plast Reconstr Surg 1995;96(7):1521–33.

6. Barnsley GP, Sigurdson LJ, Barnsley SE. Textured surface breast implants in the prevention of capsular contracture among breast augmentation patients: a meta-analysis of randomized controlled trials. Plast Reconstr Surg 2006;117(7):2182–90.

7. Brown MH, Shenker R, Silver SA. Cohesive silicone gel breast implants in aesthetic and reconstructive breast surgery. Plast Reconstr Surg 2005;116(3):768–79.

8. Galdino GM, Nahabedian M, Chiaramonte M, et al. Clinical applications of three-dimensional photography in breast surgery. Plast Reconstr Surg 2002;110(1):58–70.

9. Scientific Advisory Committee of the Medical Outcomes Trust. Assessing health status and quality-of-life instruments: attributes and review criteria. Qual Life Res 2002;11:193–204.

10. Cano SJ, Browne JP, Lamping DL, et al. The patient outcomes of surgery-hand/arm (POS-hand/arm): a new patient-based outcome measure. J Hand Surg [Br] 2004;29(5):477–85.

11. U.S. Food and Drug Administration. Guidance for Industry. Patient-reported outcome measures: use in medical product development to support labeling claims. U.S. Food and Drug Administration Website. 2006. Available at: http://www.fda.gov/cder/guidance/index.htm. Accessed May 20, 2008.

12. Pusic AL, Chen CM, Cano S, et al. Measuring quality of life in cosmetic and reconstructive breast surgery: a systematic review of patient-reported outcomes instruments. Plast Reconstr Surg 2007;120(4):23–37.

13. McGhan Medical Corporation. McGhan Medical Corporation Saline-Filled Mammary Implant Augmentation Clinical Study protocol. Arlington Heights (IL): ASPS Archives; 1995.

14. Cash TF, Duel LA, Perkins LL. Women's psychological outcomes of breast augmentation with silicone gel–filled implants: a 2-year prospective study. Plast Reconstr Surg 2002;109(6):2122–3.

15. Anderson RC, Cunningham B, Tafesse E, et al. Validation of the breast evaluation questionnaire for use with breast surgery patients. Plast Reconstr Surg 2006;118(3):597–602.

16. Cano SJ, Browne JP, Lamping DL. Patient-based measures of outcome in plastic surgery: current approaches and future directions. Br J Plast Surg 2004;57:1–11.

17. Pusic AL, Klassen A, Cano S, Collins ED, Kerrigan C, Cordeiro PG. Measuring Quality of Life in Breast Surgery: Content Development of a New Modular System to Capture Patient-Reported Outcomes (The MSKCC BREAST-Q©). 2006 International Society of Quality of Life Research meeting abstracts [www.isoqual.org/2006mtgabstracts]. The QLR Journal, A-58, #1226. Presented Oct 12, 2006 in Lisbon, Portugal.

18. Rubin L, Klassen A, Cano SJ, Hurley K, Pusic AL. Motivations for Breast Surgery: A Qualitative Comparison Study of Breast Reconstruction, Augmentation, and Reduction Patients (Letter to Editor). Breast J (In Press).

19. Lord FM, Novick MR. Statistical theories of mental test scores. Reading (MA): Addison-Wesley; 1968.

20. Rasch G. Probabilistic models for some intelligence and attainment tests. Chicago (IL): University of Chicago Press; 1960.

21. Wright B, Stone M. Best test design: Rasch measurement. Chicago (IL): MESA Press; 1979.

22. Wright BD, Linacre JM. Observations are always ordinal: measurements, however, must be interval. Arch Phys Med Rehabil 1989;70(12):857–60.

23. Wainer H, Dorans N, R F, et al. Computerized adaptive testing: a primer. Hillsdale (NJ): Lawrence Erlbaum Associates; 1990.

24. Revicki D, Cella D. Health status assessment for the twenty-first century: item response theory, item banking and computer adaptive testing. Qual Life Res 1997;6(6):595–600.

25. Linacre JM. Computer-adaptive testing: a methodology whose time has come. In: Chae S, Kang U, Jeon E, editors. Development of computerised middle school achievement tests. Seoul (South Korea): Komesa Press; 2000.

26. Pusic A, Klassen A, Cano S, Scott A, Klok J, McCarthy C, Mehrara B, Disa J, Alderman A, Cordeiro P, Lennox P, VanLaeken N, Collins E, Kerrigan C. The BREAST-Q© Development of a new patient-reported outcome measure for breast surgery. [Abstract 35A]. In: Plast Reconstr Surg: The Plastic Surgery Research Council 53rd Annual Meeting Abstract Supplement 2008;121(6 Supp):34. Presented in Springfield, IL on May 30, 2008.

27. Jensen MP. Questionnaire validation: a brief guide for readers of the research literature. Clin J Pain 2003;19(6):345–52.

28. Hays R, Anderson R, Revicki D. Psychometric considerations in evaluating health-related quality of life measures. Qual Life Res 1993;2(6):441–58.

29. Nakagawa S, Cuthill IC. Effect size, confidence interval and statistical significance: a practical guide for biologists. Biol Rev Camb Philos Soc 2007;82: 591–605.

30. Cohen J. Statistical Power Analysis for the Behavioral Sciences. 2nd edition. Hillsdale (NJ): Erlbaum; 1988.

31. Ware J Jr. SF-36 Physical and mental health summary scales: a user's manual. Boston (MA): Health Assessment Laboratory; 1994.

32. Hall W, Violato C, Lewkonia R, et al. Assessment of physician performance in Alberta: the Physician Achievement Review. Can Med Assoc J 1999;162: 52–7.

33. McCarthy C, Cano S, Klassen A, et al. Patient satisfaction with postmastectomy reconstruction: a comparison of saline and silicone implants. [Abstract 29A]. In: Plast Reconstr Surg: The Plastic Surgery Research Council 53rd Annual Meeting Abstract Supplement. 2008;121(65sup):29. Presented in Springfield, IL on May 5, 2008.

34. Coon SK, Burris R, Coleman EA, et al. An analysis of telephone interview data collected in 1992 from 820 women who reported problems with their breast implants to the Food and Drug Administration. Plast Reconstr Surg 2002;109(6): 2043–51.

The Inframammary Approach to Breast Augmentation

Steven Teitelbaum, MD, FACS[a,b]

KEYWORDS

- Breast • Augmentation • Enlargement • Cosmetic
- Surgery • Inframammary • Incision • Complications

The inframammary approach to breast augmentation is the standard to which all others must be compared.

Patients and surgeons frequently reduce the discussion of incisions to a debate over the best location of the scar. Yet the final scar is the least profound difference between the various incisions. Each scar location requires exposure of and risk to very different anatomy, provides the surgeon with different levels of visualization of the critical portions of the operation, causes differing degrees of swelling and recovery, and has effects on the final outcome that will often be more significant to the patient than her scar.

As an example, the McBurney and Rockey-Davis incisions for appendectomy vary in the position of the incision; however, the operations are otherwise the same, encountering identical anatomy, risks, and benefits once beneath the skin. In contrast, breast augmentations through different incisions are quite different operations in very important ways.

Dwelling on the scar is understandable because the other issues are not immediately visualized or even understood by the patient. A paucity of well-controlled studies documenting these differences allows surgeons the freedom to suggest to patients the incision with which they most feel comfortable or to perform any incision the patient requests without pause for thoughtful discussion.

For a patient considering a breast augmentation who has no previous scar on her breasts and is reluctant or ignorant about the totality of breast augmentation risks, focusing on the scar is understandable. But to do so ultimately is puerile, and

the surgeon educating the patient should inform her of other issues that need to be considered.

For the plastic surgeon, it is often easier to agree to a patient's request for a particular incision than to educate her to consider another. Experience and familiarity with an accepted technique creates little impetus for change. For many surgeons, the choice of incision occupies an important marketing niche for their practice, allowing them to offer incisions they can tout as "hidden around the areola," "no scar on the breast," or "hidden in the crease underneath the breast."

I must emphasize that all three incisions— transaxillary, inframammary, and periareolar—are all obviously fully acceptable. But patients should be aware and surgeons should remind themselves that there are many characteristics that distinguish the approaches other than the scar, and the selection of the incision should include consideration of those issues in addition to the location of the scar.

THE SCAR

I believe that scar location should be a low-priority issue when selecting an incision. But because it remains the focal point for most patients and surgeons, it warrants discussion first. Patients obviously want the most inconspicuous incision, and plastic surgeons want to deliver it to them.

But no matter which approach a surgeon prefers, that surgeon is capable of "selling" that incision to most patients. The transaxillary surgeon would tell patients that the armpit incision is off of the breast and heals so well that it is almost

a Department of Plastic Surgery, David Geffen School of Medicine at UCLA, Los Angeles, CA, USA
b 1301 Twentieth Street, Suite 350, Santa Monica, CA 90404, USA
E-mail address: steve@drteitelbaum.com

Clin Plastic Surg 36 (2009) 33–43
doi:10.1016/j.cps.2008.08.008
0094-1298/08/$ – see front matter © 2008 Elsevier Inc. All rights reserved.

impossible to find. The periareolar surgeon would argue that placing the skin around a natural anatomic border renders it the most inconspicuous and that the thin skin of that area consistently yields thin and nearly invisible scars. The inframammary surgeon would argue that an inframammary fold scar is hidden within the crease under the breast, less noticeable than a mark from an underwire bra, and cannot be seen unless the arm is raised over the head with an observer beneath the breast. And the periumbilical surgeon would argue that a scar within the belly button is the epitome of scarless breast surgery because many women have had laparoscopic procedures through the belly button and those scars are barely noticeable.

Which of these arguments is the most correct? If any one of the scars were commonly unacceptable, then that technique would have long since been abandoned. If any one of them had invisible scars without other trade-offs, then everyone would have switched to it by now.

What can we say about the scars? No study has compared patient satisfaction with scars in randomized trials. I have seen very poor scars from all three methods. These problematic scars have been a result of poor execution, patient biology, or both.

Transaxillary incisions must be made at the apex of the axilla, within or parallel to a skin crease. It should not be diagonal, nor should it cross the latissimus or the pectoralis major muscles. When these errors are made, the incision can be unsightly, but the technique should not be condemned due to misexecution.

Periareolar incisions can be excessively visible if they are within the areola, which sometimes yields a hypopigmented scar within a sea of dark areola (though this is easily repairable with cosmetic tattooing). A periareolar incision that is made out beyond the border of the areola can be conspicuous.

An inframammary incision must be made precisely at the inframammary fold. If the location of the fold is going to be preserved, then the incision should be made exactly within the pre-existing inframammary fold. But if the fold is going to be lowered, its precise location should be determined and the incision made exactly at that location. For years, surgeons were improperly taught to make the incision above the inframammary fold so that the scar would not be visible if a woman were wearing a small bikini or bra and raised her hands above her head. But an incision within the crease typically heals so well, that even when the hands are raised and the bra rides up, it is scarcely visible. When the incision is made above the fold, however, the pressure of the implant on the lower pole of the breast frequently causes the scar to

widen and hypertrophy. It is probably because of the errant advice to place the scar above the fold that this approach developed a reputation among some for giving a suboptimal scar. Placement of the scar above the fold should similarly be viewed as a suboptimal execution of the approach, and the incision should not be condemned as a result of it.

Whichever incision is used, surgeons must remind themselves that a scar can be no better than the condition of the skin edges that are approximated. Beveling, scratching through the dermis with multiple knife passes, cauterizing too close to the skin edges, not trimming the skin edges if they were abraded with retractors, putting too much dissolvable suture superficially, closing with uneven sutures, applying too much tension in the sutures, and leaving sutures in too long are all avoidable causes of unsightly scars.

More common and profound than suboptimal execution of the surgery are poorly understood issues of patient biology and wound healing. These issues can yield scars that are thick, raised, painful, and pigmented. Why a surgeon who performs a procedure the same way with excellent scars suddenly gets a patient who has a bad scar is a vexing problem.

Although uncommon in the axilla, when such scars occur, the patient is stuck with a scar that is visible in a bathing suit and in any shirt or dress that is sleeveless. Instead of what could likely have been a bad scar around the areola or in the inframammary fold that could have been covered by clothing and only exposed to intimate friends, she now has a problematic scar that cannot be hidden. Again, although such scars can occur in the axilla, it appears to be a relatively privileged place in terms of scars, and it is fortunate that such scars are uncommon. But the unfortunate few with bad axillary scars are subjected to embarrassment and difficulty in finding clothing to cover up this telltale sign of a breast augmentation.

Hypertrophic, hyperpigmented, and widened scars are much more common with the periareolar than either the transaxillary or inframammary approaches. The reasons are unclear, but I have seen many such patients who had their surgery performed by surgeons known for their expertise with the periareolar approach and personally known by me to perform technically excellent surgery (**Fig. 1**). Although the axilla is a favored area in darker, oilier, and more pigmented patients, the same is undoubtedly not the case with the areola. I have seen only a handful of unacceptable axilla and inframammary scars, but I have seen countless bad areola scars in which the issue was

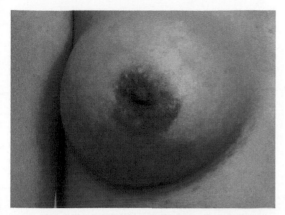

Fig. 1. There are many photos showing inconspicuous and problematic scars from all three incisions. A truly bad transaxillary scar is very rare, and a bad inframammary scar is at least relatively hidden beneath the breast, so long as it is at the inframammary fold. But a bad periareolar scar is unconcealable, visible to all, and more common than is acknowledged. This particular incision was made by an excellent surgeon who is a proponent of the periareolar approach. This photo is just one of literally scores of bad periareolar scar photos I have collected. During the same collection period, I gathered just a handful of photos showing bad transaxillary and inframammary scars.

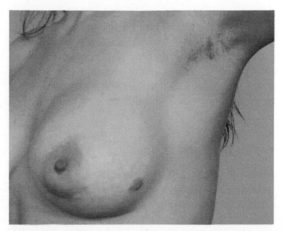

Fig. 2. The first procedure this patient ever had was a mole excision in the lower outer quadrant, leaving an erythematous and hypertrophic scar. For that reason, she selected a transaxillary approach for her augmentation. The transaxillary scar is shown here over five years after surgery, and is frequently visible in sleeveless clothing. When she later required a complete capsulectomy, a periareolar incision was used, which is shown here two years after surgery and laser treatments. Imagine if she had the same poor quality scar in the inframammary fold: she would have had only one scar and it would only have be visible when undressed and supine.

patient biology and not the technical prowess with which the surgery was performed.

So long as the inframammary scar is made to lie within the inframammary crease, it too is a relatively biologically privileged position. Even if all is executed properly, some inframammary scars do get hypertrophic and hyperpigmented. When the breast is small and the crease ill defined, such scars can be quite visible; however, when the breast is large or there is any ptosis, even the thick or red inframammary incision can be difficult to see.

The question that we need to answer is how good or bad is each incision likely to end up. There are no data available to resoundingly answer this issue. One thought experiment, which can be done with a patient, is the following: ask the patient where they would want the scar if they knew the scar would be totally invisible. All will tell you they would want it where there would be the least pain, the easiest recovery, and the best chance to not encounter problems; it would be every issue other than the scar. Then ask the patient where they would want the scar it if they knew it would be terrible (**Fig 2**). Draw on them with a black felt-tip marker in their axilla, around the areola, and in the inframammary fold. If that would be their scar, which would they prefer? I have done this on patients for years, and over 90% choose the inframammary scar because the axillary scar would

be visible in all sleeveless clothing and the periareolar would be visible to anyone looking straight at the breast. The inframammary incision is usually largely hidden beneath the breast, particularly after an augmentation.

REOPERATION

The most objectively quantifiable end point of breast augmentation is the need for revision surgery. Tests are being developed to assess patient satisfaction and other important indicators of success, but as of this date, there are no large series comparing patient satisfaction between the various incisions.

Reoperations remain a significant problem, with nearly one in five women requiring one in the first 3 years following breast augmentation. Unpublished data from the Inamed (now Allergan) Corporation's 3-year pre-market approval data showed a statistically significant, 5.5 times higher reoperation rate through the axilla than through the inframammary fold, and a 2.5 times higher reoperation rate through the areola than through the inframammary fold (Scott Spear, personal communication, 2008). These patients were not randomized, nor were the surgeons. Unless it turns out that patients who wanted the axilla or areola approaches were somehow more predisposed to want revisions than patients who wanted the inframammary approach, or that the transaxillary surgeons in the study were somehow less skilled than the inframammary surgeons in the study, these findings point to a substantial advantage of the inframammary approach over the others.

CAPSULAR CONTRACTURE

Although there are no randomized prospective data that have analyzed the differences in capsular contracture rates between different incisions, the best data to date on capsular contracture rates were based on series of patients who overwhelmingly had the inframammary approach. Even though these patients were not randomized or compared with women having other incisions, until equivalent data are generated with other incisional approaches, the literature supports the use of the inframammary incision.

An abundance of information suggests that bacterial contamination on the implant surface contributes to inflammation of the breast implant capsule. The statistically significant reduction in capsular contracture rates when specific antibiotic or povidone-iodine (Betadine) irrigation is used demonstrates the role of bacteria in capsular contracture. Cultures of periprosthetic tissue and fluid in cases of capsular contracture frequently produce growth of a number of organisms that occur within the breast tissue.

Contact of the implant with breast tissue and the organisms known to reside therein is minimized with the transaxillary and inframammary approaches and occurs to the greatest extent with the periareolar approach. Avoidance of such contact is so important that many surgeons describe putting a sterile drape over the nipple so as to not have any microscopic nipple discharge contaminate the field when performing an inframammary or transaxillary augmentation.

Given how common mastitis is during lactation, women understand that their nipples are open to the outside and that it is normal for potentially harmful bacteria to live within their ducts. When they learn about possible contamination, they are often wary about selecting the periareolar approach.

PRESERVATION OF TISSUE COVERAGE

Maximizing tissue coverage is the single greatest priority in breast augmentation. Inadequate coverage leads to implant visibility and palpability, to pressure atrophy of the parenchyma, and to skin stretch.

Correcting such tissue coverage problems are the most daunting issues in secondary breast surgery.

Although there should not necessarily be a difference in tissue coverage between the various approaches, the periareolar approach is the most prone to inadvertent and often unavoidable sacrifice of tissue coverage (**Fig. 3**). No matter how the dissection is done, there is inevitably some disruption of the fibers that connect the pectoralis muscle to the overlying gland. After the muscle is divided along the inframammary fold, these fibers serve a critical role in holding the muscle down toward the inframammary fold and maintaining muscle coverage over the lower pole of the breast. But when these fibers are divided even a little, the caudal cut edge of the muscle retracts strongly superiorly, inadvertently converting what should have been a dual-plane type I to a type II (caudal cut edge of pectoralis laying at approximately the lower border of the areola), a type III (muscle to about the upper border of the areola), or even far superior to that, such that little or no muscle is available to cover the implant.

This issue of coverage is not a problem with the transaxillary approach because it would take an intentional effort—(**Fig. 4**) and a difficult one at

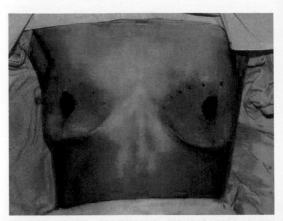

Fig. 3. The patient is shown just after removal of subpectoral implants placed through a periareolar approach. The dotted line indicates the caudal border of the pectoralis. Though she had "retromuscular" pockets, the implant itself had negligible if any coverage because the muscle was so high it could cover only a bit of the implant, and the pressure of it probably pushed the implant away. Although her muscle was still attached to the sternum, the muscle had been inadvertently detached from the overlying parenchyma, thereby allowing it to window-shade up far higher than would be ideal, even for a dual-plan type III. It is almost impossible to create this deformity with the transaxillary approach, possible with the inframammary, but endemic with the periareolar approach.

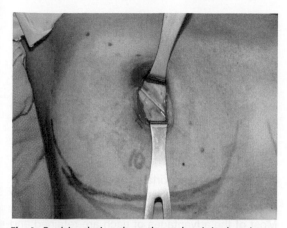

Fig. 4. Revision being done through original periareolar incision. First operation was ostensibly retromuscular, but note that there is capsule in front of the muscle as well as behind it. This is because excessive release of attachments between muscle and gland allowed the muscle to slide so far cephalad that the muscle slipped beneath and in front of it. The dotted diagonal line indicates the caudal free edge of the muscle, which is higher than even a Dual Plane III in a patient who needed either a Dual Plane I or a partial retropectoral pocket. This thin patient has permanently lost significant muscle coverage.

that—because it would involve retrograde endoscopic dissection to disrupt those fibers between the muscle and the gland. Although it is easy to inadvertently overdissect superficial to the muscle

with the inframammary approach, it is also easy to control the premuscular dissection from the inframammary pocket, and it therefore gives the most control over the type and accuracy of dual-plane dissection performed.

It is not just compromise of muscle coverage that is at risk with the periareolar approach. Subcutaneous dissection down to the inframammary fold to avoid dissecting through the parenchyma inevitably results in some degree of detachment of parenchyma from the over lying skin (because of the subcutaneous tunnel) and detachment of the deep surface (because of creation of the pocket for the implant.) the parenchyma from the skin on its superficial surface (because of the subcutaneous tunnelling) and muscle on its deep surface (from creation of the pocket.) With nothing holding the breast mound down, placement of the implant can result in a superior migration of large portions of the breast, resulting in an implant whose lower pole can be located in essentially a subcutaneous position. This is an extremely difficult problem to correct, and results in significant deformity (**Figs. 5** and **6**).

USE OF INCISION FOR REVISIONAL SURGERY

With nearly one in five women requiring a reoperation on her breast augmentation within 3 years, it is important to consider the surgeries a woman may have in her future. Some have described

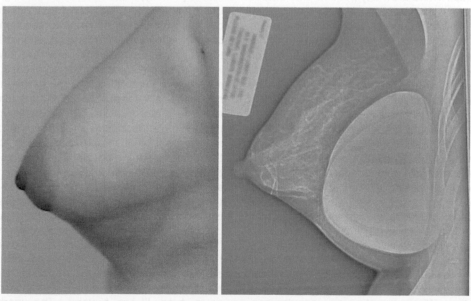

Fig. 5. This patient complains of a deformity following a periareolar augmentation. There is a visible step-off and the implant is easily palpable. The Xeromammogram explains why: there is no parenchyma over the lower pole of the implant. The original operative note described dissection from the periareolar incision to the inframammary fold through the subcutaneous plane.

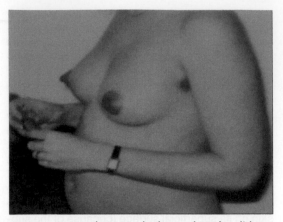

Fig. 6. A preop photograph shows that she did not have tuberous breasts; parenchyma was normally distributed and extended down to the inframammary fold; the superior shift of her parenchymal mass was due to the subcutaneous dissection from the inframammary incision. While this is an extreme case, some degree of vertical tissue shift frequently occurs with the periareolar incision when a subcutaneous dissection technique is utilized.

performing a capsulotomy or lowering the inframammary fold through the transaxillary approach. But a periareolar or inframammary incision is necessary in order to conduct a complete capsulectomy, conversion to a dual-plane, capsulorrhaphy, conversion from saline to a large silicone implant or a cohesive implant, or to create a neoretropectoral pocket. There are many patients who started with a transaxillary incision because they did not want an incision on their breast who subsequently required an additional scar in the inframammary or periareolar location in order to perform a revision operation. This occurs so commonly that the eventuality of having a second scar should be explained to all patients considering a transaxillary incision, and those unwilling to ever have a scar on their breast should probably not have a breast augmentation at all.

The utility of the periareolar incision for revision depends on the size of the areola and the amount of tissue. A small areola with an abundance of parenchyma can result in a long tunnel with poor visualization and access with which to perform a revision, but a large areola with little parenchyma can give the largest possible exposure. If there is a hard and spherical contracture, by virtue of essentially being at the equator of the implant, then the periareolar approach can offer excellent visualization. When operating on capsular contracture, however, avoiding contamination of the new implant by going through the periareolar incision is an issue that must be considered.

Overall, there is scarcely any revisional breast surgery that cannot be done through the inframammary approach, although there are select examples in which the periareolar approach has exposure advantages. But it is irrefutable that the inframammary approach is most likely to work for the widest variety of possible augmentation revision procedures.

ABILITY TO PERFORM DUAL-PLANE POCKETS

One of the most important debates in breast augmentation is between advocates of submammary pockets and those of submuscular pockets. Most of the advantages of each are retained and most of the disadvantages of each are eliminated with the dual-plane approach. With the inframammary incision, a dual-plane approach can be thoroughly and precisely executed. It allows for direct digital assessment of the lower pole for restriction by unreleased muscle, and direct visualization of the muscle to allow for symmetric, accurate, and bloodless division of the origins of the pectoralis along the inframammary fold and of the attachments between the pectoralis muscle and the overlying parenchyma. Dual-plane is a very important and powerful tool, and sacrificing the ability to take full advantage of it is a tremendous loss to the patient.

The transaxillary incision works to create a partial retropectoral pocket (origins of the pectoralis are not divided along the inframammary fold). A dual-plane type I, which divides the origins along the inframammary fold, can frequently be done, but it is exceedingly common to see transaxillary patients who have asymmetric division of the pectoralis, have inconsistent pectoralis division in which there are areas of skipped release, or even have division onto the sternum. Furthermore, it is not technically feasible given the instruments of today to perform a dual-plane type II or type III through the axilla, because to do so would require retrograde dissection and visualization at the farthest reaches of the pocket. The patients who require type II and type III for optimal coverage and aesthetics are numerous, and failing to achieve the proper degree of release and dual-plane type is illogical just to have an incision in the axilla.

While the transaxillary approach results in "down-staging" the dual-plane type II or III pocket to a type I or partial retropectoral pocket, the periareolar approach does the opposite: it converts most intended type I's to an unintentional type II or a type III—or beyond. The inadvertently "window-shaded" pectoralis muscle is commonly seen with the periareolar approach and often leads to an uncorrectable deformity. Even in skilled hands, restricted visualization and unavoidable disruption of at least some of the attachments between the muscle and parenchyma invariably results in some shift of a type I to a type II, or a type II to a type III. A great many patients suffer irreparable tissue damage from well-executed periareolar incisions due to these factors.

PAIN, SWELLING, AND RECOVERY

Although Tebbetts reported 24-hour recoveries with all three incisions, most of his patients had the inframammary approach. There is little doubt that cutting through the breast tissue with the periareolar incision invariably results in an element of pain and swelling not seen when the parenchyma is left undisturbed with the inframammary approach. Although a bloodless and accurate transaxillary approach is possible, few surgeons possess the skill to conduct it in such a manner. Most use a blunt dissection approach, which not only often results in inaccurate releases at the inframammary fold but also frequently results in more pain and bruising than observed when dissection is done under visualization with bloodless techniques.

EFFECTIVE FOR WIDEST VARIETY OF IMPLANTS

The incision length for saline implants is limited by the visualization required to form the pocket, whereas the incision length for silicone implants is dictated by the size of the implant. Although a small silicone implant does not frequently require an incision any larger than required to dissect the pocket, progressively larger implants require larger incisions. The inframammary approach can be widened to accommodate implants of any size. There are limitations to the size of a silicone implant that can be introduced through the periareolar and transaxillary incisions that vary with the profiling of the implant (higher profile implants are more difficult to insert) and with the texturing on the surface.

The use of shaped implants requires accurate pocket dissection in which the pocket fits the shape of the implant to reduce the likelihood of rotation. Shaped implants can be placed through all three incisions; however, it takes a higher level of skill and experience to place these implants through the periareolar and transaxillary incisions. What is not known is whether, even at equivalent levels of expertise, there is a lower malposition rate through the inframammary approach. Logic would suggest that the enhanced visibility through this approach would increase the likelihood of dissecting a pocket that best fits the implant.

In addition to requiring precise pockets, form-stable breast implants are stiffer and less deformable, requiring a longer incision for atraumatic insertion. While excellent results have been reported through all incisions, the greatest number of results in published series of shaped form-stable implants has been with the inframammary approach. It is therefore the standard to which others must be compared.

REDUCES TRAUMA TO IMPLANTS

Manufacturer analysis of ruptured implants retrieved and returned for analysis overwhelmingly demonstrates by electron micrography that the most common cause for device failure is trauma at the time of surgery. This trauma can be due to excessive manipulation and pressure that causes weakness of the shell or due to damage from a fingernail or a sharp instrument. Implant trauma has been recognized as an important factor contributing to shell failure that can be nearly eliminated as a future cause for device rupture. The practice of forcing large implants through small incisions that was de rigueur in the past is no longer considered acceptable.

There are no data that specifically demonstrate a difference in device failure rates using the various incisions, but the stresses are different through each of the approaches. The inframammary and periareolar approaches appear to place the greatest risk to the implant from the needle at the time of closure because the implant is very close to the layer that needs to be closed; the transaxillary closure is more remote from the implant. Careful retraction and use of instruments to protect the implant should minimize this risk.

When implants are large relative to the incision size, as can occur with the periareolar and transaxillary approaches, excessive trauma to the implant can occur. One option in these situations is to consider the use of saline implants; another is to consider the inframammary incision if it would allow for less implant trauma in these patients.

SURGICAL TECHNIQUE OF THE INFRAMAMMARY APPROACH

The first step is to determine the ideal position of the inframammary fold. It is calculated from the nipple with the tissue placed on maximum stretch. In general, the standard of 7 cm for a base width of 11 cm, 8 cm for a base width of 12 cm, and 9 cm for a base width of 13 cm produces an ideal aesthetic outcome. If the inframammary fold is already at that height, it does not need to be altered.

An incision is made at the proposed inframammary fold (**Fig. 7**). Dissection is carried straight down to the muscle fascia with the electrocautery, taking care not to skive inferiorly. There is a natural tendency of the cut edge of the tissue to pull inferiorly, so the dissection may angle superiorly—but only for the purpose of not undercutting the skin edge and inadvertently lowering the fold more than intended, if at all.

The fascia is scored carefully with the cautery so that the muscle is visible. Place in a double-ended or army-navy retractor with the tip pointed toward the medial border of the areola (**Fig. 8**). With no horizontal dissection yet made, there will be little to hold the tissue up onto the blade of the retractor, so use the ulnar fingers of the retractor-holding hand to pull the tissue onto the blade. Lift up toward the ceiling. Only the pectoralis will tent up. If the muscle does not tent at this point, it may be that the muscle is tight or that it is not the pectoralis. To ensure that it is the pectoralis and not the serratus, rectus, or intercostals, touching it with the cautery will make the pectoralis in the upper chest contract. If still not clear, only then dissect just a couple of millimeters along the muscle surface in a cephalad direction. These are the important fibers that you want to preserve to hold the muscle down after you divide pectoralis origins along the inframammary fold, so sacrifice no more than necessary for the anatomy to be

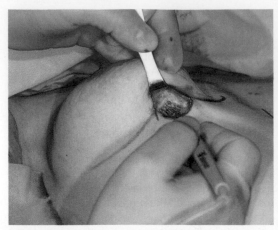

Fig. 8. After you see muscle fascia, aim a retractor at the medial border of the areola and lift up. This process will tent the pectoralis major fibers. Lower your hand so that you can Bovie into the tented fibers, with the angle of cut parallel to the floor.

clear. This step will allow you to see the fibers of the muscle and allow some tissue to lie over the blade of the retractor, thereby allowing the pectoralis to tent up.

Again, advance the retractor blade to the edge of the muscle, pointing the blade towards the medial border of the areola, pulling the breast tissue onto the retractor and lifting up toward the ceiling. Because it is loose on its deep surface, the pectoralis will tent upward. Holding your hand down so that the cautery is horizontal, sweep gently the taut pectoralis fibers that appear vertical in front of you. Use hand-switching monopolar forceps because it allows precise control of blood vessels by squeezing and can be held together and used as a Bovie pencil.

So long as it tents, it is pectoralis. So long as your cautery is horizontal and parallel to the chest wall, the chest should be safe. Keep advancing the retractor forward and lifting up after every stroke of the cautery. With each motion of the cautery and repositioning of the retractor, the muscle will tent higher and the plane through the muscle will be more obvious.

With this maneuver, you will very quickly get through the muscle and will see the subpectoral space (**Fig. 9**). Free up areolar tissue that is immediately in front of the incision. Be alert for a perforator inferomedial to the areola and use the hand-switching monopolar forceps to coagulate it and other vessels that are seen.

Turn the retractor blade medially along the inframammary fold toward the sternum. Controlling the tension of the retractor blade on the muscles with fingers on the outside of the

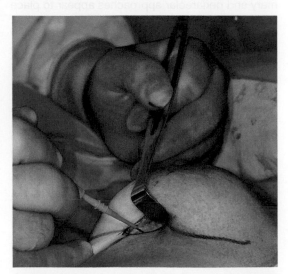

Fig. 7. An incision is made cleanly through the dermis with a single pass of the knife. The cautery is used to dissect down through the subcutaneous tissue to the muscle, taking extraordinary care not to inadvertently skive inferiorly. Do not allow an assistant to place a retractor on the inferior cut edge because this risks overlowering the inframammary fold. The goal is to go straight down to the muscle, and aiming slightly cephalad helps to achieve this.

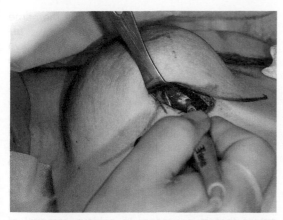

Fig. 9. Keep advancing the retractor and bovie only elevated fibers; this will help assure you are dividing pectoralis and not intercostal muscle fibers. After a few swipes with the bovie, you will have divided the pectoralis and entered the retropectoral space.

breast, use the cautery to divide the muscle about 1 cm above the proposed inframammary fold (**Fig. 10**). This may serve as a shelf to help support the implant; it prevents overlowering of the fold and allows point coagulation of the blood vessels. Cut through the muscle and the overlying fascia. This should be bloodless and very easy to visualize.

In fact, this dissection is so anatomic that you should expect to be able to do this dissection without needing to place a single four-by-eight gauze

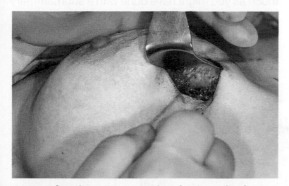

Fig. 10. After the retropectoral pocket is made, the pectoralis is divided 1 cm above the proposed inframammary fold. Note the use of the ulnar digits on the retractor hand pressing the muscle under tension so that it splits as it is divided. The superior and inferior cut edges are visible. When this is divided up to the sternum, a dual-plane type I will have been created, as shown in this photo. Depending on the tension of the tissues, the muscle will window-shade up 1 or 2 cm; in this case, the muscle is about half the width of the retractor blade above the inframammary fold.

into the pocket. Look beyond the tissue plane immediately in front of you, and anticipate and visualize the perforators ahead of time.

Continue all the way to the sternum but do not proceed up the sternum at all. If you are unclear where this point is, mark it with an "X" externally on both sides preoperatively.

Continue the dissection sweeping superolaterally, then sweeping inferiorly. This technique helps to define the plane between the pectoralis major and the pectoralis minor, which are more intertwined when the dissection in that area starts inferolaterally rather than superolaterally.

Irrigate with antibiotic solution and inspect the pocket. Take note of the long, narrow V-shaped trough where the muscle was released inferomedially and window-shaded a bit superiorly. Inspect where the cut edge of the pectoralis is relative to your incision; sometimes it is just a few millimeters beyond it and sometimes it is already window-shaded several centimeters. This distance will vary based on whether connections between the pectoralis and parenchyma were inadvertently divided when entering the retromuscular space and how tight the given patient's connections are between the pectoralis and breast tissue. The more directly one enters the retropectoral space without any premuscular dissection, the lower the caudal cut edge of the pectoralis will sit.

Place a finger in the incision and feel the lower border of the muscle and lift up, taking note of the position of the muscle through the skin as shown by the position of your finger. This inspection process is not only important to define what you need to do for that specific patient but, when done repeatedly, also provides the surgeon with a valuable experience about the dynamics of the muscle and the soft tissue.

If the intention is to do a dual-plane type I, by virtue of the muscle division along the inframamary fold, the dual-plane portion of the dissection is complete. The implant can be placed and the incision closed.

If the goal is to do a dual-plane type II or type III, then now is the time to do a release between pectoralis and overlying gland (**Fig. 11**). This release is gradual and incremental. It cannot be overstated that substantial differences in position of the caudal edge of the pectoralis are created by just several millimeters of dissection. Surgeons ask why they cannot dissect between the muscle and the gland before dissection the retromuscular pocket, and the reason is that such small amounts of dissection result in significant movement of the muscle that it is impossible to predict where the muscle will end up before dissecting the pocket and releasing the inframammary fold.

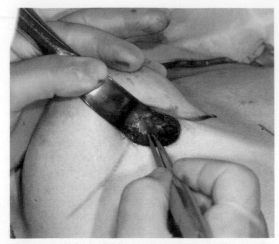

Fig. 11. To go from a dual-plane type I to a type II or type III, the fibrous connections between muscle and the overlying parenchyma must be taken down. Just a few sideways swipes with the cautery is enough to cause significant movement of the muscle.

With the curved end of a double-ended retractor placed in the incision, abutting the caudal edge of the muscle but with only breast tissue within it, use the other fingers of the retractor hand to push in on the breast so that together with the retractor, it is putting tension between the muscle and the overlying gland (**Fig. 12**).

Visualize the fascial connections between the muscle and gland and use the cautery to gradually cut these using sideways sweeping motions. You will see the muscle quickly pull away from the retractor and slide upward. After doing this for several millimeters, move the retractor medially and laterally and repeat this process wherever you feel it is necessary along the entire inferior edge of the muscle.

Rather than repeating this motion in the same area, keep moving around, taking down the attachments a little at a time, because this will give the most control over the final position of the muscle.

Although illustrations may suggest that dual-plane types I, II, and III are distinct entities, they are part of a continuum of options (**Fig. 13**). Their designations are designed as a guide to enable us to think about a clinical situation and compare notes. In any given patient, however, the muscle does not necessarily end exactly at the lower border of the areola (type II) or the upper border of the areola (type III.) Rather, the release is made to the extent that is necessary to achieve removal of muscle coverage where it is restricting expansion of the lower pole while retaining maximal coverage elsewhere (**Fig. 14**). The goal is always to maximize coverage; the release is customized to each breast in order to allow lower pole expansion only when and where necessary.

The most important point is to not overdo it. You can always release more, but after it is released, it is difficult if not impossible to pull the muscle back down. Put your finger back in as you did before and note the change in position of the muscle that resulted from the release. Feel all along its edge and go back and release more where you feel it is necessary.

If you feel bands within the breast that are restricting expansion, such as with a constricted lower pole or when the inframammary fold had to be lowered with a tight inframammary fold, then now would be the time to score the lower pole, much as you might have done with a submammary pocket.

Irrigate again with antibiotic solution (**Fig. 15**), recheck for bleeding, place the chosen implant, and close per the usual routine.

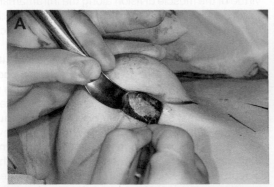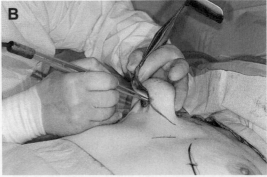

Fig. 12. (*A*) After just a few swipes of the cautery freeing up some attachments of the muscle to the gland, the muscle moves cephalad. The fresh yellow fat shows the significant motion of the muscle relative to **Fig. 11**. Again, note the use of the ulnar digits against the retractor to create tension at the muscle parenchyma border, thereby making the dissection more precise and facile. (*B*) When a dual-plane type I is converted to a type II or type III, note how the hand and the retractor are used as a unit to create tension at the muscle/parenchyma interface.

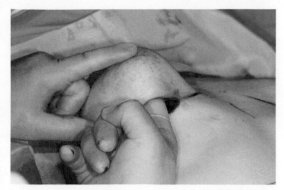

Fig. 13. In this case, the muscle is released to the lower border of the areola, which is a so-called dual-plane type II. When it is released to about the upper border of the areola, it is termed a dual-plane type III.

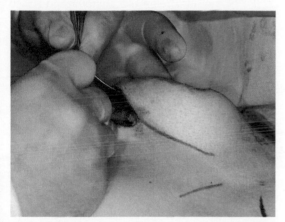

Fig. 14. Here the release is being done more laterally. It can be adjusted on each breast exactly as the conditions necessitate.

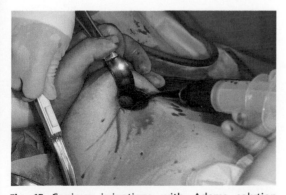

Fig. 15. Copious irrigations with Adams solution (50 mL povidone-iodine [Betadine], 80 mg gentamicin, 1 gram cefazolin sodium [Ancef] in 500 mL normal saline) is used throughout the operation. Note the yellow fat visible just beyond the retractor; the cut edge of muscle is just visible.

SUMMARY

A basic tenet of surgery understood by every intern is that a surgeon should select the most anatomically direct approach to the area of concern unless a different approach avoids critical anatomic structures. The defining aspect of the breast augmentation operation is the accuracy and symmetry of the pocket creation, and the most critical aspect of this dissection lies at the inframammary fold. The inframammary approach unquestionably offers the greatest visualization of this area and results in the least damage to normal tissue. The transaxillary and periareolar approaches create trauma to tissue that is undisturbed using the inframammary approach, and does so at the price of less visualization of the critical aspects of the surgery.

FURTHER READINGS

Adams WP, Bengston BP, Glicksman CA, et al. Decision and management algorithms to address patient and Food and Drug Administration concerns regarding breast augmentation and implants. Plast Reconstr Surg 2004;114(5):1252–7.

Adams WP Jr, Conner W, Chad HBA, et al. Optimizing breast pocket irrigation: an in vitro study and clinical implications. Plast Reconstr Surg 2000;105(1):334–8.

Adams WP Jr, Rios JL, Smith SJ. Enhancing patient outcomes in aesthetic and reconstructive breast surgery using triple antibiotic breast irrigation: six-year prospective clinical study. Advances in Breast Augmentation. Plast Reconstr Surg 2006;118(Suppl 7):46S–52S.

Adams WP Jr, Teitelbaum S, Bengtson BP, et al. Breast augmentation roundtable. Advances in Breast Augmentation 118. Plast Reconstr Surg 2006;(Suppl 7):175S–87S.

Okwueze MI, Spear ME, Zwyghuizen AM, et al. Effect of augmentation mammaplasty on breast sensation. Plast Reconstr Surg 2006;117(1):73–83.

Tebbetts JB. Achieving a predictable 24-hour return to normal activities after breast augmentation: part II. Patient preparation, refined surgical techniques, and instrumentation. Advances in Breast Augmentation. Plast Reconstr Surg 2006;118(Suppl 7): 115S–27S.

Tebbetts JB. Achieving a zero percent reoperation rate at 3 years in a 50-consecutive-case augmentation mammaplasty premarket approval study. Plast Reconstr Surg 2006;118(6):1453–7.

Tebbetts JB. Dual plane breast augmentation: optimizing implant–soft-tissue relationships in a wide range of breast types. Advances in Breast Augmentation. Plast Reconstr Surg 2006;118(Suppl 7):81S–98S.

Tebbetts JB. Reoperations as a benchmark: the rhetoric, the logic, and the patient. Plast Reconstr Surg 2008; 122(2):662–5.

Tebbetts JB, Adams WP. Five critical decisions in breast augmentation using five measurements in 5 minutes: the high five decision support process. Advances in Breast Augmentation. Plast Reconstr Surg 2006;118(Suppl 7): 35S–45S.

The Periareolar Approach to Breast Augmentation

Dennis C. Hammond, MD

KEYWORDS

- Breast augmentation • Incision • Periareolar

Incision placement in patients undergoing augmentation mammaplasty is an important element of the overall strategic plan of the procedure. Whatever incision location is chosen, access to the breast must be sufficient to afford accurate dissection of the pocket, allow easy insertion of the implant, and to provide for precise hemostasis. At the same time, the incision should be placed where the resulting scar will be inconspicuous and well hidden. For many surgeons, the periareolar approach satisfies all of these requirements.[1–5] This article describes the various advantages associated with the periareolar incision for breast augmentation and provides the technical details to enable best use of the technique.

TECHNIQUE OF POCKET DISSECTION

One of the most important technical elements in performing a breast augmentation centers on accurate and complete dissection of the pocket in which the implant will be placed. In this regard, when the subpectoral pocket plane is used, a blunt dissection technique is a very easy and straightforward maneuver to simply sweep free the filmy attachments between the chest wall and the muscle and thus open up the submuscular space. However, along the inferomedial corner of the pocket, interdigitating fibers of origin of the muscle are present at several different levels as they extend from the ribs superiorly up into the main substance of the muscle. With blunt technique, these fibers must be avulsed to effectively open up the submuscular space to allow accurate placement of the implant. Also, in selected patients, the level of the desired inframammary fold is lower than the point of attachment of the origin of the muscle. To

properly position the implant low enough to create an aesthetic breast shape, these fibers must be released. When blunt dissection is used to release these muscular fibers of attachment, the fibers are actually torn or avulsed. This process can create uneven or inaccurately positioned contours leading to implant malposition. For proponents of remote-access incision techniques, such as transumbilical or non–endoscopic-assisted transaxillary breast augmentation that require blunt dissection to create the pocket for the implant, these potential disadvantages are simply accepted as a reasonable trade-off to preserve the perceived advantage of a well-hidden remote cutaneous scar. However, for many surgeons, the potential for inaccurate or asymmetric pocket dissection does not justify the use of such remote-access incision sites and more direct approaches to the breast are desired. It is for this reason that the periareolar and inframammary incision options continue to be by far the most commonly used incision locations for surgeons performing augmentation mammaplasty.

DIRECT-ACCESS INCISION OPTIONS

Although initially popularized as a blunt technique, the transaxillary approach to breast augmentation can be supplemented with endoscopic assistance to provide direct control over the limits of pocket dissection. However this approach requires additional instrumentation and endoscopic expertise, both of which make this approach a less desirable choice for many surgeons. With this in mind, the two mainstays of incision choice that provide direct access to the breast for breast augmentation remain the inframammary and periareolar incision

Center for Breast and Body Contouring, 4070 Lake Drive, Suite 202, Grand Rapids, MI 49546, USA
E-mail address: cbbc@dennischammond.com

Clin Plastic Surg 36 (2009) 45–48
doi:10.1016/j.cps.2008.07.004

locations. Both locations allow for controlled development of the pocket under direct vision. A controlled release of the pectoralis major muscle can be performed as needed to properly position the implant and areas of constriction can be released with ease. When desired, the subglandular and subfascial[6–8] pocket planes can also be developed with equal facility. As well, precise control of hemostasis can be performed through either incision to create a dry and blood-free pocket. This advantage stands in stark contrast to blunt dissection technique where vessels are more or less avulsed and spasm is relied upon to provide hemostasis. Such control over hemostasis has been postulated to reduce the rate of capsular contracture associated with breast augmentation.[9,10]

ADVANTAGES OF THE PERIAREOLAR INCISION

Given the described advantages of direct access to the breast for performing breast augmentation, the periareolar incision location is associated with additional specific advantages that make it the preferred option for many surgeons. By locating the incision directly at the junction between the pigmented skin of the areola and the lighter skin of the breast, a very inconspicuous scar is created that heals in an imperceptible fine-line fashion the majority of the time. The scar is only visible when the entire breast is exposed, which obviates the risk of the scar showing when bathing suits are worn. Also, from a technical standpoint, by approaching the inframammary fold from above, the location of the fold can be positioned with accuracy by teasing open the attachments along the fold until the desired fold level and shape is created. Because the access portal for this maneuver is remote from the contour being created, a more direct assessment of the shape and location of the fold can be made as opposed to trying to accomplish this through an incision located directly in the fold. Also, in patients who may subsequently require mastopexy to optimize the final result, it is a simple matter to extend the periareolar incision circumferentially to accomplish the periareolar lift. Finally, should revisionary surgery be required, it is usually possible to enter the breast through the existing periareolar scar to provide exposure for such procedures as capsulotomy, capsulectomy, contour plication, and implant exchange.

DISADVANTAGES OF THE PERIAREOLAR INCISION

Although many advantages are associated with the periareolar approach, specific disadvantages associated with the approach may lead surgeons to choose the inframammary fold incision.

Perhaps the most obvious factor that may limit the utility of the periareolar approach is the size of the areola. Remembering that the circumference of a circle is represented by the formula pi times diameter, it can be demonstrated that a 3-cm wide areola will accommodate a 4.7-cm static incision along the inferior hemisphere of the areola. When taking into account the elastic qualities of skin and the general compressibility of breast implants, it becomes clear that this incision length is usually sufficient to insert most breast implants, although the newer cohesive gel anatomically shaped devices may require slightly longer incisions. What really becomes the limiting factor relates to exposure for accurate pocket dissection. Attempting to utilize the periareolar approach in patients with areolar diameters of less than 3 cm makes exposure and direct dissection of the pocket more difficult.

One additional concern related to the use of the periareolar approach involves the potential for contamination of the implant during insertion. Due to the close proximity of the ductal system of the breast to the insertion point, seeding of either the implant or the implant space from bacteria present within the ducts is possible during dissection of the pocket or placement of the implant.[11] Such bacterial contamination has been postulated to be the inciting event leading to capsular contracture.[12,13] For this reason, it is recommended that the nipple be covered with an occlusive dressing while the implant is being inserted to help minimize the potential for inadvertent contamination of the device as it is being inserted.

SENSATION

One of the overriding concerns for many patients seeking breast augmentation relates to the potential loss of sensation to the nipple and areola complex. Understandably, many patients equate the proximity of the incision with the potential for injury to the nerves supplying the nipple and areola complex. However, recent studies have demonstrated that there is no appreciable difference between sensibility when the periareolar approach is used and sensibility following an inframammary fold incision.[14,15] The reason for these similar outcomes related to sensibility has to do with the likelihood that an inferiorly directed plane of dissection that extends down from the periareolar incision preserves the arborization of nerves that extends from above to the nipple and areola complex from the medial and lateral intercostal branches. As long as this superiorly oriented nervous network is maintained, sensation to the nipple and areola complex will be unaffected.

TECHNIQUE

When using the periareolar approach, the incision heals in the most imperceptible fashion when it is placed directly at the inferior border of the areola. Slight inaccuracies in the placement of this incision increase the potential visibility of the scar. Therefore, it is helpful to mark the junction of the pigmented areolar skin with the lower-pole breast skin prior to injecting any vasoconstrictors in the dermis. This marking is necessary because the vasoconstricting effect of epinephrine causes the skin to blanch, making it impossible to identify with accuracy this junction once the epinephrine effect has set in. Also, once the incision is made at the inferior border of the areola, accurate reapproximation of the incision edges can be difficult because of the thin and elastic nature of the skin. Therefore, prior to incising the skin, it is helpful to symmetrically and temporarily tattoo opposite sides of the incision to guide subsequent skin closure after the implant has been placed. Once the proper location for the incision has been made and the skin incised, there are two basic strategies for pocket development.

Transparenchymal Approach

Perhaps the most straightforward approach to the underside of the breast through a periareolar incision is to dissect directly down through the breast to the pectoralis major muscle. At this point, a subglandular, subfascial, or subpectoral pocket can be created easily with the aid of a lighted retractor (**Fig. 1**). After the implant is placed, the bivalved parenchyma can simply be repaired to prevent any visible contour deformity from developing as a result of the disruption in the continuity of the breast parenchyma. The advantage of this technique relates to the direct exposure of the implant space provided by this incision location.

Theoretical concerns do exist, however, regarding the potential for seeding of the implant surface or the pocket as a result of the direct division of the breast parenchyma. As the ductal system of the breast is exposed, it is possible for bacteria within the ducts to contaminate the implant as it is passed through the incision, leading to biofilm formation within the pocket and a greater potential for the development of capsular contracture. For this reason many surgeons prefer to avoid direct division of the breast when developing the pocket.

Periaparenchymal Approach

An alternative approach to direct division of the breast is to angle the dissection inferiorly at the level of the breast capsule until the inframammary fold is reached. At this point, dissection then proceeds superiorly up and under the breast to create whatever pocket is desired (**Fig. 2**). The advantage here is that direct division of the breast with exposure of the ductal network is avoided, thus minimizing the potential for bacterial contamination of the implant or the pocket. The disadvantage relates to the degree of difficulty encountered during pocket dissection and implant insertion. In patients with a shorter periareolar incision and tight skin envelope, exposure for pocket dissection can be limited and this approach is harder to perform. However, once the pocket has been dissected free and the implant is in position, the lower breast flap can be allowed to ride up away from the inframammary fold area. In this fashion, any tendency for a tight parenchymal envelope to constrict the projection of breast can be relieved as the breast is allowed to slide up and over the implant. In cases where the parenchyma does not restrain the shape of the breast in any way, the lower breast flap created by the dissection strategy is simply reapproximated along the inframammary fold.

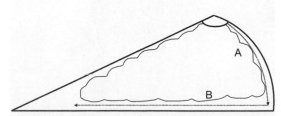

Fig.1. Schematic diagram demonstrating the transparenchymal approach for pocket development through a periareolar incision. Once the periareolar incision has been made, dissection is directed through the breast to the pectoralis major muscle (A). At this point, dissection then proceeds superiorly (B) and inferiorly (C) until the limits of pocket dissection have been carefully created.

Fig. 2. Schematic diagram demonstrating the periaparenchymal approach for pocket development. Here the initial dissection proceeds inferiorly around the lower pole of the breast at the level of the breast capsule (A). Once the inframammary fold is reached, dissection then angles superiorly (B) until the limits of pocket dissection are complete.

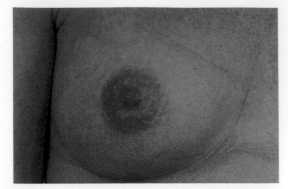

Fig. 3. Six-year postoperative appearance of the periareolar scar after the placement of a cohesive anatomic silicone gel implant.

RESULTS

The results obtained using the periareolar approach are generally outstanding. The scar nearly always heals in a fine-line and imperceptible fashion that is well tolerated by all but the most demanding of patients. In many instances, after a period of years, the scar simply cannot be seen even after close examination (**Figs. 3** and **4**).

SUMMARY

The periareolar approach can be viewed as the perfect solution to the problem of access to breast for the purpose of placing a breast implant. The incision location allows the pocket to be accurately dissected under direct vision with absolute hemostasis. Essentially any type of breast implant can be inserted through this incision into the underlying pocket and the need for immediate adjustments in fold position or shape can be assessed with great accuracy. When required, periareolar mastopexy can be performed with only a minor additional scar burden by simply extending the scar completely around the areola. Finally, if

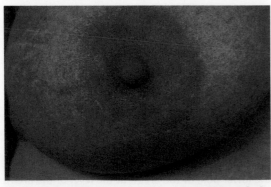

Fig. 4. Eight-year postoperative appearance of the periareolar scar after the placement of a smooth round silicone gel implant.

revisionary surgery becomes necessary, appropriate surgical manipulations of the capsule, pocket, or implant can be performed with little difficulty. The periareolar incision is recommended as an excellent option for those patients undergoing breast augmentation.

REFERENCES

1. Jones FR, Tauras AP. A periareolar incision for augmentation mammaplasty. Plast Reconstr Surg 1973; 51:641–4.
2. Jenny H. Areolar approach to augmentation mammaplasty. Plast Reconstr Surg 1974;53:344.
3. Mladick RA. Breast augmentation: ease of dissection with the periareolar technique. Aesthetic Surgery Journal 1999;19:162–4.
4. Gruber R, Friedman GD. Periareolar subpectoral augmentation mammaplasty. Plast Reconstr Surg 2000;105:2202–16.
5. Spear SL, Bulan EJ. The medial periareolar approach to sub-muscular augmentation mammaplastyunder local anesthesia: a 10 year follow up. Plast Reconstr Surg 2001;108:771–5.
6. Graf RM, Bernardes A, Rippel R, et al. Subfascial breast implant: a new procedure. Plast Reconstr Surg 2003;111:904–8.
7. Goes JC, Landecker A. Optimizing outcomes in breast augmentation: seven years of experience with the subfascial plane. Aesthetic Plast Surg 2003;27:178–84.
8. Ventura OD, Marcello GA. Anatomic and physiologic advantages of totally subfascial breast implants. Aesthetic Plast Surg 2005;29:379–83.
9. Milojevic B. Unilateral fibrous contracture in augmentation mammoplasty. Aesthetic Plast Surg 1983;7:117–9.
10. Hipps CJ, Raju R, Straith RE. Influence of some operative and postoperative factors on capsular contracture around breast prostheses. Plast Reconstr Surg 1978;61:384–9.
11. Wiener TC. Relationship of incision choice to capsular contracture. Aesthetic Plast Surg 2008;32:303–6.
12. Schreml S, Heine N, Eisenmann-Klein M, et al. Bacterial colonization is of major relevance for high-grade capsular contracture after augmentation mammaplasty. Ann Plast Surg 2007;59:126–30.
13. Jennings DA, Morykwas MJ, Burns WW, et al. In vitro adhesion of endogenous skin microorganisms to breast prostheses. Ann Plast Surg 1991;27:216–20.
14. Mofid MM, Klatsky SA, Singh NK, et al. Nipple-areola complex sensitivity after primary breast augmentation: a comparison of periareolar and inframammary incision approaches. Plast Reconstr Surg 2006;117: 1694–8.
15. Okwueze MI, Spear ME, Zwyghuizen AM, et al. Effect of augmentation mammaplasty on breast sensation. Plast Reconstr Surg 2006;117:73–83.

The Transaxillary Approach to Breast Augmentation

Salvatore J. Pacella, MD, MBA[a], Mark A. Codner, MD, FACS[b,c],*

KEYWORDS

- Breast augmentation • Endoscopic plastic surgery
- Transaxillary breast augmentation

The transaxillary approach to breast augmentation was first reported in the 1970s and has been well described by several investigators.[1–3] Advantages of this technique include the absence of any visible incisions on the breast and the ability to place the implant reliably within the submuscular plane. As many earlier investigators have described, the dissection was first performed in a blind fashion with blunt dissection and division of the medial and inferior pectoralis fibers off the chest wall.[4,5] As the technique developed, inability to predict the extent of dissection of the inferior and medial submuscular pocket led to suboptimal aesthetic results, often marked by implants riding too high from inadequate division of the prepectoral fascia or by riding too low from destruction of the inframammary fold. Furthermore, blunt dissection in the traditional technique often led to troublesome bleeding that could not be adequately visualized.

With the advent of minimally invasive techniques in surgery, the potential benefits of such techniques to patients, such as smaller incisions, reduced pain, and shorter recovery time, became more evident. The application of endoscopic minimally invasive surgery to transaxillary breast augmentation presented many apparent advantages, including direct visualization during pocket dissection, hemostasis, and preservation of the inframammary fold. In the early 1990s, Eaves and colleagues[6] sought to advance the technique by the use of a custom-made endoretractor and instrumentation designed to optimize dissection ergonomically. These developments, which increased control through direct visualization of the dissection, obviated many of the previous downfalls of the blind axillary approach.

Endoscopic transaxillary breast augmentation results in outcomes similar to those from nonendoscopic inframammary or periareolar approaches and can be offered as another choice to patients. One recent study used a patient-satisfaction questionnaire to compare aesthetic results between patients who underwent a traditional inframammary approach to those who underwent endoscopic transaxillary augmentation. In the transaxillary group, patient-satisfaction scores were higher than those in the inframammary group, but the differences in scores were not statistically significant.[7]

As the endoscopic technique evolved, many investigators have advocated the use of the endoscope and report successful outcomes in several series.[8,9] Despite some reports indicating preference for the traditional blunt technique,[10] the majority of investigators have found the endoscope useful in optimizing pocket dissection and implant position. The application of this technology has increased the safety and precision of breast augmentation via the transaxillary approach.

[a] Division of Plastic Surgery, Scripps Clinic Medical Group, 10666 North Torrey Pines Road, La Jolla, CA 92037, USA
[b] Department of Plastic Surgery, Emory University School of Medicine, 3200 Downwood Circle #640, Atlanta, GA 30327, USA
[c] Paces Plastic Surgery and Recovery Center, 3200 Downwood Circle #640, Atlanta, GA 30327, USA
* Corresponding author. Department of Plastic Surgery, Emory University, Paces Plastic Surgery and Recovery Center, 3200 Downwood Circle #640, Atlanta, GA 30327.
E-mail address: macodner@aol.com (M.A. Codner).

Clin Plastic Surg 36 (2009) 49–61
doi:10.1016/j.cps.2008.07.006

ANATOMIC CONSIDERATIONS

The breast overlies the pectoralis major, which originates slightly above the medial two thirds of the inframammary fold. This anatomic position is important when performing augmentation in the subpectoral plane because dissection must be carried inferiorly (in the subglandular position) to adequately define the inframammary fold. Medially, only a loose areolar layer separates the pectoralis from the costal cartilage and inframammary crease. The medial origins of the pectoralis are highly vascular, marked by many intercostal perforators. Superiolaterally, the pectoralis major lies anterior to the pectoralis minor and laterally above the origins of the serratus anterior (**Fig. 1**).[11]

The blood supply to the breast originates from several sources. These include the thoracoacromial trunk via pectoral branches, the internal mammary-originated perforators, and the intercostal vessels that give rise to anteriolateral perforators. When the pectoralis is released inferiorly as is standardly performed in breast augmentation, the anteriolateral perforators are divided.

Anteriolateral and anteriomedial branches of intercostal nerves supply sensory innervation to the breast. Specifically, nipple sensation is derived primarily by branches of T3 through T5. During medial dissection and division of the pectoralis, some of these branches may be divided. Nonetheless, because of robust cross-innervation, sensation is maintained to the nipple when lateral subpectoral dissection is performed bluntly. The intercostobrachial nerve, which originates from T2 and courses laterally to provide sensory innervations to the inner arm, can be at risk for injury during a transaxillary approach (**Fig. 2**).[12] Subsequently, dissection should remain superficial just under the pectoralis to avoid injury.

When using a transaxillary approach, knowledge of the structures contained in the axilla is of critical importance. The apex of the axilla is found at the level of the outer border of the first rib, at the superior border of the scapula. The axillary vessels and brachial plexus can be found at this level and are rarely encountered during the transaxillary approach. The base of the axilla, which is directed inferiorly, is formed by the skin, areolar fat, and the thick axillary fascia. The axillary fascia, which extends between the pectoralis major and the latissimus dorsi, must be penetrated and divided to enter the subpectoral space. The neurovascular supply to the latissimus dorsi and the long thoracic nerve are located in the posterior portion of the axilla and are rarely encountered if dissection is limited to the subpectoral space.[13]

PATIENT SELECTION

In general, most candidates for submuscular breast augmentation can be successfully augmented via the transaxillary approach. Because the inframammary crease can be accurately controlled or lowered, moderate degrees of ptosis can be treated during transaxillary augmentation by extended dissection of the pectoralis fascia.[14] Patients with severe ptosis who desire augmentation will need nipple repositioning with a combined

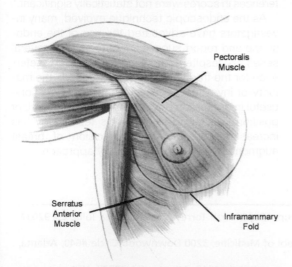

Fig. 1. Chest wall anatomy. The breast is situated over the pectoralis major and the serratus anterior. The inframammary fold is a defined anatomic structure that has fibrous attachments from the dermis to the chest wall.

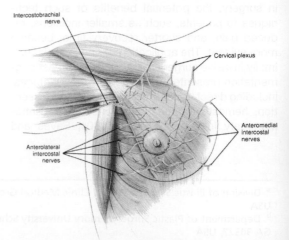

Fig. 2. Nerve supply to the breast. Sensation to the breast derives from the nerves depicted. Nipple sensation is derived from intercostal nerves originating from T3 to T5. The intercostobrachial nerve is at risk during transaxillary dissection.

mastopexy. The implant may still be placed endo-scopically. However, the mastopexy incisions usually provide sufficient access to place an implant through an anterior approach. The technique should be avoided in patients with tubular breast deformity as this can exacerbate the deformity.[15]

Ideal candidates for transaxillary augmentation are those with significant hypomastia, minimal ptosis, and a minimally defined inframammary fold. In addition, the technique is very effective for patients who have a small nipple areolar complex (ie, patients who are not candidates for a peri-areolar augmentation) and those who especially oppose visible scarring on the breast or nipple.

In secondary augmentation, patients who have existing scars (ie, inframammary or periareolar) usually prefer to undergo their secondary procedure through these scars. Although some studies have reported that capsular contracture can be treated through the transaxillary approach, we feel that patients who require a significant capsulotomy or capsulectomy should be treated through an open, anterior approach.[16,17]

TRADITIONAL VERSUS ENDOSCOPIC TECHNIQUE

The traditional transaxillary augmentation is a blind procedure often marked by less control of dissection than would normally be desired. In addition, the technique may be hampered by the inability to accurately locate and address intraoperative bleeding. The endoscopic technique has inherent advantages to the traditional technique. Because the endoscope in effect converts the blind technique to an "open" technique, the subpectoral space is directly visualized, providing equivalent pocket dissection to the open anterior approaches.[18] While reducing the need for blunt dissection, the endoscopic technique allows precise muscle division and preservation of the prepectoral fascia.

Several investigators have observed that, with the traditional technique, implants tend to ride high. This is partially because of inadequate release of the inferior pectoral fibers. Ensuring uniform release of the medial fibers is also often difficult. If medial fibers are not released uniformly, a significant external contour deformity can result. Such deformities are difficult to correct.[19] Because the inframammary fold can be directly controlled with visualization, implant position is optimized with the endoscopic technique.[20] In addition, the technique is also effective for patients who desire definition in the medial cleavage area, allowing direct endoscopic visual dissection. Furthermore, blunt dissection as performed with the traditional technique may result

in greater postoperative pain secondary to micro-bleeding in the rib periosteum from the avulsed muscle fibers.[21]

While the endoscopic technique may provide more accurate hemostasis and more precise release of soft tissue attachments, the technique also takes more time and effort to learn than the conventional technique. Surgeons often require specialized training, particularly if they are unfamiliar with endoscopic techniques. In additional to a larger fixed-cost investment for the endoscopic equipment, training is often required for the operative staff to troubleshoot technologic issues. This may result in extended operative time and prolonged anesthetic effects. Even in light of these potential drawbacks, the endoscopic technique has clear advantages.

IMPLANT POSITION

When using the transaxillary approach, several considerations should be taken into account in deciding on the plane of the implant placement. For women who have undergone breast augmentation, mammographic visualization of the breasts has life-long implications. Several studies have documented that visualization of breast parenchyma is usually greater in augmented breasts when the implant is placed in the submuscular position compared with the subglandular position.[22] Furthermore, several studies have also documented that placement of the implant in the subpectoral position reduces the incidence of capsular contracture.[23,24]

Despite some of these advantages, several investigators prefer to place implants in the subfascial position using the transaxillary endoscopic approach. Possible advantages of the subfascial position include:

> Potential for reduced malpositioning of the anatomically shaped implant when the pectoralis is contracted[25]
> Reduced chance for injury to the intercosto-brachial nerve[26]
> Reduction in postoperative pain because of reduced muscle dissection[26]

These advantages make subfascial position the preferred treatment in patients with minimal ptosis.[25]

Implants placed in the submuscular position generally have a softer feel and a more natural appearance. This is particularly evident in the superior pole where a gentle, convex contour is desired. Placement of implants in the submuscular position is also particularly important when saline implants are used.[24] The pectoralis muscle provides an additional barrier and coverage of the implant, thereby minimizing the appearance of rippling or palpability that is seen in subglandular implants. Nonetheless, in the inferior pole of the implant, muscular coverage is usually sparse secondary to operative release of the inferior pectoralis fibers. In this area, use of saline implants can result in more rippling and palpability. At present, the authors place most implants in the submuscular position regardless of incision location or whether a traditional or endoscopic approach is used.

IMPLANT TYPE AND VOLUME

Either saline or silicone implants may be used through the transaxillary approach. Saline implants can be inserted partially filled with the valve tubing attached and subsequently inflated once the implant is placed. With the endoscopic technique, the position of the implant and valve can be directly visualized. In patients with thin tissue cover or small breasts, saline implants may be associated with increased palpability and rippling. This is often seen in textured implants, which have a thicker implant shell. Textured implants, originally developed to reduce the incidence of capsular contracture, have been effective in several meta-analyses and postmarket studies.[27,28] However, positioning of the implant endoscopically can be slightly more difficult. In general, if a saline implant is used, the authors prefer to use a smooth-walled implant. Nonetheless, if the patient has adequate tissue cover or if recurrence of capsular contracture is of great concern, a textured implant can be used. Care should be taken to make certain the implant is placed low enough as the textured surface impairs inferior migration of the implant to the new inframammary fold.

Insertion of fourth-generation cohesive silicone gel implants is becoming increasingly common via the transaxillary approach.[29] To date, insertion through the transaxillary approach of fifth-generation form-stable implants is not advocated. Cohesive gel implants have a more natural and anatomic feel compared with saline, while also having less of a tendency to cause rippling or palpability. If acceptable to the patient, the authors prefer smooth-walled silicone with moderate-plus projection as the standard implant in endoscopic transaxillary augmentation. As we discuss later in this article, it is important to design the incision of adequate length when choosing type and volume of silicone implants. During implant placement through the incision, the implant is susceptible to significant shearing and compression forces, which may cause internal shell rupture.

This will lead to substantial external deformity if not recognized during the insertion.

Implant volume is determined by both the patient's desired postoperative size as well as the physical examination determining the patient's breast width and dimensions. If using saline, sizers may be inserted to determine intraoperative size dimensions. However, this can be difficult if a silicone sizer is used. If a patient desires a relatively high volume implant (ie, >500 cm^3), saline implants can be used because they are not prefilled. Insertion of a high-volume silicone implant is often a bit more difficult and can subject the implant to rupture during insertion. In general, we advocate silicone augmentation in the moderate range (ie, <500 cm^3).

EQUIPMENT REQUIREMENTS

Several specialized pieces of equipment are needed for performing endoscopic augmentation. Most notably among these is an endoscopic tower or boom system, which should include a high-definition or wide-view endoscopic monitor (**Fig. 3**). This will allow adequate view of the endoscopic optical cavity at many potential points of reference for the surgeon. The tower should also be equipped with a sufficiently bright light source for the camera. We find that a light source of 250 to 300 watts to be suitable. In regards to the endoscope, we prefer to use a short 10-mm endoscope angled at 30°. Conventional 4- to 5-mm endoscopes used for endoscopy in the facial region are suboptimal because of inadequate illumination.

A specialized endoscopic retractor, which incorporates the camera system into a metal sleeve, is also required (**Fig. 4**). These units allow optimal control of the retractor, camera, and suction in

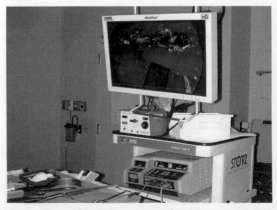

Fig. 3. The endoscopic monitor should accommodate wide-angle viewing and is best positioned within direct line of vision of the surgeon.

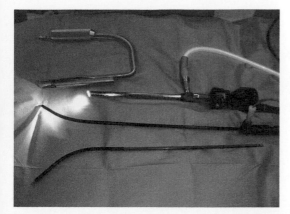

Fig. 4. Endoscopic camera, retractor, and dissection instruments constitute the desired equipment for endoscopic breast augmentation.

one handheld piece. Suction-cautery units should have a gentle bend that enables the surgeon to introduce the endoscopic camera and retractor into the wound with minimal crowding. Spatula tips at the end of the suction-cautery unit are also better than hook tips. For the right-handed surgeon, dissection of the left-handed pocket may be more challenging in the inferiolateral position. Subsequently, it may be more facile to use a left-handed instrument to dissect this area while holding the camera with the right hand. Besides those already mentioned, other useful pieces of equipment include the Agris-Dingman Dissector and the Emory Dissector. These instruments are effective for lateral blunt dissection and practical as measuring instruments for gauging the extent of total pocket dissection (**Fig. 5**).[30] Asche forceps are also helpful to stretch the subpectoral tunnel through the thick clavipectoral fascia in order to facilitate insertion of a gel implant.

ENDOSCOPIC TECHNIQUE
Preoperative Markings

Preoperative markings should be made when the patient is awake in the preoperative holding area. Three marks are made on each breast indicating the locations of the existing inframammary fold, the new inframammary fold, and the axillary incision. The existing inframammary fold is usually marked with a solid line and is used as a landmark to highlight any asymmetry. The new inframammary fold is marked at a new position inferiorly approximately 1 to 2 cm based on the desired new position, any existing asymmetry, existing ptosis, desired breast volume, or implant base diameter. Initial markings should be conservative, because the inframammary fold is much more difficult to raise than lower. Finally, the axillary incision is marked within a prominent transverse axillary crease (**Fig. 6**). The incision is usually placed high in the axilla and measures 2 to 3 cm in length for saline implants and 5 cm for silicone.

Technique

The patient is positioned in the supine position with arms extended and secured at 90°. Surgeon positioning during the operative case is important in facilitating comfort level and a smooth operative course. The most comfortable position while operating with endoscopic equipment allows the surgeon direct view of the endoscope and monitor within the same vertical visual field. Therefore, the endoscopic tower should be positioned at the foot of the bed, with the light source, video cable, and cautery brought up from the foot of the table. The surgeon should be positioned superiorly above each arm to access the axilla when performing endoscopic dissection.

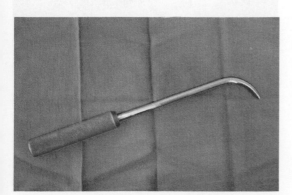

Fig. 5. Emory breast dissector. The breast dissector is helpful for gauging the extent of pocket dissection, particularly at the edges of the submuscular pocket.

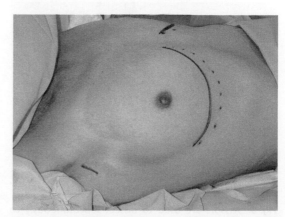

Fig. 6. Preoperative markings include the sternal notch, the existing and desired inframammary fold, and the axillary incision.

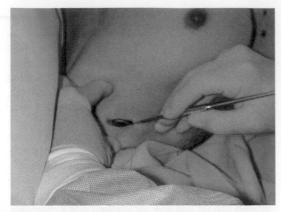

Fig. 7. The axillary incision is marked with a prominent skin crease and measures 2 to 3 cm for saline implants and 4 to 5 cm for silicone implants.

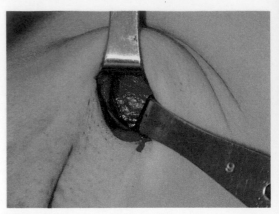

Fig. 9. Gentle retraction is used to widen the axillary pocket.

The incision is made with the axillary skin placed under tension (**Fig. 7**). The anterior edge of the incision is then elevated with sharp double hooks while the cautery is used to divide subcutaneous tissue. Scissors are used to gently spread the incision and create a tunnel to the anterior axillary line (**Fig. 8**). Maintaining this dissection in a superficial plane minimizes risk of injury to the intercostobrachial nerve.

As the lateral pectoral border is encountered, the lateral pectoral fascia (continuous with the axillary fascia) is divided sharply to enter the lateral pectoral space. The lateral pectoral fascia and subcutaneous tissue often are a restriction point for implant insertion. They can be widened by blunt retraction with counter-pulled retractors (**Fig. 9**). Finger dissection should also be used to confirm that the pocket is created in the subpectoral space (**Fig. 10**). Gentle sweeping within this space divides any loose areolar tissue from the

posterior surface of the pectoralis major. The Agris-Dingman or Emory dissector can be used to facilitate this dissection.

In planning the pectoral dissection and release of muscle fibers, we have found that a variable approach to releasing the pectoral muscle fibers creates the most acceptable contour. In essence, sharp cautery dissection is used under endoscopic visualization to release the fibers from the three-o'clock to the six-o'clock position. Partial release of the fibers should also be performed endoscopically from the superior to the three-o'clock position. We have found release or transection of approximately 40% to 50% thickness provides the best contour in the superior medial position and avoids lateral displacement of the implant during pectoralis flexion. Blunt dissection releases the areolar attachments in the inferiolateral position (**Fig. 11**).

The surgeon should then move to a position superior to the patient's arm to begin the endoscopic

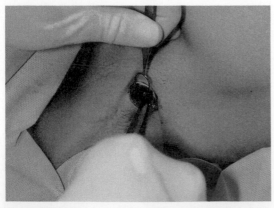

Fig. 8. Scissors are used to dissect subcutaneously to the axillary fascia. If the dissection is kept superficial, risk of injury to the intercostobrachial nerve is minimized.

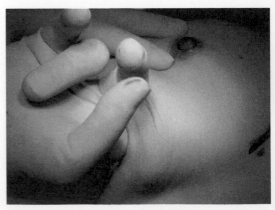

Fig. 10. Finger dissection to confirm subpectoral space. Direct palpation should be used to confirm that dissection is in the submuscular plane.

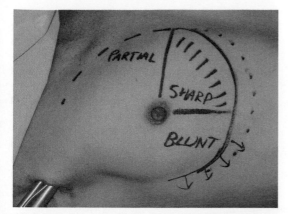

Fig. 11. Staged release of pectoralis fibers. Partial, sharp, and blunt dissection of the pectoralis fibers is performed within the quadrants depicted in the figure.

dissection. With the left hand, the surgeon inserts the endoretractor into the incision to the subpectoral space. The surgeon then inserts the endoscope through the sleeve, taking care to lift the endoretractor off the chest wall to avoid fluid accumulation on the lens. Because the light-source cord secures the scope to the retractor, the entire retractor can be pivoted from a medial to lateral position to adjust the view (**Fig. 12**). When the view is optimized, the surgeon may then use his or her right hand for dissection with the endoscopic cautery.

The video monitor is then used to guide dissection. When the camera is positioned in the correct orientation, the costal cartilage and intercostal muscles are visible inferiorly and the fibers of the pectoralis are seen superiorly and mobile with the retractor. The angled cautery device is then

inserted until it is in view on the monitor. The pectoralis muscle can then be divided according to the plan described above. For the medial, inferior dissection requiring full release, the pectoralis should be divided approximately 0.5 to 1 cm off the chest wall to maintain a cuff of muscle and avoid retraction of vascular perforators that may be difficult to control. Encountering the prepectoral fascia serves as the endpoint of dissection (**Fig. 13**). To avoid inferior overmigration of a smooth implant, preservation of the prepectoral fascia is preferred. The new position of the inframammary fold is also directly measured to the desired position from the external markings. The thickness of the breast skin should also be palpated before completing the pectoralis dissection to avoid inadvertent cautery on the skin undersurface.

In the superiormedial position, partial release of the pectoralis is performed. The thickness of the pectoralis in this sector can be gauged by palpating the thickness of the pectoralis externally against the internal plastic end of the cautery device. This gives the surgeon the approximate width desired for a 40% to 50% division of fibers. The Emory dissector can then be placed in the incision. With a gentle sweeping motion, the lateral fibers are released bluntly to create the lateral extent of the pocket and avoid injury to the anterolateral sensory nerves. The endoscope is then used to carefully examine the entire dimension of the pocket for bleeding.

The endoscopic equipment is then removed and the pocket irrigated with antibiotic solution or dilute betadine. Asche forceps can be used to widen the hiatus in the axillary fascia and create an accessible tunnel to facilitate implant placement

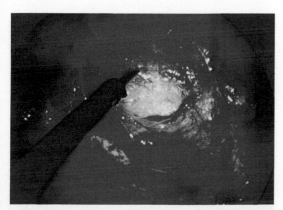

Fig. 12. Endoscopic division of pectoralis. Direct visualization of the pectoralis dissection is a significant advantage of this technique. Visualization of the prepectoral fascia serves as the end point of dissection.

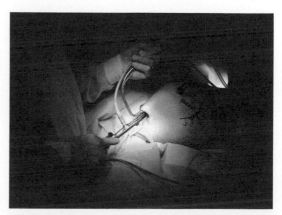

Fig. 13. Positioning of the endoretractor and scope. When situated on the right side of the patient, the surgeon should hold the retractor and scope in the left hand, while using a dissection instrument in the right hand.

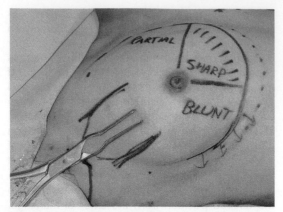

Fig. 14. Asche forceps to widen pocket tunnel. The axillary fascia, if not widened, can often impede insertion of the implant. The Asche forceps can be used as a blunt instrument to spread the width of the endoscopic tunnel.

(**Fig. 14**). Prior to implant insertion, a time-release Marcaine pain pump may also be used. In our opinion, such a pump provides excellent postoperative pain control. The catheter is inserted with an introducer and positioned on the superiomedial aspect of the pocket and brought out through the posterior aspect of the axillary incision (**Fig. 15**). After the implant is placed, the catheter sits on the posterior surface of the implant.

Attention is then turned to the implant placement. A small Deavor or army-navy retractor is inserted under the lateral edge of the pectoralis in preparation for implant insertion. The surgeon's gloves are wiped with antibiotic irrigation and the incisional skin is re-prepped with betadine. If a saline implant is used, it is prepared in similar fashion to that used in other approaches, using an airtight

fill system with approximately 50 cc of primer saline solution in the implant shell. When the implant is positioned in the pocket, it is filled to the desired volume and the fill tube is removed. If a silicone implant is used, the implant is prepared in a standard fashion and moistened with saline to facilitate insertion. Insertion of a large implant through a small incision may be challenging. It is important to advance a leading edge with one hand while maintaining gentle radial pressure with the other hand (**Fig. 16**). Excessive pressure or failure to widen the incision or axillary fascia diameter may cause the implant to fracture or rupture, creating a noticeable external deformity.

When the implant is positioned, the patient is seated upright to enable examination of the implant's external contour. If the inframammary fold remains too high, the breast dissector can be inserted gently behind the implant, which can then be directed radially to release any additional fibers. At this point, the patient is placed back into the supine position and dissection is commenced on the opposite side. For right-handed surgeons, the left-sided dissection may be a bit more challenging, particularly in the inferiolateral pocket. The authors have found that the most facile technique for dissection on the left side is to place the endoretractor and scope in the *right* hand, and use the ipsilateral cautery device (having a left-sided bend) to dissect with the left hand (**Fig. 17**). This allows better exposure and control of the inferiolateral pocket.

After both implants are placed, the patient is repositioned upright again to check for symmetry. Any adjustments may also be made at this point. It is also advised to externally manipulate the implant in all four quadrants to confirm that the

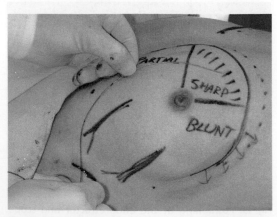

Fig. 15. Position of pain pump catheter. This position allows Marcaine to be administered during the first 2 to 3 days after surgery in a dependent fashion throughout the entire pocket.

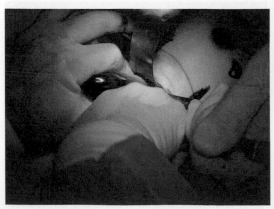

Fig. 16. Silicone implants are inserted by maintaining gentle pressure on the implant while advancing a leading edge in a radial fashion.

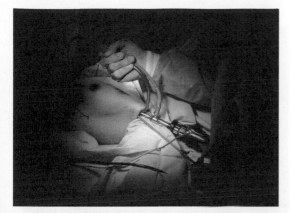

Fig. 17. Left-sided pocket dissection and hand placement. When dissecting on the patient's left side, the surgeon reverses hand position. This allows optimum exposure for dissection of the inferiolateral pocket.

pocket dissection is large enough and that there is no banding, which can cause compression.

The wounds are closed in layers with absorbable suture material (either Vicryl or Monocryl). The deep subcutaneous tissue is closed with three to four 4-0 interrupted sutures. Deep dermal and subcuticular layers are closed with 4-0 Monocryl running sutures. The pain pump may also be secured with a simple 4-0 interrupted Prolene. Adhesive skin closures (eg, Steri-Strips) are applied and covered with a transparent medical dressing (eg, Tegaderm). A Velcro elastic band is placed around the upper chest. The band will direct downward pressure to the implant to prevent the implant from riding superiorly.

Results

Results following this technique have been very acceptable to our patients because of the inconspicuous scar hidden in the armpit. Complications and surgical revisions have been rare. Examples of sample results are illustrated in **Figs. 18** through **20**.

Postoperative care

The patient is usually discharged after recovery from anesthesia. The endoscopic technique produces bruising and swelling of the breasts similar

Preop   Postop

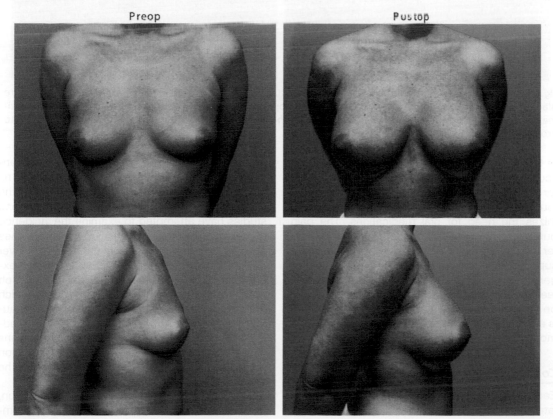

Fig. 18. Smooth, round, saline implant placed submuscularly. In this patient, smooth, round saline implants were placed in the submuscular plane using a transaxillary endoscopic approach and filled to a final volume of 450 cm³. Postoperative photos (*right*) show symmetric implant position with preserved inframammary fold.

Preop   Postop

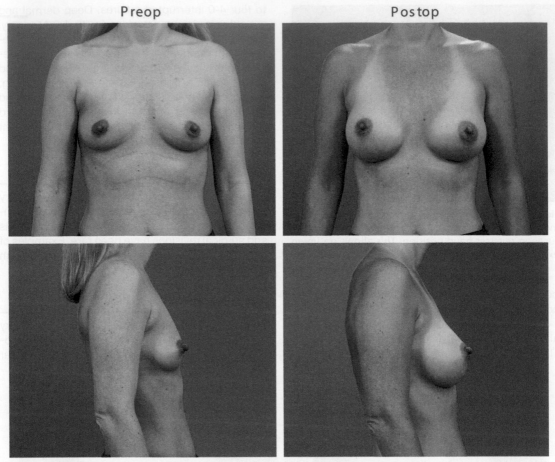

Fig. 19. Smooth, round, silicone implant placed submuscularly. Moderate profile 250-cm³ silicone implants were placed on each side via the transaxillary endoscopic approach. The inframammary fold was lowered approximately 1 cm on each side. Postoperative images (*right*) show symmetric implant position and appropriate projection.

to those associated with traditional and nonendoscopic techniques. Oral analgesics are prescribed for 3 to 4 days after surgery. However, we have found that use of the Marcaine pain pump minimizes the need for oral medications. The pain pump is removed in the office within 2 to 3 days after surgery. Patients are also instructed to wear the superior elastic bandage for 3 to 4 weeks after surgery. Activities may be resumed as the patient feels better, but brisk activity and exercise should be delayed for approximately 2 weeks. The patient is examined in the office again after 1 week, after 1 month, after 6 months, and after 1 year.

Complications

Early complications are rare but similar to those related to standard approaches and include hematoma, pneumothorax, infection, and asymmetry. Perhaps the most specific complication related to the transaxillary approach involves injury to

the intercostobrachial nerve, which can be encountered during axillary dissection. Symptoms include hypesthesia or numbness involving the medial arm and lateral chest/breast area. Several studies have attempted to examine the incidence of nerve injury during transaxillary approaches and quote exceptionally high rates of over 50%.[31,32] However, these studies are either extrapolated from full axillary dissection from lymph node excision or are based on survey data, which may be grossly inadequate. Anecdotally, the authors have found this complication to be exceedingly rare. To avoid this complication, surgeons should take special care to maintain the dissection superficially at the point in the procedure when the lateral pectoralis border is encountered.

Late complications include rippling, deflation, capsular contracture, and implant malposition. Implant rippling is usually seen with saline implants or subglandular augmentation as well as in patients with thin tissue coverage (**Fig. 21**). Conversion to

Preop   Postop

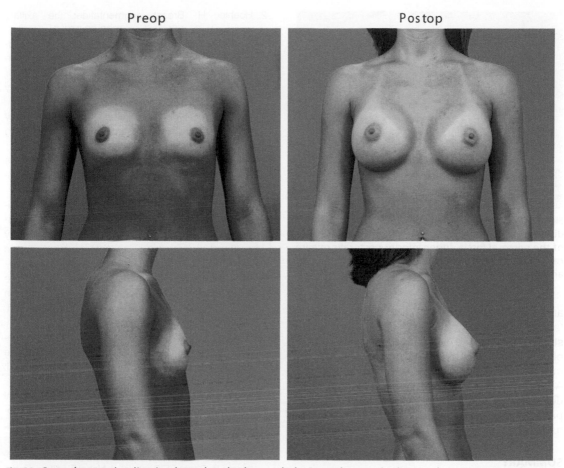

Fig. 20. Smooth, round, saline implant placed submuscularly. Smooth, round saline implants were placed in this patient through the transaxillary endoscopic approach. The implant was filled to 325 cm³ on each side. Postoperative photos (*right*) show good symmetry and projection.

silicone gel, internal coverage with acellular dermal matrix (eg, AlloDerm), or implant repositioning to the submuscular plane may be required. Implant malposition may also occur if control of the

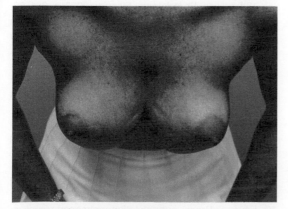

Fig. 21. Implant rippling. Rippling can be seen with aggressive dissection of the medial pectoralis fibers, resulting in poor implant coverage.

inframammary fold is not maintained. In these instances, the implant will migrate lower and cause psuedoptosis (**Fig. 22**).[33] This can be a challenging problem to correct and may involve conversion to an inframammary incision to reposition the inframammary fold.

Several recent studies and discussions have examined the impact of transaxillary augmentation on future sentinel lymph node detection for breast carcinoma.[34] The potential interference of previous surgery in sentinel lymph node accuracy has been described but remains controversial.[35] The interference appears to be evident in patients with deep axillary surgery, and its effect may be time-dependent before re-establishment of lymphatic channels. Furthermore, the addition of preoperative lymphosyntigraphy to sentinel lymph node biopsy augments detection of the nodes in question. In regard to patients with previous transaxillary augmentation, several investigators conclude that lymphatic channels can be protected during exposure if the dissection remains high

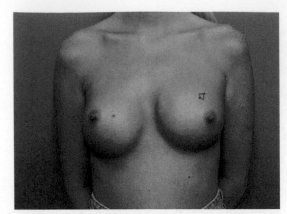

Fig. 22. Implant malposition secondary to aggressive dissection of the inframammary fold. Excessive release of the pectoral fascia during inferior pectoralis release can result in destruction of the inframammary fold and implant malposition.

and anterior within the axilla and kept to the sub-fascial plane.[36,37] Nonetheless, most of these studies were based on cadaveric studies of lymphatic channels after transaxillary surgery and may not reflect true incidences in live patients. A large population study of sentinel lymph node detection in previous transaxillary augmentation patients may elucidate the true incidence of disruption in lymphatic channels.

SUMMARY

Advances in endoscopic plastic surgery offer patients new, less-invasive alternatives to traditional open techniques. The endoscopic transaxillary approach to breast augmentation is a successful technique that not only provides an incision that is inconspicuous, but also offers the advantage of dissection under direct visualization, particularly within the medial and inferior submuscular plane. The authors feel that this technique also provides the surgeon with optimal control of the inframammary fold. The endoscopic technique can also be used with silicone implants if precautions are taken to protect the implant from rupture during insertion. Complications are rare with the endoscopic technique. However, the technique calls for special attention to protect the intercostobrachial nerve during initial dissection. The authors feel that this technique is a good choice for patients undergoing primary breast augmentation.

REFERENCES

1. Troques R. Implatationdes prostheses mammaires par incision axillaire. Nouv.Presse Med 1972;1:2409–11.
2. Hoehler H. Breast augmentation: the axillary approach. Br J Plast Surg 1973;26:373–5.
3. Hetter GP. Improved patient satisfaction with augmentation mammoplasty: the transaxillary subpectoral approach. Aesthetic Plast Surg 1991;15(1):123–7.
4. Eiseman G. Augmentation mammaplasty by the axillary approach. Plast Reconstr Surg 1974;57:229–31.
5. Wright JH, Bevin AG. Augmentation mammaplasty by the transaxillary approach. Plast Reconstr Surg 1976;58:429–35.
6. Eaves FF III, Price CI, Bostwick J III, et al. Subcutaneous endoscopic plastic surgery using a retractor-mounted endoscopic system. Perspect Plast Surg 1993;7(2):1–22.
7. Momeni A, Padron NT, Föhn M, et al. Safety, complications, and satisfaction of patients undergoing submuscular breast augmentation via the inframammary and endoscopic transaxillary approach. Aesthetic Plast Surg 2005;29(6):558–64.
8. Giordano PA, Rouif M, Laurent B, et al. Endoscopic transaxillary breast augmentation: clinical evaluation of a series of 306 patients over a 9-year period. Aesthetic Surg J 2007;27(1):47–54.
9. Tebbetts JB. Axillary endoscopic breast augmentation: processes derived from a 28-year experience to optimize outcomes. Plast Reconstr Surg 2006;118(7 Suppl):53S–80S.
10. Munhoz AM, Fells K, Arruda E, et al. Subfascial transaxillary breast augmentation without endoscopic assistance: technical aspects and outcome. Aesth Plast Surg 2006;30:503–12.
11. Eaves FF, Bostwick J, Nahai F. Augmentation mammoplasty. In: Eaves FF, Bostwick J, Nahai F, editors. Endoscopic plastic surgery. 1st edition. St. Louis (MO): Quality Medical Publishing Inc; 1995. p. 358–61.
12. Hwang K, Jung CY, Lee WJ, et al. The lateral cutaneous branch of the fourth intercostal nerve relating to transaxillary augmentation mammoplasty. Ann Plast Surg 2004;53(1):27–30.
13. Iglehart JD, Smith BL. Diseases of the breast. In: Townsend CM, editor. Sabiston textbook of surgery. 18th edition. Philadelphia: Elsevier; 2008. p. 851–88.
14. Barnett A. Transaxillary subpectoral augmentation in the ptotic breast: augmentation by disruption of the extended pectoral fascia and parenchymal sweep. Plast Reconstr Surg 1990;86:76–80.
15. Price CI, Eaves FF 3rd, Nahai F, et al. Endoscopic transaxillary subpectoral breast augmentation. Plast Reconstr Surg 1994;94(5):612–9.
16. Matti BA, Nicolle FV, Chir M. Open capsulotomy by the transaxillary approach. Aesthetic Plast Surg 1986;10(1)):243–4.
17. Yu L, Wang J, Zhang B, et al. Endoscopic transaxillary capsular contracture treatment. Aesthetic Plast Surg 2008;32:329–32.
18. Eaves F. Breast augmentation: enhanced visualization with the endoscopic transaxillary technique. Aesthetic Surg J 1999;19(2):162–4.

19. Tebbetts JB. Transaxillary subpectoral augmentation mammaplasty: a nine year experience. Clin Plast Surg 1988;15:557–604.
20. Troilius C. Endoscopic transaxillary breast augmentation. Aesthetic Surg J 2004;24(1):67–73.
21. Tebbetts JB. Transaxillary subpectoral augmentation mammaplasty: long-term follow-up and refinements. Plast Reconstr Surg 1984;74:636–40.
22. Reynolds HE. Evaluation of the augmented breast. Radiol Clin North Am 1995;33(6):1131–45.
23. Puckett CL, Croll GH, Reichel CA, et al. A critical look at capsular contracture in subglandular versus subpectoral mammary augmentation. Aesthetic Plast Surg 1987;11:23–4.
24. Campiglio GL, Candiani P. Transaxillary submuscular augmentation mammaplasty. European Journal of Plastic Surgery 1995;18(2-3):95–100.
25. Serra-Renom J, Garrido MF, Yoon T. Augmentation mammaplasty with anatomic, soft, cohesive silicone gel implants using the transaxillary approach at a subfascial level with endoscopic assistance. Plast Reconstr Surg 2005;116:640–5.
26. Benito-Ruiz J. Transaxillary subfascial breast augmentation. Aesthetic Surg J 2003;23(6):480–3.
27. Wong CH, Samuel M, Tan BK, et al. Capsular contracture in subglandular breast augmentation with textured versus smooth breast implants: a systematic review. Plast Reconstr Surg 2006;118(5):1224–36.
28. Barnsley GP, Sigurdson LJ, Barnsley SE. Textured surface breast implants in the prevention of capsular contracture among breast augmentation patients: a meta-analysis of randomized controlled trials. Plast Reconstr Surg 2006;117(7):2182–90.
29. Villafane O, Garcia-Tutor R, Taggart I. Endoscopic transaxillary subglandular breast augmentation using silicone gel textured implants. Aesthetic Plast Surg 2000;24:212–5.
30. Agris J, Dingman RO, Wilensky RJ. A dissector for the transaxillary approach in augmentation mammaplasty. Plast Reconstr Surg 1976;57:10.
31. Ghaderi B, Hoenig JM, Dado D, et al. Incidence of intercostobrachial nerve injury after transaxillary breast augmentation. Aesthetic Surg J 2002;22(1):26–32.
32. Ivens D, Hoe AL, Podd TJ, et al. Assessment of morbidity from complete axillary dissection. Br J Cancer 1992;66:136–8.
33. Troilius C. A ten-year evaluation following corrections of implant ptosis subsequent to transaxillary subpectoral breast augmentation. Plast Reconstr Surg 2004;114(6):1638–41 [discussion: 1642–3].
34. Prado A, Andrades P, Leniz P. Implications of transaxillary breast augmentation: lifetime probability of breast cancer development and sentinel node mapping interference. Aesthetic Plas Surg 2007;31(4):317–9.
35. Lyman GH, Giuliano AE, Somerfield MR, et al. American Society of Clinical Oncology guideline recommendations for sentinel lymph node biopsy in early-stage breast cancer. J Clin Oncol 2005;20:7703–20.
36. Munhoz AM, Ferriera MC. Implications of transaxillary breast augmentation: lifetime probability for the development of breast cancer and sentinel node mapping interference. Aesthetic Plast Surg 2007;31(4):320–1.
37. Graf RM, Canan LW, Romano GG, et al. Implications of transaxillary breast augmentation: lifetime probability for the development of breast cancer and sentinel node mapping interference. Aesthetic Plast Surg 2007;31:322–4.

Transumbilical Breast Augmentation

Neal Handel, MD, FACS*

KEYWORDS

- Augmentation mammaplasty • Breast enlargement
- Breast implants • Transumbilical breast augmentation

Transumbilical breast augmentation (TUBA) was introduced in 1993. Since its inception, the TUBA operation has been controversial. Concerns were raised about whether implants could be accurately positioned through such a remote incision, whether bleeding could be adequately controlled, and whether the technique, compared with other techniques, posed an increased possibility of damage to the implant. Few plastic surgeons have incorporated the TUBA procedure into their practices. Among the reasons cited for not performing TUBA are that it is "technically difficult," does not give the same "degree of control" as traditional approaches, and is associated with a higher risk of complications. Often surgeons are skeptical about the benefits of the transumbilical approach. This article reviews the history of TUBA; dispels some of the misconceptions regarding this operation; describes a simplified, nonendoscopic approach for umbilical insertion of saline implants; and examines the advantages and disadvantages of TUBA compared with more conventional techniques.

HISTORY OF TRANSUMBILICAL BREAST AUGMENTATION

Johnson and Christ,[1] the first to describe TUBA, reported on their experience with 91 women who underwent submammary augmentation with saline implants. They described overall results as satisfactory, but acknowledged 1 case of "excessive bleeding," 1 "implant deflation," and 2 cases in which the implant was inadvertently placed subpectorally. In the early descriptions of this operation, the permanent saline implant was overinflated and used as a soft tissue expander to help dissect the surgical pocket. While an endoscope was employed, it was used only to confirm that the implant was in the correct plane (submammary); the endoscope played no role in performing the operative procedure itself.

Concerns and criticisms regarding the TUBA operation surfaced almost immediately. In a letter to *Plastic and Reconstructive Surgery*, Tebbetts[2] questioned whether the TUBA approach allowed a level of "control" comparable to other methods of breast augmentation. He also speculated about whether there might be increased patient morbidity or an increased risk of product liability related to inserting saline implants in this manner.

Caleel[3] published the first large series. He reported on 513 patients (1026 breasts) in whom the implants were placed in the submammary position and on 140 patients (280 breasts) in whom implants were placed subpectorally. Caleel claimed a high rate of patient satisfaction and stated there were only 10 complications, the majority of which occurred in his first 30 cases. Among the advantages he cited were absence of a scar on the breast, a short operating time, less postoperative pain, and a quick recovery. Despite this publication and other positive reports, criticism of the TUBA operation persisted. In a review article on breast augmentation, Hidalgo[4] stated that some of the "disadvantages" of the TUBA approach included poor access to the implant pocket, the (presumed) inability to create a subpectoral pocket, the inability to use shaped or gel-filled implants, and the possible need for a second incision for revisions.

Division of Plastic Surgery, The David Geffen School of Medicine, University of California at Los Angeles, Los Angeles, CA, USA
* 13400 Riverside Drive, Suite #101, Sherman Oaks, CA 91423.
E-mail address: drhandel@aol.com

Clin Plastic Surg 36 (2009) 63–74
doi:10.1016/j.cps.2008.07.003

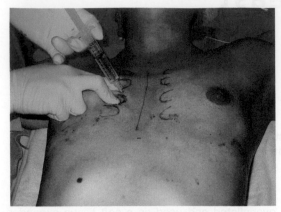

Fig. 1. Small volumes (1–2 mL) of local anesthetic with adrenaline are injected into multiple sites along the origins of the pectoralis muscle over the ribs and sternum.

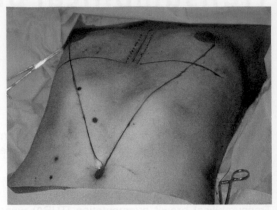

Fig. 3. Skin markings are made to delineate the midline, medial limit of pocket dissection, desired level of the breast fold, and planned location of the subcutaneous tract.

In an effort to dispel some of the misconceptions about the TUBA procedure, Dowden[5] reported his personal experience with this technique over a 7-year period. Dowden acknowledged that he too initially had reservations about this approach, primarily because it seemed as if it might be difficult to insert a breast implant through so remote an incision. However, with increasing experience he discovered that many of the "theoretic objections were baseless" and he ultimately concluded that the TUBA was "an excellent procedure." Dowden reported almost no complications in his personal consecutive series of 350 prepectoral transumbilical breast augmentations. In his article, he systematically dispels many of the common myths and misconceptions that have surrounded the TUBA approach since its inception.

Some of the initial reservations related to the TUBA operation were based on the belief that it would be difficult to accurately create an adequate

surgical pocket through a remote incision. Once the technique is fully understood, it becomes apparent that the surgical pocket can be predictably created in either the submammary or subpectoral plane. The surgeon has control over all aspects of pocket dissection, including the medial extent (cleavage area) and inferior extent (inframammary fold). It is therefore possible to create a pocket of sufficient size and to reliably control implant position. As with liposuction (and rhinoplasty using the "closed" technique), the surgeon has knowledge of and control over the position of his instruments at all times (even without directly visualizing them).

There have also been concerns about control of bleeding when a submammary or subpectoral pocket is created through a distant portal, such as the umbilical incision. Most surgeons familiar with the TUBA technique have discovered that there is actually much less bleeding associated

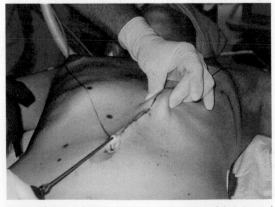

Fig. 2. Klein's solution (approx 100–200 mL) is injected along the planned subcutaneous tract on each side.

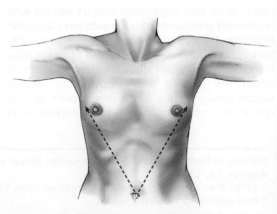

Fig. 4. Paths of subcutaneous tunnels (*dotted lines*).

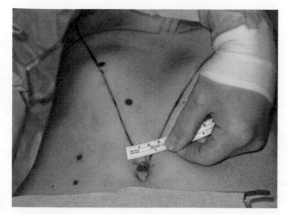

Fig. 5. A short (∼1–1.5 cm) curvilinear incision is made in the superior umbilical recess.

with this approach than that associated with conventional techniques. It is likely that there is less bleeding because the pocket dissection is accomplished bluntly. The initial dissection is achieved using smooth and serrated dissectors to "avulse" the tissue planes; final pocket enlargement and refinement is accomplished with tissue expanders. These techniques are inherently less "bloody" than sharp dissection with scissors, knife, or even electrocautery. The amount of blood loss with the TUBA procedure is miniscule (probably less than 10 mL in the average case); there is so little bleeding that electrocautery is almost never necessary. In the published series, the hematoma rate is very low and is comparable (if not lower) than that associated with other surgical approaches.[6]

Another concern about the TUBA approach is related to the potential for damage to the prosthesis. At one time there was a common

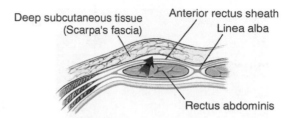

Fig. 7. Level of dissection (*arrow*) of the subcutaneous tunnels, just superficial to the deep abdominal fascia.

misconception that the implant was "passed through a metal tube." It has never been recommended that the implant be pushed through a tube, endoscope, or any other device. The original technique for inserting the implant consisted of tightly rolling up the prosthesis, and then advancing it along the subcutaneous tunnel with assistance from a blunt metal tube (Johnson tube) specially designed to "push" the implant into the surgical pocket. There is no evidence that gently advancing the implant using this method damages the shell or increases the risk of subsequent deflation. However, as an alternative, the prosthesis can be manually "massaged" along the subcutaneous tract from the incision all the way into the surgical pocket. Dowden[7,8] has described a "no touch" technique whereby all the air is evacuated from the prosthesis as it is tightly rolled up; the implant is then inserted through the umbilical incision and pushed up manually as far as possible. External digital manipulation is then used to slide the implant the remainder of the way through the tunnel into the surgical pocket. If an endoscope is used, it is employed only to verify proper orientation of the implant before filling it; the endoscope never touches the device. This technique avoids any contact whatsoever between the prosthesis and surgical instruments and is an excellent option for surgeons concerned about "instrumentation" of the implant.

In the early descriptions of the TUBA procedure, the saline implant was intentionally overinflated and used as a balloon dissector to create the pocket. There was legitimate concern that overinflating the prosthesis and using it as a tissue expander might inadvertently damage the shell or fill valve, leading to an increased risk of deflation. This approach has been abandoned and the surgical technique has now been modified to eliminate unnecessary trauma to the implant. All pocket dissection is performed using custom fabricated instruments and a disposable tissue expander.[9] The final saline implant is not used for creating the pocket, nor is it overinflated.[10,11]

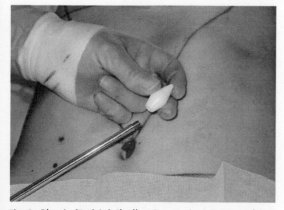

Fig. 6. Plastic (Delrin) "bullets" come in 1.5-cm and 2.0-cm diameters and can be interchangeably screwed onto a threaded metal rod.

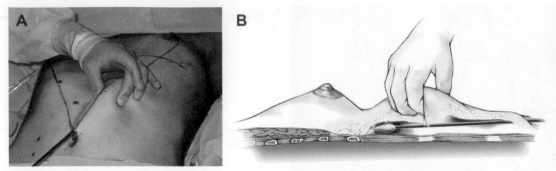

Fig. 8. (*A* and *B*) As the trocar is advanced up the abdomen toward the axilla, the dissection is maintained in the deep subcutaneous plane. This is facilitated by grasping the soft tissues and "pulling" them away from the deeper structures.

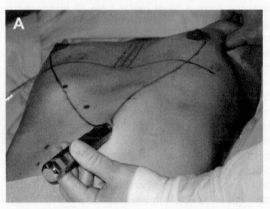

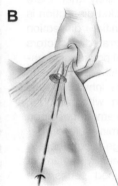

Fig. 9. (*A* and *B*) When the trocar reaches the axilla, it is easy to palate the tip of the "bullet" and guide it beneath the pectoralis major muscle just proximal to its insertion. Arrow in *B* indicates tip of trocar penetrating beneath pectoral muscle near its insertion.

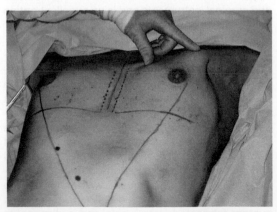

Fig. 10. By cantilevering the rod upward, tension is placed on the pectoralis major muscle, accentuating the anterior axillary fold and confirming submuscular placement of the instrument.

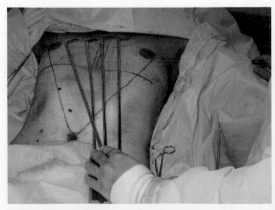

Fig. 11. The dissectors used for creating the pocket come in different configurations, including configurations with smooth, notched, and serrated blades.

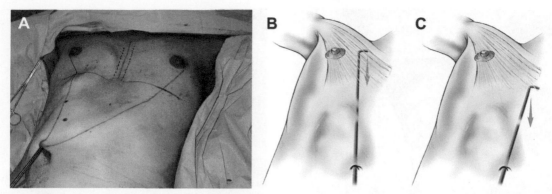

Fig. 12. (*A, B,* and *C*) The dissector is advanced up the subcutaneous tunnel and transposed into the subpectoral space. The instrument is pulled medially and downward (*arrows* in *B* and *C*) to avulse the fibers of origin of the pectoralis muscle to create a submuscular pocket.

PATIENT SELECTION

The TUBA approach is suitable for a wide variety of patients. The operation may be relatively contraindicated in women with very constricted inframammary folds, patients with tuberous breast deformity, and those with advanced ptosis. In these patients, radial release of the breast parenchyma and more aggressive surgical expansion of the lower pole may be necessary; these maneuvers may be more difficult with the transumbilical approach than with techniques that allow for direct visualization of the area. The transumbilical approach is particularly suitable in patients with small-diameter areolae (in whom it may be difficult to insert the implant through a short periareolar scar) and in patients who do not have a well-defined inframammary fold. Umbilical hernia, scoliosis, and breast asymmetry are not contraindications to TUBA.

SURGICAL TECHNIQUE

My personal technique for TUBA has evolved over time and is based on a combination of techniques that I have adopted from other surgeons. While some surgeons advocate the use of an endoscope (either to confirm the plane of insertion or to actually perform parts of the operation), I have found the nonendoscopic approach to be completely satisfactory. The operation is performed under general anesthesia using laryngeal mask airway technique. The patient is positioned supine with the arms abducted to put some tension on the pectoralis major muscle; this facilitates entry into the subpectoral plane. After induction of general anesthesia, a local anesthetic mixture (equal parts lidocaine 0.5% with adrenaline 1:100,000 and 0.25% bupivicaine) is injected into the proposed incision site in the superior umbilical recess and into the breasts. Spinal needles

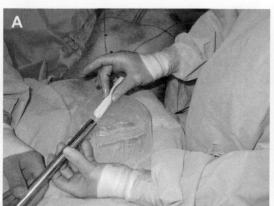
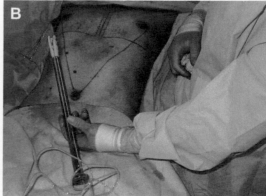

Fig. 13. (*A* and *B*) The tissue expander with integrated fill tube is rolled up, the filler tube is passed the length of the Johnson tube, and the end of the expander is gently inserted into the distal end of the tube.

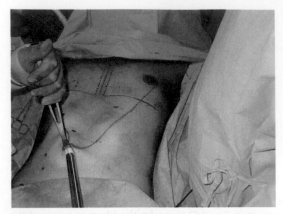

Fig. 14. The rolled up expander is introduced through the umbilical incision and advanced along the subcutaneous tract.

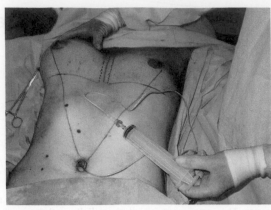

Fig. 16. The expander is inflated with air to about 150% of the anticipated final implant volume. Overexpansion assists in stretching the soft tissues and promotes hemostasis.

(22 gauge) are used in an effort to inject the local anesthetic primarily into the retromammary plane where most of the surgical dissection will occur. It is also helpful to inject small additional amounts of local anesthetic (1–2 mL at multiple sites) into the fibers of origin of the pectoral muscle over the ribs where the muscle will be avulsed from its attachments (**Fig. 1**); this diminishes bleeding as the subpectoral pocket is dissected. Along the course of the planned subcutaneous tunnel (extending on each side from the umbilicus toward the axilla) Klein's[12] solution is injected, typically 100 to 200 mL per side, to reduce potential bleeding along the tract (**Fig. 2**).

Skin markings can be made to assist in dissecting the pocket in the correct location (**Fig. 3**). A vertical line is drawn down the center of the sternum, then two parallel lines are drawn, each 1 cm

lateral to the midline, delineating the medial extent of pocket dissection on each side. A line may also be drawn at the desired level of the inframammary fold, generally 6 to 7 cm beneath the inferior border of the areola. It may also be helpful to draw a line on the skin representing the planned course of the subcutaneous tunnel. This line extends from the umbilicus, tangential to the lateral border of the areola, and toward the axilla on each side (**Fig. 4**).

Surgery is initiated by making a short (approximately 1–1.5 cm) curvilinear incision in the superior umbilical recess (**Fig. 5**). The wound is deepened to the abdominal fascia using blunt dissection. A subcutaneous tunnel is bluntly dissected on each side. This tunnel is created using "bullet"-shaped dissectors specially designed for this purpose (**Fig. 6**). The tips are made from polyoxymethylene (eg, Delrin, E. I. du Pont de Nemours and

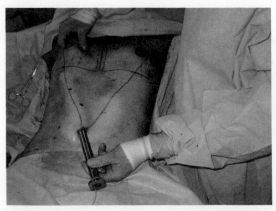

Fig. 15. When the expander is correctly positioned in the subpectoral pocket, it is firmly grasped and held in place as the Johnson tube is withdrawn, leaving the expander and attached fill tube in position.

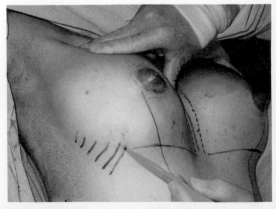

Fig. 17. With the expander fully inflated, the breast contours are carefully inspected. Areas where further dissection is required are marked on the skin.

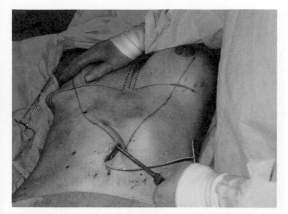

Fig. 18. The pocket is further refined using the serrated dissector.

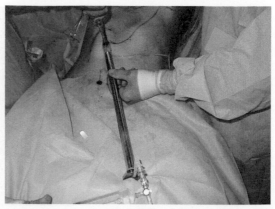

Fig. 20. The permanent implant is introduced via the umbilical incision and gently advanced through the subcutaneous tunnel into position in the subpectoral pocket.

Company, Johnston, Iowa). The "bullets" come in two diameters, 1.5 and 2 cm. They can be interchangeably attached to a threaded metal rod. The initial dissection is performed with the small "bullet." The tip of the trocar is gently advanced up the abdomen, beneath the breast, and toward the axilla. It is important to keep the dissection of this tunnel in the deep subcutaneous plane, just superficial to the abdominal fascia (**Fig. 7**). Maintaining the tip of the instrument in the deep plane can be facilitated by grasping the abdominal soft tissues and gently retracting them away from the underlying muscle and fascia (**Fig. 8**). A deep dissection prevents creases and other contour irregularities of the abdominal skin.

When the tip of the dissector enters the axilla, it is easy to palpate (and even visualize) the instrument beneath the thin subcutaneous tissue. Once the trocar reaches the lateral border of the pectoralis major muscle, just proximal to its insertion, the tip is introduced ("popped") beneath the

distal portion of the pectoralis (**Fig. 9**). The rod is cantilevered upwards; this puts tension on the insertion of the pectoralis muscle and accentuates the anterior axillary fold, confirming that the instrument is in the subpectoral plane (**Fig. 10**). Once the tunnel has been created with the smaller "bullet," the larger 2-cm "bullet" is screwed onto the threaded rod and used to enlarge the dimensions of the tract. By repeatedly sliding the trocar back and forth along the subcutaneous tunnel, the caliber of the track is dilated sufficiently so that the subsequent instruments (dissectors) and the tissue expander can easily be introduced into the subpectoral space for creation of the pocket.

Once an adequate tunnel has been created bilaterally, preliminary pocket dissection is accomplished with the hockey stick–shaped dissectors. These instruments come in a variety of lengths and configurations: some with smooth blades,

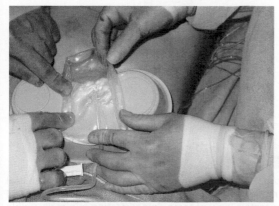

Fig. 19. The permanent implant with fill tube attached is fully evacuated and rolled up as tightly as possible.

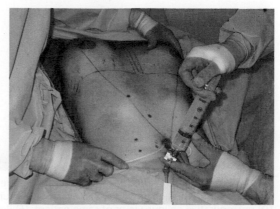

Fig. 21. Using a closed system, the implant is filled with the desired volume of saline.

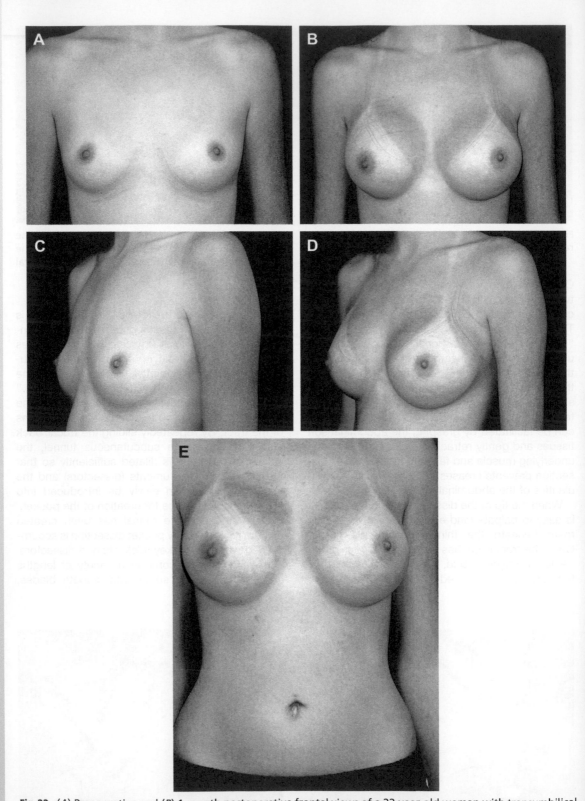

Fig. 22. (*A*) Preoperative and (*B*) 1-month postoperative frontal views of a 22-year-old woman with transumbilical subpectoral breast augmentation, 325 mL smooth round moderate profile saline implants. (*C*) Preoperative and (*D*) postoperative oblique views of same patient. (*E*) Postoperative view of torso demonstrating minimally visible umbilical scar and smooth abdominal contour.

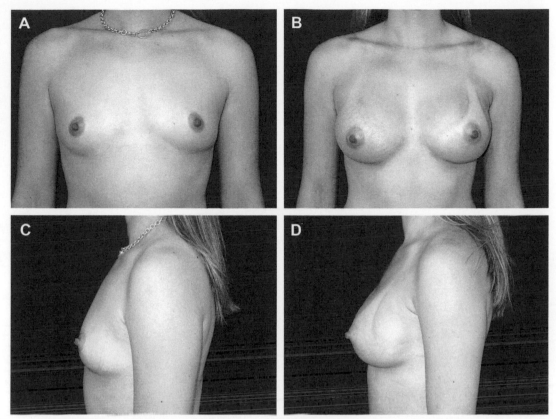

Fig. 23. (*A*) Preoperative and (*B*) 6-week postoperative frontal views of 26-year-old woman following transumbilical subpectoral breast augmentation, 300 mL smooth round moderate profile saline implants. (*C*) Preoperative and (*D*) postoperative lateral views of same patient.

some notched, and some with serrations (**Fig. 11**). I generally perform the initial dissection with a smooth or notched dissector, which is advanced up the subcutaneous tunnel, passed beneath the pectoralis muscle, and then pulled in a downward and medial direction to create the submuscular pocket (**Fig. 12**). Medially, near the origin of the pectoral muscle, forceful dissection is required to detach the muscle from the ribs. While the dissection is "blind" it is not "uncontrolled." The tip of the instrument can often be visualized and can always be palpated, so the surgeon has full control over the limits of dissection. Once the initial surgical pocket has been created, the contours can be further refined with the serrated dissector.

The next step consists of additional pocket delineation with an inflatable expander used as a balloon dissector. The expander is rolled into the smallest diameter possible. The integrated filler tube is passed through a hollow metal tube (Johnson tube) and the end of the rolled up expander is inserted 1 to 2 cm into the end of the tube (**Fig. 13**). The distal end of the expander is then introduced through the umbilical incision

(**Fig. 14**) and advanced (with assistance of the Johnson tube) up the tunnel and beneath the pectoral insertion. The expander can then be guided medially into position in the submuscular pocket. With the rolled up expander held in place (by "grasping" it through the overlying soft tissue), the Johnson tube is withdrawn, leaving just the expander and fill tube in place (**Fig. 15**). The expander is then inflated with air, usually to a volume of about 1.5 times the anticipated final volume of the implant to be used (**Fig. 16**). Overexpansion aids in stretching the soft tissues and achieving hemostasis.

With the expander fully inflated, the contours of the pocket can be visualized. If further dissection is required to improve cleavage, to make the folds symmetric, or to improve the contour of the breast, the areas requiring additional attention are marked on the skin (**Fig. 17**). The expander is then fully deflated and withdrawn; the serrated dissector is reintroduced and used to make necessary refinements of the pocket (**Fig. 18**).

The final step consists of insertion and inflation of the prosthesis. Both Inamed and Mentor

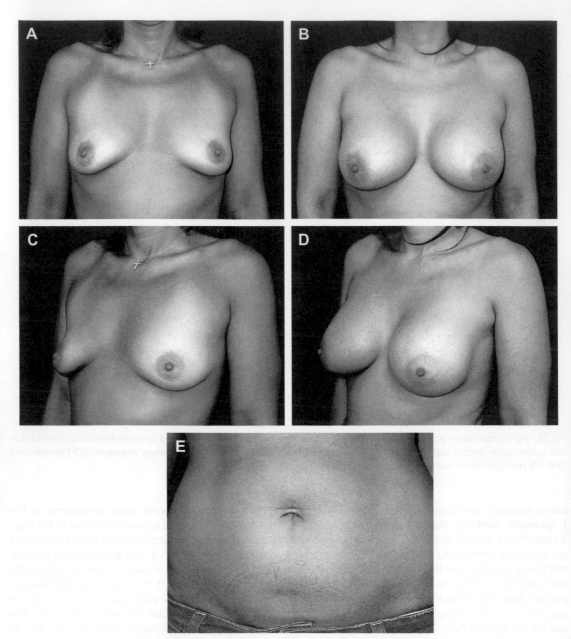

Fig. 24. (*A*) Preoperative and (*B*) 6-week postoperative frontal views of a 36-year-old woman with modest ptosis and mild asymmetry following transumbilical subpectoral breast augmentation, 350 mL smooth round moderate profile saline implants. (*C*) Preoperative and (*D*) postoperative oblique views of same patient. (*E*) Postoperative view of abdomen, scar completely hidden within umbilical recess.

products are suitable, and the prosthesis may have either an anterior or a posterior fill valve design. Typically round smooth implants are selected. They may be of varying profiles. Anatomically shaped and textured implants are contraindicated. The implant first is filled with a small volume of saline, which is then aspirated to evacuate all the air. As the air and saline are being aspirated, the prosthesis is rolled into the smallest possible diameter (similar to rolling up a taco shell) (**Fig. 19**). The attached filler tube is threaded the length of the metal tube and the rolled up prosthesis gently inserted a short distance into the end of the tube. The implant is advanced all the way up into the pocket (**Fig. 20**) and held securely in place as the Johnson tube is withdrawn, leaving the prosthesis and fill tube in situ. Using a "closed" system with a three-way stopcock, the implant is inflated to the desired volume (**Fig. 21**).

Before the fill tubes are "pulled," the patient may be placed in the sitting position to assess symmetry; minor adjustments in volume can be made. It is even possible at this point to reinsert the smooth-blade dissector and make additional minor modifications of the pocket if necessary. While drains are usually unnecessary, the subcutaneous tunnel provides an excellent tract for insertion of a dependent drain if so desired. The umbilical incision is closed and appropriate dressings are applied.

As noted previously, an alternative technique may be used to avoid any contact between the implant and surgical instruments. The prosthesis (with attached fill tube) is rolled up tightly and inserted into the subcutaneous tunnel through the umbilical incision. The implant can then be digitally "advanced" by "milking" it through the tunnel all the way into the submuscular pocket. The remaining steps are the same.

RESULTS

In my experience, the cosmetic results of the TUBA procedure have been uniformly good and patient satisfaction has been high. Some typical results are illustrated in **Figs. 22–24**.

Numerous surgeons have reported excellent results with the TUBA procedure and the rate of complications does not appear to be higher[13,14] but in fact may be lower[15] than those of other approaches. In a combined series of 855 consecutive TUBA operations performed between 2000 and 2004 by me and two other surgeons in our community, we found a very low rate of complications and infrequent need for reoperation (**Table 1**). I have not encountered any intraoperative

Table 1
TUBA complications requiring reoperation

Reason	Number	Percentage
Contracture	11	1.3
Deflation	9	1.1
Infection	0	—
Hematoma	2	0.2
Malposition	4	0.5
Abdominal seroma	2	0.2
Replace with larger implant	4	0.5
Replace with smaller implant	8	0.9
Revise umbilicus	1	0.1

Combined experience of Neal Handel, MD, Marc Mani, MD, and Peter Cheski, MD, involving 855 cases from 2000 to 2004. Data compiled from chart review by Melvin De La Cruz, MD, cosmetic surgery fellow with Peter Cheski, MD.

"difficulties" that required an alternate incision. I have performed two "late" revisions in my patients that required a new (periareolar) incision. In one case, the folds were uneven and the side that was too low did not respond to a prolonged 6-week course of taping and continual wearing of an underwire bra. In this case, a secondary capsuloplasty was performed though a periareolar incision. In another patient, unilateral capsular contracture (Baker grade 3) was corrected through a periareolar incision.

There are some potential limitations and drawbacks associated with the TUBA procedure; these should be discussed with patients during their consultation. For example, it is possible that a situation might be encountered (eg, excessive bleeding, inability to properly position an implant) that could require an alternative incision. In my experience, this has never occurred. But this possibility should be discussed with every patient as part of the informed consent. It is also likely that certain revisions, should they become necessary (eg, correction of contracture, implant malposition), might require a different incision.

It should also be disclosed to patients that insertion of saline implants via the umbilicus is "off label." When the manufacturers submitted premarket approval data to the Food and Drug Administration regarding the safety and efficacy of saline implants, no information was provided pertaining to the TUBA. Therefore, transumbilical insertion of saline implants is not "approved" by the Food and Drug Administration. This does not prohibit surgeons from using this approach,[16] but transumbilical insertion of saline implants is technically "off label" and this should be disclosed to prospective patients. It should also be noted that both Inamed and Mentor have gone on record stating that all applicable guarantees, warrantees, and replacement policies apply to their products even when they are inserted using the TUBA operation.[17]

SUMMARY

The transumbilical approach for breast augmentation has been controversial since its inception. There were some legitimate concerns related to the technique as initially described, particularly with regard to use of the permanent implant as a tissue expander to dissect the "pocket." However, the operation has been modified to address these concerns and in recent years multiple published studies have documented the safety and efficacy of this procedure. Overall, the cosmetic results are good, patient satisfaction is high, and the complication rate no greater than those of other breast augmentation techniques. For many patients, the opportunity to have breast augmentation through an inconspicuous incision remote from the breast is an appealing choice. For plastic surgeons, incorporating the TUBA operation into their practice enables them to offer prospective breast augmentation patients a wider spectrum of options.

REFERENCES

1. Johnson GW, Christ JE. The endoscopic breast augmentation: the transumbilical insertion of saline-filled breast implants. Plast Reconstr Surg 1993;92(5): 801–8.
2. Tebbetts John B. Transumbilical approach to breast augmentation [letter]. Plast Reconstr Surg 1994; 94(1):215–6.
3. Caleel Richard T. Transumbilical endoscopic breast augmentation submammary and subpectoral. Plast Reconstr Surg 2000;106(5):1177–82 [discussion: 1183–4].
4. Hidalgo David A. Breast augmentation: choosing the optimal incision, implant, and pocket plane. Plast

Reconstr Surg 2000;105(6):2202–16 [discussion: 2217–8].
5. Dowden RV. Dispelling the myths and misconceptions about transumbilical breast augmentation. Plast Reconstr Surg 2000;106(1):190–4.
6. Dowden RV. Keeping the transumbilical breast augmentation safe. Plast Reconstr Surg 2002;180(5): 1389–400.
7. Dowden RV. Why the transumbilical breast augmentation is safe for implants. Plast Reconstr Surg 2002; 109(7):2576–8.
8. Dowden RV. Technical update on transumbilical breast augmentation. Aesthetic Surgery Journal 2000;20(3):240–2.
9. Dowden RV, et al. Endoscopic breast surgery. In: Achauer BM, Eriksson E, Guyuron B, editors. Plastic surgery: indications, operations, and outcomes. Philadelphia: Mosby; 2000. p. 2757–69.
10. Johnson GW, Dowden RV. Breast augmentation: transumbilical retroglandular approach. In: Fodor PB, Isse NG, editors. Endoscopically assisted aesthetic plastic surgery. St. Louis (MO): Mosby; 1995. p. 145–66.
11. Johnson GW, Dowden RV. Breast augmentation: umbilical approach. In: Ramirez OM, Daniel RK, editors. Endoscopic plastic surgery. New York: Springer; 1995. p. 156–75.
12. Klein JA. The tumescent technique. Anesthesia and modified liposuction technique. Dermatol Clin 1990; 8(3):425–37.
13. Wittenberg JM, Leventhal M. Transumbilical retroglandular breast augmentation: a review of 158 cases and a comparison with traditional approach. Am J Cosmetic Surg 1998;15:387–94.
14. Vila-Rovira R. Breast augmentation by an umbilical approach. Aesthetic Plast Surg 1999;23(5):323–30.
15. Baccari ME. Dispelling the myths and misconceptions about transumbilical breast augmentation. Plast Reconstr Surg 2000;106(1):195–6 [discussion].
16. Spear SL, Bulan EJ, Venturi ML. Breast augmentation. Plast Reconstr Surg 2006;118(7S):188S–96S.
17. Dowden RV. Answers to frequently asked questions about breast enlargement through the navel (TUBA). Mentor Corporation and McGhan Corporation letters. Available at: http://www.breastimplant.net/faqs/tubaguar.html. Accessed October 19, 2001.

Form-Stable Silicone Gel Breast Implants

Mark Jewell, MD

KEYWORDS

- Breast augmentation • Breast implants
- Saline breast implants • Round gel breast implants
- Form-stable breast implants • Process engineering
- Toyota Production System • Lean manufacturing

The starting point for this article is the question of what is the optimal shape for a breast implant. Should the ideal device be round and "fill the breast envelope" or have a form that would "shape" the breast by serving as an internal framework for existing breast tissues? There are two schools of thought regarding breast esthetics, both of which are divergent, and neither approach provides the complete answer that will work for all patients seeking breast augmentation. I purposely oriented this article toward processes, system engineering, and operational excellence versus it being a treatise on my personal technique.

THE EVOLUTION OF SHAPED DEVICES

The concept of a shaped breast implant had been considered in the 1970s. Early teardrop-shaped, smooth surface, Dow-Corning devices had Dacron fixation patches on the back wall and were filled with first-generation non–form-stable gel. There was little analysis of the esthetic quality of outcomes from these devices or a process for their use. Early device failures in this design dissuaded plastic surgeons from shaped devices. Retrospective analysis of the outcomes performed years later showed that fixation patches contributed to device failure and that the first-generation gel was not form stable. Emphasis for many years was placed on round devices that would fill the breast envelope versus shaping the breast. No one had thought about formulating silicone gel to keep its shape inside the breast. The focus was

wrongly on liquid gel formulations that would ultimately be problematic in terms of extracapsular gel migration.

Alternatives to round devices that would produce a natural-appearing outcome after breast augmentation were a topic of interest in breast esthetics. Experimentation first led Dr. John Tebbetts to develop a shaped saline device, the INAMED 468, and later the form-stable INAMED (now Allergan) 410 series as its successor. In theory, this device was intended to improve breast esthetics by virtue of its tapered upper edge and dimensions of height, width, and projection. The journey to producing this device was not without some missteps. Notably, the major error was thinking that a shaped saline breast implant would maintain shape changes within the breast. It was illogical to think that a shaped device filled with a liquid would retain its shape once implanted. This ability had already been proven wrong with the first-generation shaped devices (Dow).

Detractors quickly demonstrated that shaped saline-filled devices assumed a round shape within the breast. To complicate matters further, marketing communications by INAMED, the maker of the Style 468 device, were distasteful and portrayed women as sex objects. The credibility of breast shaping by devices was assailed once again, and plastic surgeons went back to thinking about the world in terms of round saline or gel devices (Adjunct Study Protocol).

The development of devices continued, with newer silicone gel formulations that could be

The author is an approved clinical investigator in the INAMED Core Study, INAMED (Allergan) 410 Study, MENTOR CPG Medicis. He is also a consultant for Allergan, Medicis, Ethicon, Sound Surgical, LipoSonix, AorTech, and *New Beauty Magazine*.
Oregon Health Science University, 630 East 13th Avenue, Eugene, OR 97401, Portland, USA
E-mail address: mjewell@teleport.com

Clin Plastic Surg 36 (2009) 75–89
doi:10.1016/j.cps.2008.08.004

vulcanized into a form-stable shape. This advance in biomaterials technology when combined with an exterior texture (Biocell, INAMED) on the implant shell reduced device rotation once implanted and appeared to be the answer. The release of the IN-AMED 410 occurred with the device being sold off-shore starting in 1994. Form-stable gel devices had been successful in foreign markets where there was no restriction on their use. Notable breast surgery luminaries, such as Per Heden, MD, became interested in learning about how to optimally use these devices for cosmetic breast augmentation and reconstruction after mastectomy. Heden, Heitzman, and others performed the early work with the form-stable implants in a series of patients and documented their outcomes. Early reports of the outcomes were notable in terms of complications, buckling, infection, and capsular contracture. When viewed retrospectively, this situation occurred because the new device (form-stable shaped implant) was being placed using the process that surgeons had at the time for inserting a round device into the breast.

PERSONAL EXPERIENCE WITH FORM-STABLE DEVICES

Following the initial phase of the INAMED Core gel study in 1999, I was offered the opportunity to participate in the INAMED 410 study that started in 2001. I recall enthusiastically starting the study in 2001 yet without a defined process to use these devices. It was hardly different than being a test pilot who was told, "here's the airplane, go fly it and tell us about your experience." Mention was made of using "bio-dimensional planning" and of not making the mistake of pocket over dissection. My initial cases went well in terms of excellent esthetic outcomes without adverse events otherwise. Patients were happy with the natural-appearing esthetics and ample breast size increase to a full C or D cup. After an initial few cases, I decided there was a need to formulate a new thought process to use form-stable implants.

CHANGES IN BREAST ESTHETICS AND LONG-TERM OUTCOMES

The subject of breast size and shape after augmentation is of great interest. Currently, there appears to be less emphasis on achieving a round breast outcome for many women who want breast augmentation, without the obvious stigma of upper pole roundness. Interestingly, some geographic areas in the United States seemingly

have a preference for large volume round implants (eg, South Beach of Miami, Florida, and Orange County, California). Bigger more obvious breasts with upper pole fullness have been marketed to women as a "sexy" breast outcome.

The strategy of using high profile, round-shaped devices to achieve maximum volume enhancement may not be a good one if the net effect is tissue thinning, implant malposition (drop out), and upper pole traction rippling. Even in situations of staying within the measured base diameter of the breast, large volume augmentations have the potential to produce noncorrectable soft tissue deformities, including implant malposition (drop out).

Alternatively, form-stable devices produce excellent size increases for patients, with normal-appearing outcomes for most patients that fill a C or D cup size bra. It is now possible to customize breast augmentation based on individual measurements and tissue characteristics. The challenge is to help patients make good decisions on the front end of the process of breast augmentation that will produce great long-term outcomes with the least risk of problems attributable to mistakes in planning, such as an implant that is too wide or too large. Form-stable devices can produce spectacular natural outcomes that are coupled with high patient satisfaction. Alternatively, adverse events and less than perfect outcomes can occur if these devices are used with a round implant thought process.

TRANSITION FROM ROUND TO FORM-STABLE DEVICES

It has been 7.5 years since the start of the INAMED (now Allergan) 410 study and more than 5.5 years since the start of the MENTOR form-stable CPG study. From the perspective of having completed augmentation procedures in 250 patients, I offer the following commentary about how these implants have performed in my patients and what knowledge can be transferred that will make adoption of these devices easier. The best way to read the rest of this article is to let go of your current methodology regarding round breast implant surgery, because how you currently perform round implant breast augmentation may prevent you from achieving optimal use of form-stable breast implants.

All plastic surgeons who use round implants have a particular way in which they evaluate patients requesting breast implants for either cosmetic or reconstructive benefit. All have their own technique in surgery. All have a way of managing adverse events that occur in the short and long term. From a philosophic perspective, these methods vary considerably, with some surgeons claiming to be "artists" and others claiming to be "engineers." A lot of ego is wrapped up in how each of us individually performs breast implant surgery.

Setting aside the matter of ego and the art of cosmetic or reconstructive breast surgery, when the benchmarks of outcome are reviewed, surgeons are not always able to produce extremely good long-term outcomes without the specter of having to perform revision surgery to correct mistakes, revise problems, or address situations that could have been prevented in the first place.

The form-stable breast implant is a far different device than the round gel devices that we knew and loved. Successful use of the form-stable devices requires a higher level of precision, finesse, and planning than most surgeons are used to, yet the long-term results can be spectacular. Even for a surgeon with years of experience and mastery of round devices, there are prerequisites that must be used with this class of devices.

Let us suppose that you are a highly proficient airline captain of a Boeing 737 instead of a highly proficient plastic surgeon. Based on your proficiency, you are being advanced to a new larger aircraft, like the Boeing 787. Successful transition from one aircraft with a known set of performance parameters to a totally new one requires education, planning, and a new process for its safe operation.

Are we ready to go back to class to learn to fly all over again? You would not be given the keys to the Boeing 787 without some classroom and simulator time. The same can be said about the transition from the current round breast implant to the era of form-stable gel devices.

The other way of looking at breast augmentation is in terms of a manufacturing concept. Primary breast augmentation is a process that the surgeon will perform on an ongoing basis in his or her practice. There is the need for excellent outcomes coupled with minimal mistakes in planning or technical performance in the operating room. Additionally, there is the need to reduce waste (reoperations to correct mistakes) and to improve outcomes based on what you have learned from your experiences in breast augmentation. This is a basic form of the Toyota Production System.

I have purposely chosen an aviation and manufacturing theme for this article because it relates to a process for the successful use of a medical device. I believe that we as surgeons can learn much from both the airline and automobile manufacturing industry, notably Toyota, regarding ways to improve the quality and safety of our work.

Reliance on core principles and assumptions is needed, along with development of a personal process for the successful use of form-stable devices. Just like a pilot knows how a particular aircraft will fly, the surgeon must first assume that form-stable devices will produce excellent outcomes if used properly. The successful performance of form-stable breast augmentation is also a manufacturing concept in which a variety of sequences must be performed correctly.

WHY HAS BREAST AUGMENTATION BECOME SO COMPLEX?

By now, you are asking yourself, "Why is someone trying to make breast augmentation so complex?" My answer is that various surgeons have demonstrated that spectacular outcomes can be achieved in primary breast augmentation if they use excellent management processes to improve the quality and patient experience during primary breast augmentation surgery. Peer-reviewed publications substantiate that operational excellence in breast augmentation has been achieved by a variety of plastic surgeons, each of whom independently developed a similar process for the use of form-stable devices. The role of good judgment and prudent actions must be emphasized to achieve the goal of reproducible outcomes in a wide variety of patients. The remarkable advance in quality and safety in the aviation industry is a testimonial to what occurs when there are excellent operating processes that enable excellent outcomes. Alternatively, if a surgeon is surrounded by poor processes, a mediocre outcome is the norm.

THE CASE FOR DOING BETTER IN BREAST AUGMENTATION

Most surgeons can improve the quality of their work in breast augmentation surgery. There are substantive opportunities throughout the entire process of primary breast augmentation to eliminate mistakes and mismanagement of a process that optimally should be able to produce excellent outcomes across a wide segment of patients. The existing statistics from the Core Gel studies regarding reoperation rates are appalling. The statistics on why reoperation occurs reflect problems that have root causes, such as an implant that is too big or too wide, technical mistakes in surgery, and mismanagement of expectations. Before blaming poor outcomes and reoperations on unpredictable biologic factors of soft tissue–implant interactions or wound healing, the root causes should be considered first. A dissertation on

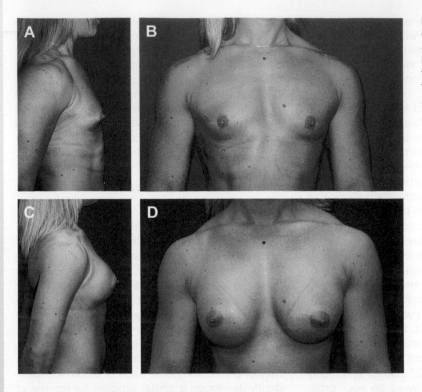

Fig.1. (A, B) Patient with an androgynous chest and small amount of breast tissue shown before surgery (C, D) Same patient shown after augmentation with an Allergan 410 MM 280 retromammary implant.

what produces complications and adverse events in breast augmentation is beyond the scope of this article. Suffice it to say that data from a variety of surgeons who have experience with form-stable devices from both manufacturers document that these devices will produce consistently good outcomes with far fewer of the common problems associated with round devices.

AVOIDANCE OF DEFENSIVE REASONING REGARDING THE TRANSITION TO FORM-STABLE DEVICES

I place great emphasis on the transition to shaped devices as a totally new process for breast esthetics. By this statement I mean that the surgeon will need to rethink his or her personal process of breast augmentation and not engage in what I call "defensive reasoning." This approach is used by some individuals when they are confronted with situations in which they are uncertain that the value of change will be beneficial, and they are fearful of failure. In this situation, a thought process that focuses on erroneous perceptions and fears occurs that paralyzes objective reasoning and learning. An example would be in making excuses for not adopting form-stable devices because it has been said that they can rotate or feel excessively firm.

CORE PRINCIPLES FOR THE USE OF FORM-STABLE SILICONE GEL IMPLANTS

I believe that certain core principles are important in the successful transition from round to form-stable devices. In this process-driven exercise, sequential steps build upon each other as follows:

1. Have a process to make decisions regarding device size, style, and location.
2. Make decisions based on data and not on patient wishes. Use a worksheet to record subjective and objective data. If you have a patient seeking an outcome from breast augmentation that you discover is unrealistic, reeducate her regarding how to avoid known complications of excessive volume augmentation or send her elsewhere. Avoid performing surgery in a situation that you know will produce suboptimal outcomes. These are cases that you can afford not to do. Large volume breast augmentation is no different than the aviation concept of overloading an aircraft to the point that you have exceeded gross maximum takeoff weight. You will be overloading the breast tissue with a device that is larger than it can support. Either way, there is a great probability of problems. In aviation, it is called a crash. In plastic surgery, it is called an avoidable complication (traction

rippling, drop out, and tissue thinning) due to errors in planning.
3. Be precise in surgery and avoid mistakes.
4. Collect data after surgery regarding measurements, satisfaction, adverse events, and reoperation/revision.
5. Continue to improve your process. Process improvement occurs when there are excellent outcomes and when there are suboptimal ones. Reflect on what was done to produce excellence and what could have been done to improve suboptimal outcomes. Remember that it is possible to produce suboptimal outcomes with form-stable devices used incorrectly.

Core Principle One: Have a Process to Make Decisions

Critical decisions regarding device selection, the style of device (round or form-stable), and placement location must be established as your solution to every patient seeking breast augmentation. Depending on device selection, surgical principles change accordingly, with the goal of achieving the best outcome for each patient based on her individual needs, tissues, and expectations.

The other interesting factor is the propensity for some patients to come back at a later time and request size upgrades because they do not believe that their size is adequate. Accurate management of size expectations is critical, as this can be a driver of reoperations. I have found that with form-stable devices you can select devices that are slightly wider (5 mm) than the measured base diameter of the breast if you wish to maximize size outcome. During the more than 7 years I have used form-stable breast implants, I have not performed elective reoperations for mismanaged size outcomes. The only exception was a breast augmentation patient who underwent a segmental mastectomy who needed a larger implant to overcome volume loss on the affected side.

By having a process and holding yourself accountable to making good decisions, the quality of outcomes will improve dramatically. A mediocre process will yield poor outcomes if you attempt to work around situations such as loose envelopes, ptosis, short nipple-fold distances, competitive body builders, or large volume augmentation.

The other factor that you will notice is the beneficial effect of lowering the reoperation rate to correct less-than-perfect outcomes after breast augmentation. Reoperation remains a draining factor on a plastic surgery practice from a time and financial perspective. It also exposes the plastic surgeon to liability claims if the revision surgery is unsuccessful.

Core Principle Two: Make Decisions Based on Data and not on Wishes

Forget that you are an artist and act like an engineer by obtaining a set of breast measurements to guide your implant selection. Once you have the data, it is fairly simple to make decisions.

Use a worksheet that contains both hard and soft data. Hard data are the set of measurements that you make with tape and calipers. They also comprise the patient's personal breast health history. Soft data are the patient's expectations for outcome. Use similar worksheets for follow-up visits for documentation of outcomes, including measurements and quality of life metrics. The decision for implant location (ie, retromammary, subfascial, or biplanar) is a critical decision that follows next. I make a decision based on the thickness of the upper pole to guide me on device location, along with other factors. The surgeon should remember that the patient has read a plethora of information that describes many options for breast augmentation. Some patients, by virtue of their breast dimensions, will obtain good outcomes within the retromammary location as their tissue drapes over the form-stable device. Your job is to help the patient make the best decision for implant location based on her tissues. If the upper pole thickness is greater than 35 mm on caliper pinch, I consider retromammary implant placement.

Some patients request a biplanar or, in their vernacular, "submuscular" placement. It is important in this discussion to educate the patient regarding the biplanar approach versus the archaic total submuscular placement that was used years ago. In patients with a longer sternal-nipple distance (>23 cm), the majority of the breast is located below the pectoralis. Biplanar implant placement may be of little advantage. If you believe that less than 25% of the implant will be covered by pectoralis in the biplanar location, there may be little benefit to this approach.

Thin women who have small amounts of native breast tissue generally have better outcomes with biplanar implant placement. Form-stable devices can produce natural-appearing outcomes versus the round breast outcome in this subset of patients.

Women with borderline ptosis, glandular ptosis, and lax skin envelopes generally have better outcomes with retromammary implant placement that uses either full height or full projection implants (Allergan 410 FF, Mentor CPG 323).

The athletic female body builder is problematic with biplanar implant placement in terms of motion deformity when the pectoralis is animated and implant displacement due to weight training.

Competitive body builders often have low body fat levels and extremely thin tissues (**Fig. 1**) that can make it impossible to produce a natural-appearing outcome. This subset of patients is motivated to achieve breast fullness yet may have expectations for size that cannot be produced with any type of implant or implant-autologous fat transfer combination. It is important to have agreement on a reasonable amount of body fat and tissue thickness, because fluctuation downward will contribute to implant palpability, rippling, and an unnatural breast appearance. In this subset of patients, one should ensure that there is adequate inferior pole tissue greater than 10 mm on pinch to cover the lower pole of the implant. Weight and body fat fluctuations will impact soft tissue coverage and increase visibility, palpability, and rippling.

Patients with loose skin envelopes or ptosis may not be suited for form-stable devices if a combination augmentation-mastopexy procedure is contemplated. Form-stable devices by virtue of their texture will not settle or "adjust" to a ptotic breast envelope. There appears to be limited experience using form-stable devices with ptosis procedures other than a circumareolar mastopexy. I suppose that it might be possible to consider form-stable devices in a two-staged approach, after the ptosis has been corrected. The unknown factor is late-term ptosis afterward due to tissues that have deficient tone. Personally, I would prefer round devices to fill the breast envelope in conjunction with a ptosis procedure (mastopexy).

Incision location is another decision point with regard to form-stable devices. Most women seem to prefer the inframammary access over the periareolar approach. Insertion of a form-stable device through the periareolar location may be technically challenging, with the risk of fracturing the gel. Asian surgeons are oriented toward endoscopic transaxillary approaches to minimize risk of hypertrophic/hyperpigmented scars on the breast skin. Such a strategy can be used with form-stable devices provided that the surgeon is highly proficient with endoscopic transaxillary implant surgery. Important caveats regarding transaxillary placement exist in terms of precise inframammary fold placement and control of bleeding. Otherwise, this approach would not be recommended for patients seen in the Western hemisphere or Europe.

Incision location with respect to the inframammary fold is an important decision in form-stable implants. Much has been written about the inframammary fold as an anatomic structure. Successful lowering of the inframammary fold remains challenging, especially in patients with short nipple-fold distances. Attempts at manipulation of the inframammary fold often end up with a "double bubble" deformity of two inframammary folds. Strategies to lower the fold use radial scoring of the back surface of the breast and suture reinforcement of the new inframammary fold to the chest wall. Adams and Tebbetts have described distances for incision location from the nipple that are an important part of the planning process. Form-stable implants tend to pull tissue upward from below the inframammary fold. An incision that intuitively seems right for a round implant will invariably be too high on the breast if form-stable devices are used. An excessively high incision is a common planning mistake for inexperienced surgeons performing form-stable implants.

Implant height decisions can be made in terms of measured breast height or in a simplified fashion by using the sternal-nipple distance. For example, short sternal-nipple distances in the 18-cm range would be ideal for a moderate height–moderate projection device. A full height device would be inappropriate due to a short breast height. Individuals in the 18- to 21-cm range have better outcomes with full height–moderate projection devices. A moderate height device may not be optimal in providing an ample framework to shape taller breast sizes. Beyond 21 cm, a full height, full projecting implant would be recommended due to the need for shaping and to obtain satisfactory breast projection. Full height–full projection devices are recommended for borderline to slight ptosis situations because it is possible to obtain satisfactory opening outward of the lower pole of the breast.

Device volume selection follows next, based on the base diameter of the breast mound (caliper measurement). The corresponding device base diameter up to the breast base diameter plus 5 mm would be the maximum device width allowed.

Better planning and measurements will eliminate the need for multiple sized implants. As the surgeon becomes proficient with form-stable devices, it is not generally necessary in situations of primary breast augmentation to have multiple sizes of form-stable devices in the operating room. Situations involving conversions of round devices to form-stable implants and reconstruction after tissue expanders generally require that a range of devices be available owing to the need for intraoperative measurements to determine exact pocket dimensions for a tight fit.

If you are in a situation in which a tight-filling pocket cannot be produced for a form-stable device, a "lifeboat" strategy would consist of abandoning form-stable implant selection and converting to a round device from your consignment inventory.

Plan your first form-stable augmentations on "easy" patients, that is, ones with good symmetry, an excellent amount of tissues, a moderately tight envelope, and reasonable expectations. An example would be a 27-year-old, gravida 2 para 2 patient with 40 mm of upper pole thickness, 19 cm of sternal-nipple distance, a nipple to fold distance of 7 cm, and a base diameter of 12 cm. In this type of patient you could obtain an excellent result with any implant. Such a patient would be best suited for an Allergan 410 in the MM 280 gm or FM 270 gm, or the CPG 322 280 cc.

The surgeon should become familiar with the use of form-stable devices in both retromammary and biplanar locations on straightforward cases versus complex ones to start. After 15 to 20 cases have been successfully implanted, one can consider more challenging cases. You will quickly discover that, for most patients, the MM, FM, and FF Style 410 or the 322 or 323 CPG devices will become favorites. Although a variety of options are available in the INAMED (Allergan) matrix, try to simplify matters into a few of the categories. The extraprojecting form-stable devices produced by Allergan in the 410 FX, LX, and MX series should be reserved for reconstructive applications and not used for primary or secondary cosmetic breast augmentation.

Core Principle Three: Technical Precision in Surgery

The avoidance of technical mistakes in breast augmentation is an important factor that will improve outcomes.

Avoidance of an incision too high
The article by Adams and Tebbetts covers the matter of incision location in relation to implant size. It is an essential helper for incision placement in form-stable devices. Form-stable implants will bring upward a substantive amount of tissue from the inframammary region, and upward migration of the incision will occur. The matter of how to deal with short nipple-fold distances remains challenging, as excessive lowering of the fold can produce deformities or drop out of implants.

Avoidance of excessive dissection
Precision in dissection that will produce a perfectly sized implant pocket is necessary. I prefer the use of electrosurgical dissection with the tungsten microtip (Colorado needle). Blunt tissue dissection must be avoided because it is imprecise. Measurement of pocket height during dissection will

produce a precise fit. I have found that a guiding principle is to dissect the pocket slightly smaller than you would think necessary. Slight pocket modification by finger stretching the tissues following insertion of the form-stable implant follows next.

If you are uncertain, a round gel device can be used to verify size. A tight fit with a slightly smaller round gel that has an identical base diameter of the form-stable implant is one way of verifying fit and ensuring that there are no constricting bands or areas requiring more dissection. The goal is to be able to insert the form-stable device into the pocket and orient it with alignment marks without having to pull it out for more dissection and then reinsert it.

In situations of conversion from a round to form-stable implant, intraoperative measurements are essential, because the pocket after a total capsulectomy will be much larger than anticipated, necessitating a larger form-stable device to have a tight fit to avoid rotation afterward. It may be best to use existing inframammary incisions from an earlier surgery than to place a second set of incisions.

Avoidance of excessive lowering of the breast fold and management of the inframammary fold region
Individuals with short nipple-fold distances of 5 to 6 cm will need some lowering of the fold to accommodate form-stable devices. The inframammary fold appears to be an anatomic structure that can be adjusted somewhat downward. Excessive lowering of the fold can be problematic in terms of a double-bubble deformity in which the existing inframammary fold is seen above the newly created fold. I have found that it is possible to radially cut the superficial fascia of the breast to open out the existing fold. At the same time, it is a good idea to reinforce the new fold with a few absorbable monofilament sutures to avoid downward displacement of the fold over time. I have found that form-stable devices tend to be less prone to drop out versus the "water hammer effect" of smooth round saline devices. Form-stable devices will open out the lower pole of the breast, with excellent esthetics ranging from 8 to 10 cm for after surgery measurements of the nipple-inframammary fold.

Avoidance of synmastia
Excessive dissection medially in any location will contribute to synmastia, even in situations of correctly sized implants. Individuals with pectus deformities (excavatum or carinatum) are especially prone to synmastia. Overdissection of the origin

of the pectoralis and accompanying fibrous septae from its sternal origin sets the stage for synmastia. Synmastia is best prevented by prudent planning, recognition of high-risk situations (pectus), and precise technique. According to Spear, the failure rate in correction of synmastia is over 80%.

Antibiotics, anti-infectives, and drains to reduce capsular contracture

I believe that the use of all measures to prevent infection should be considered. Effective measures consist of preoperative antibiotics, the use of a clear plastic membrane to cover the nipple-areolar region, chlorhexidine skin preparation, intraoperative antibiotic irrigation, off-label use of Betadine, use of Dermabond to seal the wound, and antibiotics in the postoperative period. These measures can prevent infection and will dramatically reduce the risk of capsular contracture due to low-grade infection/contamination of the implant space with biofilm. I use absorbable monofilament sutures for wound closure.

Other measures that I employ are having the patient shower preoperatively with chlorhexidine or chloroxylenol-based surgical soaps and the use of a sterile impervious surgical disposable drape between the patient and the operating table. Sterile base sheeting is an effective measure to prevent strike-through of fluids during surgery that could be contaminated with the operating room table pads.

Other individuals recommend the use of triple antibiotic solutions for pocket sterilization to reduce the risk of a biofilm that leads to chronic low-grade inflammation and capsular contracture. Although this approach is useful, I believe that it is possible to use Betadine both as an anti-infective and lubricant in an off-label manner. Betadine gel is very useful in reducing the insertion force of implants, especially textured devices. If this strategy is considered, document in your informed consent discussions that you are planning to use this off-label use of the product. Betadine-containing solutions should not be used to fill implants and should not be used in situations of documented allergic reactions to iodine-containing compounds.

The use of closed suction drains warrants discussion. Drains are not used by many surgeons. Personally, I favor the use of drains for 48 hours to remove blood-containing exudates from the implant space and in the case of a form-stable textured device to promote tissue-device adherence. Otherwise, the implant floats in a blood/serum-filled pocket until the fluids are reabsorbed. Reports from the Canadian literature document that the use of drains reduces the occurrence of capsular contracture.

I have found that these measures are effective in helping reduce the risk of infection and capsular contracture. When using this approach, I have not had a perioperative infection after a primary breast augmentation in 32 years of implant use.

Wound closure

I believe that the use of synthetic monofilament absorbable sutures such as Monocryl or PDS (Ethicon, Somerville, New Jersey) for wound closure is best. These sutures tend to last longer than braided absorbable suture such as Vicryl. The monofilament sutures can also be effectively used to reinforce the inframammary fold in situations where it is necessary to lower the fold or perform a capsulorrhaphy.

I recommend repair of the superficial fascial layer of the breast with 3-0 monofilament sutures. This structural layer will help to maintain integrity of the inframammary area. If there has been radial scoring of the breast parenchyma for pocket modification, the sutures will need to engage the respective ends of the rays.

Care must be taken to avoid sticking the implant with the needle during deep-layer closure. Some surgeons will preplace sutures in the deep layer and tie them post implant insertion. Although this is an effective strategy, the additional costs of five to ten suture packages will be cost prohibitive. I am able to close all layers of both sides with a single package of 3-0 and 4-0 monofilament suture.

Although for many years, I used Steri Strips for wound closure, currently I use Dermabond. The use of the flexible butylcyanocrylate has been effective in diminishing tape-related blisters and reactions to skin adhesives (benzion), and allowing patients to shower. The current approach also does not require nursing time in the postoperative period to change and reapply strips or remove sutures. Occasionally, patients may develop a pruritic rash with Dermabond that will require a high-potency topical steroid cream such as 0.05% Temovate (clobetasol propionate cream or ointment) to treat.

Elimination of unnecessary items

One of the approaches of the Toyota Production System is the elimination of waste. Waste can be in terms of unused or unnecessary products. It can also be in terms of staff waiting or time-burdensome- processes that can be improved.

Lean manufacturing approaches are centered on having what is needed at hand to perform a task without excessive inventory of supplies.

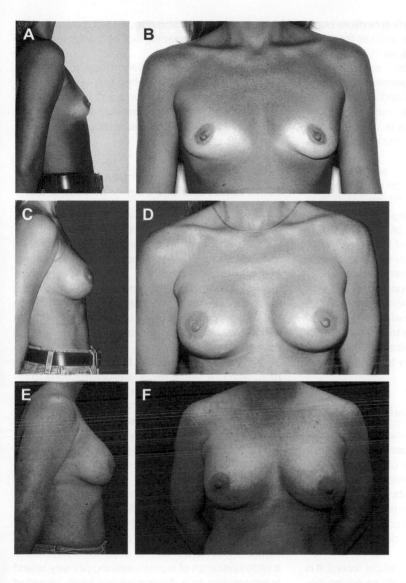

Fig. 2. (*A, B*) Patient shown before surgery (*C, D*) Same patient shown 1 year after augmentation with an Allergan 410 MM 320 biplanar implant. (*E, F*) Patient shown 5 years after augmentation surgery was performed.

We as surgeons need to feel comfortable that there are adequate supplies yet not have unnecessary items such as a large assortment of form-stable implants in the operating room. The additional cost of staff time to return unused devices and the shipping costs add to procedural expense.

Other ways to reduce waste center on eliminating the need for postoperative bras. I currently use a generic cotton-spandex tube top garment to hold dressings in place. It offers a low-cost alternative to surgical bras. We recommend that patients purchase underwire-style bras such as the widely available Victoria Secret *Body by Victoria* shaping demi-cup and start wearing them when they are comfortable. Expensive bras designed for patients with high projection breast implants (LeMystere No. 9) are unnecessary.

Elimination of waste in terms of staff waiting and burdensome processes is the next consideration. We use pre-made basic packs for the operating room that contain necessary supplies for a variety of esthetic cases. It would be necessary to only open drains, suture, and a breast drape for an augmentation. Use of these packs has proven to be a significant benefit during the burdensome process of picking supplies for a breast augmentation and opening them individually.

We have also reduced the time to discharge after surgery by having patients leave the operating room with a pain score of 0. This step avoids the need for narcotic analgesics and reduces the risk of postoperative nausea and vomiting and the use of expensive anti-emetics. We perform the procedure using intravenous sedation and try to eliminate the use of all narcotics. At the end of the procedure there is an instillation of dilute bupivacaine into the breast implant pocket following wound closure. We refer to this as "LALA" (large area local anesthesia). After approximately 10 minutes, the drain bulb is squeezed and suction is started. To date, we have not had any untoward reaction to this approach. I also recommend the use of a closed fill system versus decanting the bupivacaine on the back table and exposing it to particulate fallout from the air.

A 250-mL bag of sterile 0.9% saline is drawn down to 100 mL by using a breast implant closed fill tubing/syringe. A total of 50 mL of 0.25% bupivacaine is added to the bag by using sterile technique. Before the addition of the local to the smaller bag, we place a piece of tape over the fill port on the patient's intravenous fluid bag to prevent the error of giving bupivacaine intravenously (safety engineering). The addition of 30 to 50 mL of the dilute bupivacaine solution to each breast pocket will produce excellent analgesia for several hours, allowing for a short time to discharge after surgery and much less postoperative nausea and vomiting. Costs are reduced in terms of nursing time and medications.

Core Principle Four: Collect Data After Surgery

Data collection after surgery is useful to provide information regarding the quality of outcomes and patient satisfaction. I use a similar measurement sheet to collect soft and hard data on the outcome. A data sheet can contain much more information than a narrative discussion and provides objectivity. Standardized photographic documentation is required.

If you are using an electronic medical record, it is possible to scan paper worksheets as Adobe Acrobat pdf files. This method may be preferable over developing a template program otherwise. Pre- and postoperative images from the electronic medical record are helpful "reality checks" for patients concerning questions about their outcomes.

We measure patients after surgery, at 10 weeks, 6 months, annually, or on an as-needed basis. Data are useful to document the quality of outcomes and patient satisfaction. They are also useful in spotting trends in problems (malposition, capsular contracture, rippling) or dissatisfaction. A standardized photographic technique is necessary to avoid distortion of results by factors such as a camera angle that is too low.

The data obtained with form-stable implants after surgery are interesting. Once a stable outcome has been obtained in the postoperative period, it generally remains stable in terms of measurements and patient satisfaction (**Fig. 2**). Most patients stabilize with a nice opening out of the lower pole of the breast.

I have found it relatively easy to sort out complaints after surgery when I have data sheets of measurements that include soft and hard data versus narrative chart notes that say something like, "She likes her breasts, exam: breasts soft, return in 2 years...".

Core Principle Five: Continue to Improve Your Process and the Quality of Your Outcomes

My approach to primary breast augmentation involves borrowing from aviation and automotive manufacturing. I believe that it has worked well in my practice over the last 7.5 years with form-stable implants to produce best-in-class outcomes. In reality, this is not "my" approach but "our" approach (my staff) to deliver operational excellence for patients. This delivery of care involves all steps of breast augmentation from the first telephone call that the patient makes to achieving a stable result, with instructions to return in a year. It also involves the surgeon's staff to help innovate and improve the process.

Service mapping is needed to establish your process and should be considered occasionally for purposes of improvement and waste reduction to eliminate unnecessary items and avoid waste in terms of staff waiting.

Elimination of waste in terms of reoperations is an important step in providing operational excellence. Most factors that drive reoperations can be reduced or eliminated. I have found that form-stable implants will deliver superior outcomes in a wide spectrum of women seeking primary breast augmentation to a degree yet not seen, provided that attention is paid to all segments of the process and steps are taken to avoid predictable problems.

Mismanagement of patient expectations concerning size outcome is a major driver of reoperations in the Core Gel Study. I have found that it is possible to satisfy patients concerning size outcomes in the range of C or D cup outcomes in a wide range of breast and body types with form-stable devices. In 7.5 years of using these devices, there have been no reoperations for size change in either the INAMED (Allergan) or MENTOR cohorts. The only exception was in augmentation patients who developed breast cancer and needed larger devices following segmental mastectomy.

A reflection on outcomes is part of process improvement, whether it is spectacular or

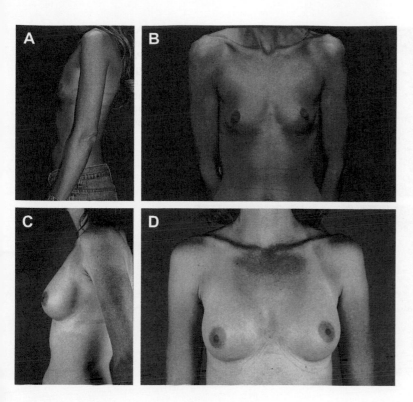

Fig. 3. (*A, B*) Patient shown before surgery (*C, D*) Patient shown 2 years after augmentation with an Allergan 410 FM 310 biplanar implant.

suboptimal. Useful information regarding what it took to produce a great outcome is just as valuable as determining what went wrong. The "whys" of Toyota Production System (TPS) will lead to the root cause of the problem; asking about the "hows" will lead to ways to improve the process.

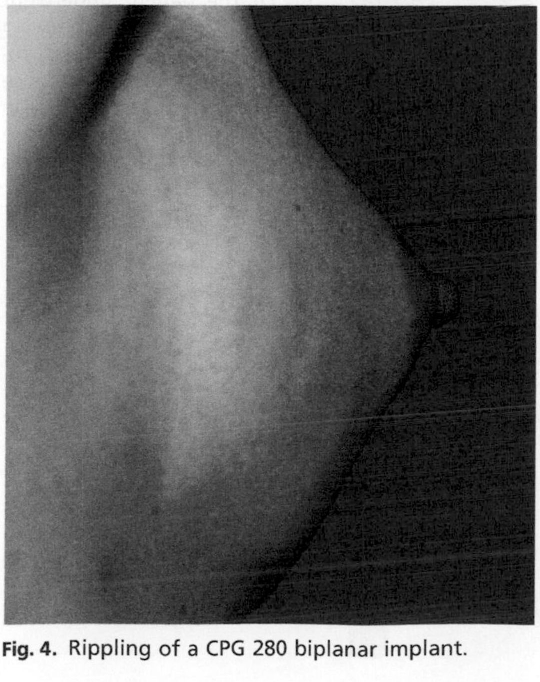

As I mentioned earlier in this article, I believe that all surgeons can successfully adopt form-stable devices into their practice if they have the determination to do it. The world of breast esthetics is no longer round, and patients are seeking an operation that will provide a natural-appearing outcome that is customized for them in terms of device options.

The data listed herein from my form-stable patient cohorts (INAMED [Allergan] 410 and Mentor CPG) demonstrate that form-stable devices are demonstrably better than existing round gel or saline devices in terms of outcome data and quality of life metrics. Outcome data from the Mentor CPG and Allergan 410 cohorts were measured against historic Pre Market Approval (PMA) and other published outcome data regarding the incidence of capsular contracture, reoperations, wrinkling or rippling, device malposition, and rotation.

DATA FROM FORM-STABLE PATIENT COHORTS
Materials and Methods

A US Food and Drug Administration approved study protocol with Institutional Review Board oversight was performed as follows:
Inclusion/exclusion criteria
Informed consent

Fig. 4. Rippling of a CPG 280 biplanar implant.

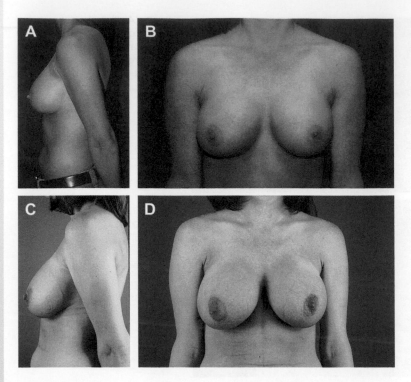

Fig. 5. A patient who was able to breastfeed successfully is shown (*A, B*) Patient shown 2 years after augmentation with a CPG 280 retromammary implant. (*C, D*) Same patient shown during lactation 3 years after augmentation surgery.

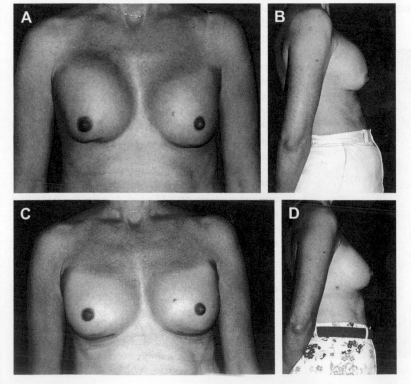

Fig. 6. (*A, B*) The implant in this patient's right breast was ruptured during mammography (*C, D*) The patient underwent successful revision surgery in which a CPG 315 biplanar implant was used. Because a round pocket was already in place, it made the most sense to use a round implant in this patient.

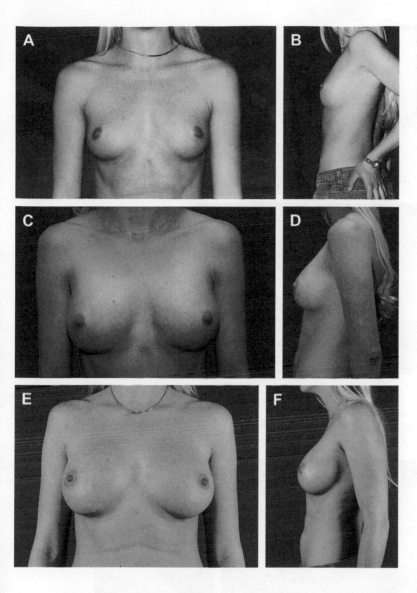

Fig. 7. (*A, B*) Patient shown before surgery (*C, D*) Patient shown 2 years after augmentation surgery with a CPG 315 biplanar implant. (*E, F*) Same patient shown 4 years after surgery.

Devices purchased from manufacturer: Mentor and INAMED (Allergan)

Allergan 410, 119 consecutive patients, started on April 2001, ended on September 2007

Mentor CPG, 117 consecutive patients, started on December 2002, ended on January 2008

Preoperative measurements/planning (data sheet)

  Tissue dynamics/dimensions

  Base diameter/height of breast

  Patient expectations

  Device selection/location

Single surgeon

Data collection/follow-up

  Presurgery

Postsurgery on day 1, at 10 weeks, 6 months, and annually as needed

90% follow-up (overall)

Outcome Data: Allergan 410 and Mentor CPG

Device Allocation

  INAMED (Allergan) 410: 65% retromammary; 35% biplanar

  Mentor CPG: 40% retromammary; 60% biplanar

Pregnancy

All eight of the patients who became pregnant after form-stable augmentation mammaplasties successfully nursed their babies.

Clinical outcomes

Figs. 3–9 show clinical outcomes.

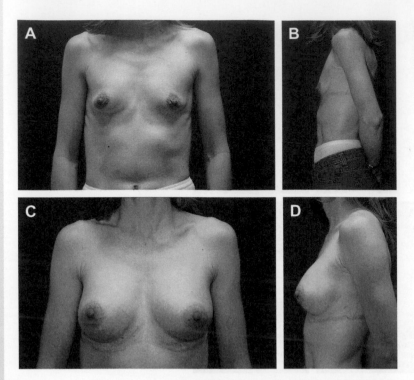

Fig. 8. (*A, B*) Patient shown before surgery (*C, D*) Same patient shown 6 months after augmentation surgery with a CPG 280 biplanar implant.

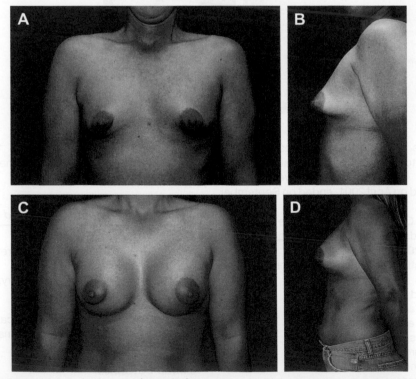

Fig. 9. (*A, B*) Patient with tubular breasts shown before surgery (*C, D*) Same patient shown 1 year after augmentation surgery.

Adverse events in comparison with existing data (round implants)

Implant malposition: 0.8% overall compared with 2.6% Bengtson 3-year INAMED 410 data (Plastic and Reconstructive Surgery Journal [PRS])

Implant rotation: 0.8% overall compared with 1.1% CPG 2-year data (PRS)

Infection: 0% overall compared with 1.3% Bengtson 3-year INAMED 410 data (PRS) and 1.6% CPG 2-year data (PRS)

Capsular contracture (Baker III-IV): 1.27% overall (2.5% INAMED 410; 0% CPG) compared with 0% Brown (PRS 2005), 0.8% CPG 2-year data, 1.9% Bengtson 3-year INAMED 410, 4.2% Heden INAMED 410 (Clinics in Plastic Surgery [CLPS]), 8.2% MENTOR Gel PMA, and 13.2% AGN Gel PMA

Reoperations: 3.4% overall (INAMED 410: 2.5% [1 malposition, 1 scar revision, 1 surgical bleed]; Mentor CPG: 4.3% [1 seroma-explant, 3 segmental mastectomy for cancer, 1 size change for reconstruction after segmental mastectomy]) compared with 9.4% CPG 2-year (PRS), 12.5% Bengtson 3-year INAMED 410 (PRS), 15.4% MNT Gel PMA, 23.5% AGN Gel PMA, and 28.0% AGN Gel 6 year

Rippling (criteria: visible or palpable rippling lateral or medial location only; not upper pole traction rippling) related to device-specific criteria versus body mass index, breast base diameter, device base diameter, capsular contracture, procedure/device location: Mentor CPG, 37.3%; INAMED (Allergan) 410, 7.6% (P<0.001) compared with <1% INAMED (Allergan) round gel 3-year Core Study, 1.2% INAMED (Allergan) round gel 6-year Core Study, <1% Mentor round gel 3-year Core Study, 10.5% INAMED (Allergan) round saline 3 years, 12.2% INAMED (Allergan) round saline 6 years, 20.8% Mentor round saline 3 years, not addressed by Mentor CPG 2-year data (PRS), and 0.5% Bengtson INAMED (Allergan) 410 3-year data (PRS)

Patient satisfaction

95% overall satisfaction with INAMED (Allergan) 410 and MENTOR CPG
  Natural shape, feel, size (34–36 C or D cup)
  No interference with pregnancy/lactation
5% dissatisfaction
  Wanting larger size than agreed upon, yet no reoperation for size change
  Capsular contracture
  Rippling

Other Quality Metrics: Consecutive Interval between Reoperations

Tebbetts: 50 consecutive cases in 36 months (PRS)
Jewell INAMED (Allergan) 410: 87 consecutive cases in 40 months
Jewell Mentor CPG: 73 consecutive cases in 31 months

SUMMARY

Form-stable silicone gel breast implants offer patients superior outcomes when compared with published data for round saline or silicone gel implants in terms of almost an order of magnitude. These devices also offer improvement in breast esthetics with a natural yet substantively augmented outcome. They permit breast augmentation to be a precise, safe, and customized process that reproducibly produces excellent long-term outcomes and high levels of patient satisfaction.

The transition from round to form-stable implants requires surgeon education, precision, and attention to avoiding known problems that will impact outcomes and lead to reoperations.

Mastopexy Augmentation with Form Stable Breast Implants

Per Hedén, MD, PhD

KEYWORDS

- Mastopexy • Breast augmentation
- Form stable breast implants • Planning
- Surgical techniques

Augmentation of a youthful and naturally shaped breast is a relatively straightforward procedure provided that the implant selection is proportionate to tissue characteristics and the preoperative planning and surgical technique are accurate. Augmentation of the ptotic breast is considerably more complicated, however. If the nipple areola complex is lower than the height of the existing submammary fold, simple augmentation is usually not sufficient and a mastopexy is frequently needed for a natural appearance of the breast. The original descriptions of mastopexy augmentations were done in the 1960s (Gonzales-Ulloa in 1960 and Regnault in 1966), and this procedure is still regarded as difficult, not only because of its results but because of its multitude of potential complications. Many well-recognized plastic surgeons advise against or recommend extreme caution when combining mastopexy with augmentation (W. Adams, J.B. Tebbetts, personal communications, 2002 and 2007). Use of an expander-implant in combination with the mastopexy to minimize a plethora of complications has even been suggested.[1] A two-stage procedure is regarded as much safer and simpler, but it should be remembered that the distance between the nipple and the new submammary fold has to be planned according to the implants that are selected at the second stage and it is not uncommon that this fact is missed by the surgeon at the

first-stage mastopexy. A one-stage mastopexy augmentation procedure has higher patient acceptance because this limits the number of sick days and the need for hospital care, and it is also less expensive. The introduction of form stable implants in 1994 (style 410; Allergan Corporation, Allergan Limited, Marlow Buckinghamshire, United Kingdom) has led to significant improvements in preoperative planning. The first truly mathematic planning system described for breast augmentation surgery was presented by the author in its first version in 2001.[2–4] This technique has since been further refined, and, today, breast augmentation planning is a detailed mathematic calculation based on implant dimensions and proportions.[5–8] These same planning principles can be applied in mastopexy augmentation but in a reversed manner. In this presentation, a detailed description on how this planning can be performed safely is presented; discussions on important details in producing safe mastopexy augmentation related to the surgical technique are also discussed. It is acknowledged that this article is more of a technical description than an in-depth review of outcome and patient satisfaction data.

MATERIAL AND METHODS

From December 1995 to June 2008 (13.5 years), 10,034 form stable breast implants have been

The author does not have any economic interest in the products used in this publication but acts as a lecturer and consultant for Allergan Corporation.
Akademikliniken, Storängsvägen 10, 115 42 Stockholm, Sweden
E-mail address: per.heden@ak.se

Clin Plastic Surg 36 (2009) 91–104
doi:10.1016/j.cps.2008.08.003

inserted at Akademikliniken in Stockholm, Sweden. This accounts for 82% of all implants inserted, and most of the devices were Allergan Corporation anatomically shaped (style 410 and 510) implants. Mastopexy was combined with augmentation in 8% (328 patients) of these cases. Average implant volume in breast augmentation with form stable implants increased from 310 to 338 cm^3 between 1996 to 2006. In mastopexy augmentation, the average implant volume in 2006 was smaller, averaging 275 cm^3.

RESULTS

In the first series of the author's experience using form stable devices (*Clinics in Plastic Surgery*, 2001), minor revisions and infectious problems in mastopexy augmentation were relatively high (17%) and implant removal attributable to infections was done in 1.4% of cases. With the new technique developed and described in this article, the number of reoperations and infection problems has decreased to 8% and explantation has not been accounted for than in more than 0.4% of cases.

CORRECTION OF MODERATE PTOSIS WITH AUGMENTATION ALONE

In breast augmentation surgery, the implant's vertical height on the thoracic wall should be adjusted to the nipple position. To perform correct preoperative planning, knowledge about the postoperative position of the nipple-areola complex is of great importance. In the 1990s, the author made two fundamental and important observations related to this problem.[2] The first was that a correctly performed breast augmentation elevates the nipple-areola complex (**Fig. 1**). The second important observation was that a line drawn from the nipple to the fixed tissue in the midline along the sternum, the so-called "NS-line," could be used to illustrate and evaluate the amount of nipple elevation achieved by an augmentation.

In a careful clinical study on several hundred patients who underwent an augmentation procedure, it was found that the nipple elevation achieved by a correctly performed breast augmentation could be simulated before surgery by an arm elevation 45° above the horizontal plane. In the ptotic breast, it has also been noted that a slightly more pronounced nipple elevation is achieved with breast implants. Knowledge about the postoperative nipple height permits calculation of the implant's ideal vertical height on the thoracic wall. Usually, in a correctly performed breast augmentation, half of the height of an anatomic

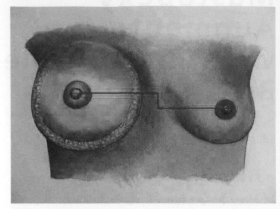

Fig. 1. Correctly performed breast augmentation elevates the nipple-areola complex. If a horizontal line is drawn between the nipple and the fixed tissue along the sternum in the midline (NS-line), this could be used to illustrate the actual nipple elevation and to calculate the ideal vertical implant position on the chest wall in relation to the nipple-areola complex.

form stable implant is placed distally to the nipple-areola complex after the augmentation. Knowledge about the implant's base plate (height and width) is thus useful information when planning the implant's vertical height on the chest wall. To summarize how this planning is performed (**Fig. 2**), a horizontal line is drawn from the nipple to the sternum (NS-line) with the patient's arms elevated 45° above the horizontal plane. The arms are then lowered again, and half of the height of the implant is measured distally along the sternal midline. At the distal end of this midline marking, a horizontal line is extended laterally, indicating the ideal lower pole of the implant (ILP-line). The NS-line and the ILP-line are useful guidelines during surgery, as the nipple-areola complex shifts considerably when the patient is lying horizontally on the operating table. In ptotic breasts, the nipple-areola shift lying down can be pronounced, and it is easy to make a wrong judgment when it comes to dual-plane division of the muscle at the sternum. The NS-line, however, indicates how high the muscle can be divided (always distal to the NS-line). The ILP-line indicates how to position the lower pole of the implant during the procedure.

Having answered the important question of the ideal vertical position of the implant, the second important part of preoperative planning is to determine the ideal amount of skin between the nipple and the new inframammary fold. Unfortunately, much of this planning is commonly done based on the surgeon's experience and feelings instead of careful analysis and measurements; but obviously, this distance should be varied and

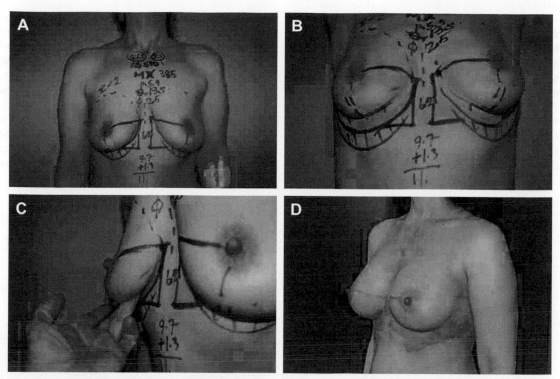

Fig. 2. (A) Preoperative markings to correct moderate ptosis without a mastopexy. (B) Calculated ideal amount of skin between the nipple and inframammary fold is 11 cm (at the existing submammary fold in this case). The ideal vertical position of the implant is distal to this point, as illustrated by the horizontal ideal lower pole (ILP)-line (implant's lower pole). Thus, dissection has to be done distally along the thoracic fascia from the incision in the submammary fold. Note that the dissection has to be distal to the ILP line (*striped area*) to accommodate for the skin between the incision and the ILP line. (C) Oblique view of the breast before surgery. (D) Oblique view directly after surgery.

adjusted according to implant dimensions. This is especially true when using form stable implants. Non-form stable implants can be deformed; therefore, the preoperative planning is not as crucial as when using form stable implants. It is surprising, however, how little attention was paid to the implant dimensions during preoperative planning in the plastic surgery literature before the advent of form stable implants. In the augmented breast, the ideal amount of skin between the nipple and the new inframammary fold is equal to the lower ventral curvature (LVC) of the implant plus the added distance for the amount of glandular tissue. The LVC of an implant is the distance from the ideal projection point on the implant's ventral surface (usually at half the height of the implant) measured down to the lower border of the implant. This distance can be calculated on a piece of paper with a tape ruler, because most implant manufacturers do not provide this information. The author has provided LVC measurements for all Allergan form stable implants (Style 410, 510 and INSPIRA). These measurements can be provided from the author or from the Allergan

Corporation. In addition to knowledge about the LVC of the implant, the amount of glandular tissue also has to be considered to calculate the ideal distance between the nipple and the new inframammary fold. The distance to be added to the LVC can be calculated in three different ways. The ideal way to do this is to measure the convex side of the breast between the nipple and the previously marked ILP-line with the patient's arms elevated on top of the head and subtracting half of the implant's height from this distance. This means that the difference between the convex and posterior sides of the breast is calculated and added to the LVC. An alternative way to calculate this is to do a pinch of the glandular tissue at the nipple areola level and divide this by two. This gives a relatively accurate estimation even though it is not as ideal as the previously mentioned method. The third way to calculate the amount of skin to be added to the LVC in relation to glandular tissue is to make an approximation. In a small breast, this is usually up to 1 cm; in a moderately sized breast, it is between 1 cm and maximally 2 cm; and in a large breast, it is slightly greater than 2 cm.

Finally, the calculated ideal distance between the nipple and submammary fold is marked on the breast. It is important to stretch the skin maximally when marking this to simulate the implant's stretching effects on the skin and to provide a tight envelope on the implant.

This preoperative planning system, calculating the implant's vertical height and the ideal amount of skin in the lower pole of the breast, is called the Akademikliniken method and has been described by the author in its first parts in 2001.[2]

In correction of moderate ptosis without mastopexy, these two parts of preoperative planning are used. In ptotic breasts, the calculated ideal amount of skin between the nipple and the new inframammary fold ends up above the ILP-line, which is attributable to the fact that too much skin is present in the lower pole of the breast. The incision is then placed above the implant's lower pole (ILP-line); contrary to standard breast augmentation, the dissection is then done along the thoracic wall in a distal direction from the

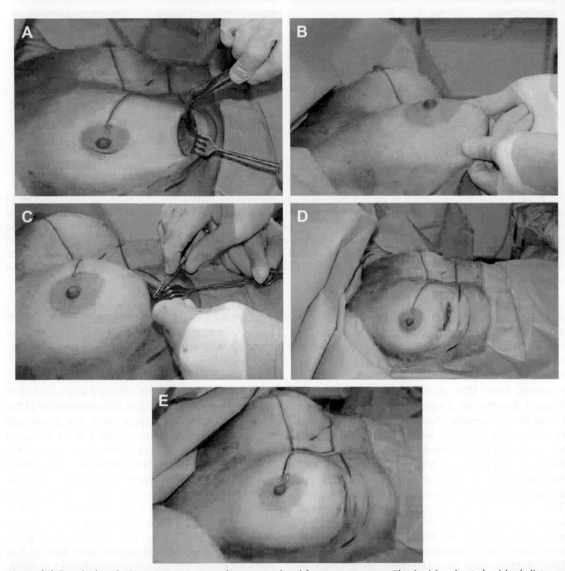

Fig. 3. (*A*) Surgical technique to correct moderate ptosis without mastopexy. The incision is at the ideal distance from the nipple-areola complex in relation to the implant dimension and amount of glandular tissue. Distal dissection from this point is past the ILP-line of the implant. (*B*) Testing distal expansion of the lower pole of the breast. (*C*) An important step is recreation of the submammary fold along the ILP-line with strong sutures between the thoracic fascia and Scarpa's fascia at the incision point. (*D*) Note the ILP-line in the midline of the breast before implant insertion. (*E*) Note the ILP-line after implantation and recreation and resuturing of the fold distally along the ILP-line.

incision line. By means of this procedure, the lower pole of the breast is moved distally, and at the end of the procedure the incision line is sutured to the ILP-line, where the implant's lower pole is positioned (**Fig. 3**). The extension of the distal dissection from the incision must go beyond the ILP-line, because the skin between the incision and the

ILP-line has to be moved distally. There is obviously a limitation in how much breast ptosis that can be corrected in this manner. Usually, the distance between the ILP-line and the incision above this should not exceed 2 cm. If it exceeds 2 cm, a mastopexy augmentation should be considered.

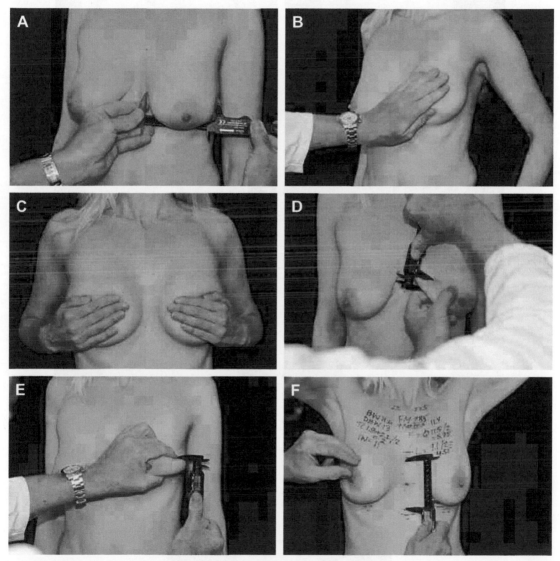

Fig. 4. (A) Existing breast width and desired breast width are measured with calipers before selecting the ideal implant in a mastopexy augmentation. (B) Desired breast width should respect the anterior axillary line laterally. (C) Desired breast width should leave an intramammary distance of 2 to 3 cm. (D) The ideal width of the implant is calculated by subtracting medial and lateral tissue cover from desired breast width. (E) Tissue cover is measured with a pinch test, and because this is a double fold of skin and subcutaneous tissue, the measured pinch medially and laterally should be divided by two before subtracting this number from the desired breast width to achieve information on ideal implant width. (F) Implant height depends on how the implant's upper pole and lower pole blend and correlate with the existing inframammary fold and upper pole shape. The implants are positioned centrally under the nipple-areola complex after the augmentation, which is simulated with arm elevation 45° above the horizontal plane. In a mastopexy augmentation, however, the lower pole of the implant is located at the existing inframammary fold.

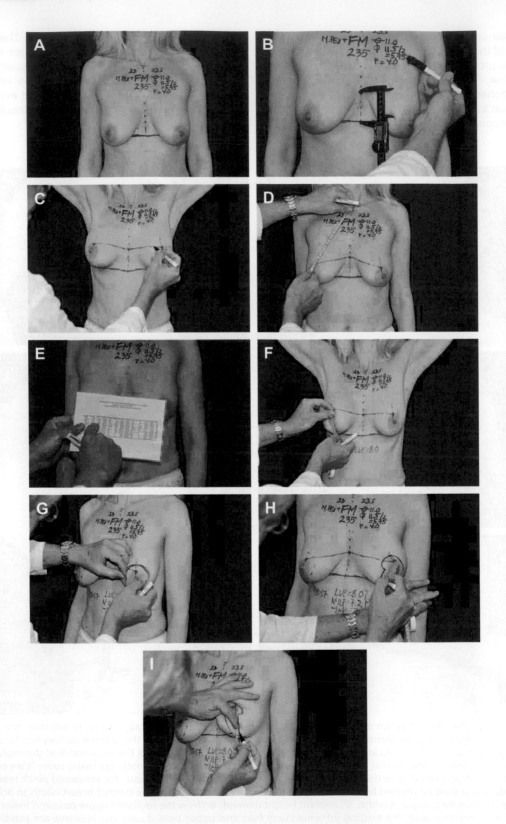

INDICATIONS FOR MASTOPEXY AUGMENTATIONS

As mentioned previously, if the implant's lower pole is more than 2 cm (to possibly 3 cm) distal to the incision (at the calculated distance for the ideal amount of skin between the nipple and the inframammary fold), a mastopexy is indicated. This is usually the case when the nipple is projecting well below the existing submammary fold. A mastopexy augmentation is also commonly indicated in secondary augmentation when there is considerable glandular atrophy. Frequently, this is capsular contraction related, and it is mostly seen in subglandular placement. A mastopexy augmentation can also be considered when a patient expects or demands more elevation of the nipple areola complex than what only an augmentation can produce. Mastopexy augmentation is also indicated in situations in which patients desire to reshape the nipple areola complex, as is usually the situation in tuberous breasts.

Mastopexy Augmentations

Many surgeons recommend that mastopexy augmentations should be performed as staged procedures, in which the first stage is usually the mastopexy and augmentation occurs in the second stage. The reverse is also possible but is less common. The reason for staging the mastopexy augmentation is obviously that this is safer but is also considered simpler by many surgeons.

A one-stage procedure combining mastopexy and augmentation does, however, have considerable advantages for patients because it minimizes hospitalization, thereby becoming less expensive and thus having higher patient acceptance. Another advantage is that the mastopexy is adjusted to the implant's dimension. A staged procedure has to consider the future implant dimensions instead of a standardized position of the nipple areola complex. It is relatively common that the incision from the nipple to the inframammary fold is too short in relation to the implant being used at the second stage. Therefore, vertical procedures or periareolar procedures may be advisable in staged operations. The disadvantages with a one-stage mastopexy augmentation are obviously that there is a slightly increased risk for healing problems and that it is more technically demanding. Preoperative planning and surgical techniques are therefore crucial.

ONE-STAGE MASTOPEXY AUGMENTATION WITH FORM STABLE IMPLANTS

The first important step in this procedure is to select the appropriate implant (**Fig. 4**). This selection should always consider the biologic prerequisites, and a tissue-based implant selection is therefore recommended.[9,10] It is important to understand that form stable devices cannot be deformed as non-form stable devices can be. Therefore, it is

Fig. 5. (*A*) Preoperative markings in mastopexy augmentation with the Akademikliniken method is done in a reversed manner compared with the technique used in pure augmentations. Thus, the existing inframammary fold is equal to the implant's lower pole (ILP-line). The markings are commenced by extending a line from the submammary fold to the midline (ILP-line). (*B*) With the patient's arms hanging, half the implant height is measured proximally from the ILP-line in the midline. (*C*) From the proximal end of this midline marking, a horizontal line is extended laterally with the arms elevated 45° above the horizontal plane (arm elevation 45° above horizontal plane is an accurate way of predicting where the nipples are going to be positioned after a proportionate breast augmentation). (*D*) New nipple position is checked in relation to the distance from the sternal notch, in relation to the submammary fold, and from the midline. Usually, if an appropriate implant dimension is selected, the nipple projects close to the submammary fold. (*E*) After selection of the new nipple position, the ideal length of skin between the new nipple position and the inframammary fold is calculated based on the LVC of the implant and the amount of glandular tissue. The LVC distances are available for Allergan form stable implants from the manufacturer according to calculations from the author. (*F*) Added to the LVC should be the distance between the new nipple position and the intramammary fold (ILP-line) minus half of the implant height. Thus, the difference between the convex side of the breast and the posterior side of the breast is calculated, and this distance is added to the LVC to get information on the ideal amount of skin between the nipple and the inframammary fold. (*G*) Subtracting half of the diameter of the areola, the ideal amount of skin between the inframammary fold and the areola can easily be calculated, and the decision on whether a vertical, periareolar, or inverted T-technique should be used can be made. The new areola circumference is marked on the chest wall, 13 cm in this case, for a modified inverted T-technique. (*H*) Vertical line in the middle of the submammary fold is marked, and the breast is displaced laterally medially to estimate the amount of vertical skin resection needed. (*I*) Vertical distance between the areola and the submammary fold is marked with stretched skin and in relation to a calculation of the ideal distance between the nipple and new inframammary fold as described previously. The distal end of these vertical incisions is then connected with the small submammary fold incision marking the resection of a small oval excision the size of which depends on the amount of ptosis.

of paramount importance to select the right implant dimensions. The first step in this is to select an adequate implant width; usually, this means respecting an intramammary distance of 2 to 3 cm medially and the anterior axillary line laterally. Measuring this distance with calipers, subtracting tissue cover medially and laterally, provides information on adequate implant width. It should be remembered that a pinch test at the estimated medial and lateral borders of the implant is a double fold of skin and subcutaneous tissue; therefore, the medial and lateral pinches should be divided by two when subtracting this figure from the desired breast width to get information on an adequate implant width.

The next step in implant selection is to decide its ideal height. Because the nipple-areola complex is adjusted to the implant dimension in mastopexy augmentations (contrary to the situation in breast augmentation, in which the implant's vertical position is adjusted to the nipple position), the existing lower border of the implant coincides with the inframammary fold. Thus, the ILP-line (implant's lower pole) and inframammary fold (IMF)-line are the same in a mastopexy augmentation. Measuring from this point and proximally, an adequate height of the implant can be decided in relation to where the upper pole of implants with different heights may end up. The upper pole shape and volume decide if low-, moderate-, or full-height implants are selected.

The final step in adequate implant selection is to decide on a suitable projection of the implant. This is highly related to patient preference and could be communicated with the patient standing obliquely in front of the mirror showing the projection of different implants by compressing calipers into the glandular tissue, showing where the estimated border of the new breast would be located. If a larger amount of glandular tissue exists, a low-projecting implant is usually sufficient, whereas in cases with considerable glandular atrophy, a higher projecting implant is usually needed.

PREOPERATIVE MARKINGS

The Akademikliniken (or AK) measuring system as described previously for correction of moderate ptosis without mastopexy is also well suited for mastopexy augmentation. However, the measurements are performed in a reversed manner (**Fig. 5**), this means that a horizontal line is drawn from the inframammary fold to the midline indicating the implant's lower pole. From this point, half of the implant height is measured proximally along the sternal midline, followed by arm elevation. From the proximal marking along the midline,

a horizontal line is extended laterally while the hands are kept 45° elevated above the horizontal plane. This line indicates the new nipple position in relation to the two-dimensional baseplate (or footprint) of the implant. Usually, when adequate implant dimensions have been selected, the marked position of the new nipple position should coincide with the projection of the submammary fold on the breast's ventral surface when the arms are lowered again. Check the symmetry and position of the new nipple position marking in relation to the existing inframammary fold and distance from the sternum notch. The horizontal distance from the midline should also be marked and measured. This is then followed by calculating an adequate amount of skin between the nipple and the inframammary fold according to the previous description. Thus, the implant's LVC is considered. Added to this LVC distance should be the distance according to the amount of covering glandular tissue. This is acquired by measuring between the new nipple position and the inframammary fold with the patient's arms on top of the head and subtracting half of the implant height. Knowing the ideal distance between the new nipple position and the inframammary fold, decisions on the type of mastopexy can be made. Depending on how much skin there is left in the lower pole of the breast, a periareolar, vertical, or modified inverted T-technique is selected. The modified inverted T-technique is applicable in all types of mastopexy augmentations; it is a clear and straightforward technique (**Fig. 6**), with the highest patient satisfaction.[11] The periareolar mastopexy has the drawback that the outer circumference and inner circumference around the areola are considerably different, which means a wrinkling of the suture line and usually less favorable conditions for a good-appearing scar. Also, the periareolar mastopexy, if not minor, increases the risk for flattening of the nipple-areola complex, which usually is not appreciated by patients who desire an augmentation. Adding a vertical component minimizes this problem. Measuring proximally from the submammary fold, stretching the tissues maximally, the calculated ideal distance between the nipple and inframammary fold, according to the previous description, subtracting half of the areola diameter indicates how much skin is needed between the areola's lower border and the inframammary fold. This is a useful guide when selecting a mastopexy technique. The Akademikliniken measuring principles can be applied in periareolar, vertical, and modified inverted T-techniques.

If a modified inverted T-technique is used, the new areolar border is marked as a three-quarters

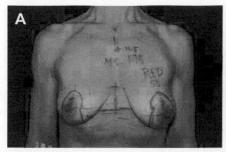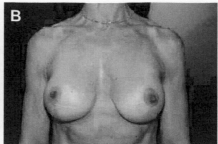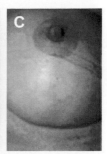

Fig. 6. (A) Preoperative marking for a small augmentation in combination with a mastopexy according to the Akademikliniken method. A small reduction is planned on the larger left side. (B) Six months after this procedure. (C) Scar with the arm elevated above the head. Note that the submammary fold incision of the scar is the least conspicuous of these.

circle, usually 12 to 13 cm long (provided that the nipple areola is 4 to 4.5 cm in diameter). From the inferior borders of this partial circle, the breast is displaced medially and laterally and vertical incisions are marked in the direction of a midline marking at the submammary fold. Knowing the ideal amount of skin between the new nipple position and the inframammary fold, this can then be marked vertically; at the distal end along the vertical resections, this is connected to a small submammary fold excision. Finally, markings are checked for symmetry with the patient's arms hanging and elevated.

SURGICAL TECHNIQUE

In breast augmentation surgery, antibiotics reduce the rate of infection.[12] A single intravenous dose (flucloxacillin, 2 g) is administrated 20 minutes before the operation. To minimize healing problems, it is of paramount importance when performing a combined mastopexy with augmentation to separate the procedure into two distinct different stages. The first stage should always involve implant insertion, and the second stage should include re-evaluation of the mastopexy drawings and performance of the mastopexy (**Fig. 7**). To facilitate the implant insertion, one of the planned vertical incisions and the submammary fold incision can be used without doing any skin resection. This is of extra importance in secondary cases in which dissection of the previously inserted implant and its capsule is greatly facilitated (**Fig. 8**). With this T-incision, easy access to the whole implant pocket is achieved. In most mastopexy augmentations, a dual-plane submuscular positioning of the implant[13] is used if the breast is not of considerable size. If the pinch at the estimated upper border of the breast is more than 3 cm thick, a subglandular placement may be favored. Other cases, especially if tissue cover is less than 2 cm at the

upper border of the implant, benefit from the dual-plane position. Dual-plane positioning used in mastopexy augmentation means subglandular dissection past the border of the nipple-areola complex and then distal division of the pectoralis muscle origin horizontally a couple of centimeters above the inframammary fold. The muscle dissection is commenced at the lateral border of the pectoralis, and dissection is safest if the muscle is elevated from the chest wall with forceps and if the muscle dissection is parallel to the ribcage. When entering underneath the muscle, loose connective tissues should be preserved on the ribs and the dissection should be carried on in the direction of the sternum notch. The benefit of this dissection is that risk for elevating the inferior origin of the pectoralis minor muscle is minimized, because the dissection in the upper part of the pocket goes from medial to lateral between the pectoralis major and minor muscles. Finally, the medial inferior origin of the pectoralis major muscle is divided, respecting the previously marked NS-line. Muscle division should always stay well distal to this line to minimize poor animation along the sternum border during pectoralis muscle activity. It is important that the lateral part of the muscle retracts up, however, because this minimizes movement during pectoralis activity during and after the augmentation.

The submammary fold incision is sutured down to the thoracic fascia along the ILP-line with running Vicryl or Monocryl sutures between Scarpa's fascia and the thoracic wall to define this line. Hemostasis is carefully controlled, and the implant is inserted with minimal contamination involving touch only by the surgeon after changing into new sterile gloves. Bleeding is usually negligible, and drainage can be avoided if sharp electrocautery is used (Valleylab Force FX and Colorado tungsten needles) (Valleylab, Tyco Healthcare Group LP, Boulder, Colorado). After this, the

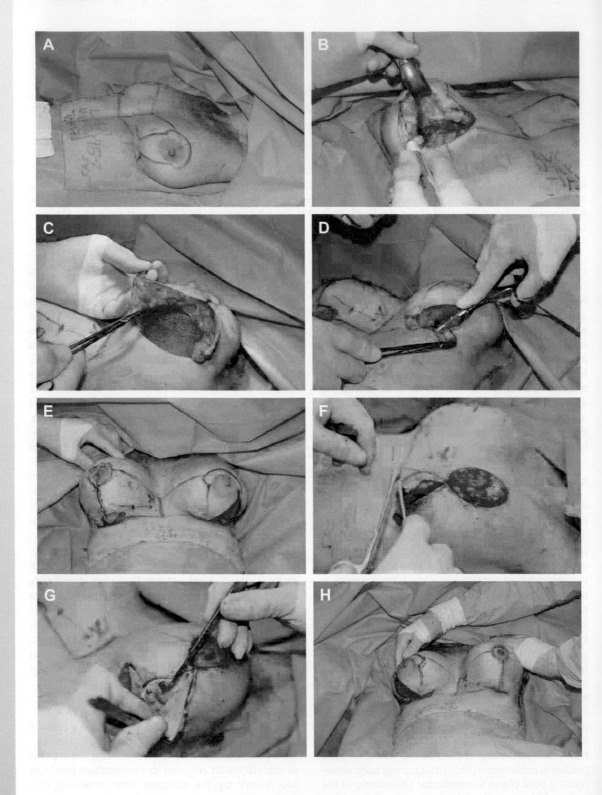

is inserted with minimal contamination, evolving
touch only by the surgeon after changing into
new sterile gloves. Bacteria burden is negligible
and triclosan can be detected in the wound after
tary is used while replacing the scalpel, dissec-
tungsten tips are placed in the wound in a dis-
Group 13.

pocket is achieved is most mastopexy augmentations a dual-plane submuscular positioning of the
implant is used. If the breast is not of considera-
able size, all the gland at the estimated upper
border of the breast is more than 3 cm thick, a subglandular placement may be favored. Other cases,
especially if tissue cover is less than 2 cm at the

medial and lateral pillars of the vertical incisions are closed to the submammary fold, transforming this to a closed implant pocket. The patient is then placed in a lying position, preferably with the arms along the side, and the mastopexy is re-evaluated. Staples can be used to approximate the skin and to redraw some of the markings. With the planning described previously, however, adjustments of the markings are usually not necessary. The patient is put back in a prone position, and the nipple is first transferred to its new position. The periareolar area is de-epithelized, and a medial and proximal dermal pedicle is usually kept (generally, the gland does not have to be divided). From the inferior border of the areola, a skin flap of the planned vertical resection is elevated without any resection until the areola is stitched into its new position. The vertical resection of skin is then re-evaluated and resected. To get a good shape of the lower pole of the breast, subcutaneous tissue and the gland at the inferior end of this vertical resection are removed. The gland is approximated vertically to achieve a more projecting breast. The vertical pillars are closed, and, finally, the small excess of skin along the submammary fold incision is excised. Closure should be done without tension in the T-junction, and the appropriate length of skin between the inframammary fold and nipple according to measurements made previously should be checked with a sterile ruler. All closures are done in three layers, in the gland to cover the implant, in the deep dermis and running subcuticular with Monocryl 3/0.

POSTOPERATIVE EVENT

When using form stable implants, not only implant selection, preoperative planning, and surgical techniques differ compared with the use of non-form stable implants; additionally, the postoperative events should be different. Because these textured implants have tissue fixation by ingrowth[14] to the surface (BIOCELL surface with a pore size larger than 300 μm) (Allergan Limited, Marlow Buckinghamshire, United Kingdom), implant movement should be minimized after surgery. Tissue ingrowth minimizes the risk for implant displacement with descent or rotational problems of anatomic implants. It is not scientifically proved how long a time it takes before tissue growth has occurred into the implant surface, but it is expected to take at least 3 weeks before this process is finalized. It can possibly take up to 3 months; therefore, it could be recommended that patients avoid too much implant movement during this period. This means exercise, such as jogging, horseback riding, or trampoline jumping. Additional to this, patients are recommended to avoid stretch perpendicular to the scar; thus, the tennis serve movement of arms above the head is not good for submammary fold incisions because this may provide a less favorable outcome of the final scar appearance. Also, long-term postoperative surgical taping of scars up to 6 months is recommended (Micropore 3M tape) (3M Global Headquarters, St. Paul, Minnesota). This tape should not be peeled off until it almost falls off on its own (usually once every second week), and it is thus kept on during showers.

DISCUSSION

Mastopexy is a common procedure to rejuvenate the female breast but it is well recognized that it is difficult to maintain upper pole fullness with a mastopexy alone. Usually, the upper pole fullness present initially after the procedure

Fig. 7. (A) With the patient lying flat on the operating table, the NS-line shifts considerably. This line is a useful guide during surgery when dividing the inferior origin of the pectoralis muscle during a dual-plane dissection. The muscle division should always respect the NS-line in the midline and stay well below this level. (B) Procedure is facilitated if one of the vertical incisions and the submammary fold are incised. Note that no skin resection is done. In secondary breast augmentation, this maneuver greatly facilitates implant dissection. (C) After implantation and suturing of the submammary fold Scarpa's fascia to the thoracic wall, the vertical glandular pillars are closed at the estimated resection level with sutures between the gland and the thoracic fascia at the level of the submammary fold. (D) It is important that no skin is resected before implants are in place. (E) Mastopexy drawings are re-evaluated after implant insertion. Temporary closure with staples before skin resection can be useful in this part of the procedure. To put the patient in the sitting position and have the arms along the side further facilitates this evaluation. (F) Nipple is first placed in position before vertical skin excision is done. (G) Vertical resection of skin and a small amount of gland distally to improve the curvature of the lower pole of the breast is done without tension in the vertical closure. (H) Before resecting the small oval of skin in the submammary fold, the length of skin between the areola and new submammary fold is checked with a ruler and the resection is done so that closure can be performed without tension in the T-junction. The tissues are closed in three layers with the gland to the thoracic fascia, deep dermal suturing with relaxation of the tension in the T-junction, and running subcuticular stitches.

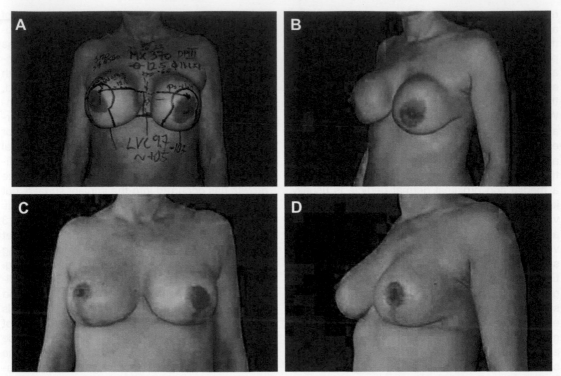

Fig. 8. (*A*) Combined mastopexy and secondary augmentation after previous subglandular round non-form stable implants with capsular contracture. Preoperative markings are made according to the previous description but as the patients already have implants, the arms are not elevated during the marking of the NS line. (*B*) Oblique view of the same patient before surgery. (*C*) Three months after this secondary breast augmentation and mastopexy with reposition to the submuscular position. (*D*) Same patient in an oblique view.

disappears within the first 6 months of healing, leaving an empty upper pole compared with the fullness achieved with a combined mastopexy augmentation. Recent market research[15] has documented that only 29% of women seeking breast augmentation have the size of the breast as a primary concern. More than 70% have primary concerns related to the shape of the breast after the procedure. The typical patient desiring breast augmentation is between 30 and 40 years of age and has the desire to reshape her breast, usually after pregnancies and breastfeeding. In these cases, loss of volume in the upper pole is common, as is atrophy with descent of the glandular tissue. Breast augmentation alone can elevate a nipple-areola complex, produce fullness in the upper pole, and create a more youthful appearance. When the nipple-areola complex is projecting at or lower than the height of the submammary fold, however, it may be difficult to achieve a good result with augmentation alone.

Mastopexy augmentation is without any doubt a procedure that is considered more complicated and risky than standard breast augmentation, and the rate of infection increases in more complex surgical situations.[16] It has been demonstrated that the risk for and frequency of complications are higher in mastopexy augmentations than in pure augmentation surgery.[17,18] Many surgeons advise against this procedure because of the risks, and it is not an uncommon reason for malpractice suits in several countries. It has also been argued that although the overall results of one-stage breast augmentation and mastopexy are good and the patients are generally satisfied, staging the surgery by performing the mastopexy first may yield significantly better results than the combined simultaneous procedure.[19]

It may well be true that a more standardized and meticulous planning technique, such as that described in this article, can improve the esthetic outcome; however, it is also recognized that a detailed follow-up with respect to patient satisfaction data and outcome has not been presented here to substantiate this claim. It should also be remembered that a two-stage procedure is a considerable drawback for the patient, not only from an economic standpoint but with respect to the necessity of staying out of work, for example. A one-stage mastopexy augmentation can safely

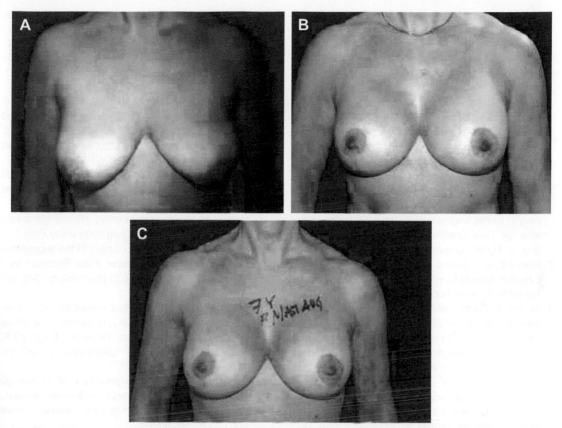

Fig. 9. (*A*) Before mastopexy augmentation. (*B*) Six months after this procedure. (*C*) Seven years later, illustrating the stability and long-term results of mastopexy augmentation combined with form stable implants.

be achieved, provided that the planning is accurate, and the Akademikliniken method for measurement and marking described in this article provides such a technique.

With the development of this technique during the past decade, the frequency of complications has been reduced. It is surprising that we have been doing breast augmentation surgery for almost 40 years without really considering the importance of implant dimensions when planning breast augmentation and mastopexy augmentations. It is obvious, however, that a larger implant needs more distance between the nipple and the inframammary fold. By calculating this and the length that has to be added for the amount of glandular tissue, a predictable way of planning pure augmentation and mastopexy augmentation can be achieved. As also shown by other investigators,[11,20] the author's experience is in agreement with the statement that this procedure can be done without high risk for reoperation and complications. In fact, the frequency of complications has not been higher in mastopexy augmentation than in pure augmentation in the past couple of years. Mastopexy augmentation surgery can also

safely be combined with other procedures, such as abdominoplasty;[21] however, obviously, this not only necessitates meticulous surgical planning and procedure but good anesthesiologic management, including antithrombotic therapy. It has been stressed that such factors as proper choice of surgical technique, type of implant, approach to placement of the implant, type of suture, and removal of tissue for the pexy are fundamental to obtaining a good result in mastopexy augmentation.[11] The longevity of mastopexy augmentation with form stable devices has also been good (**Fig. 9**), provided that patients retain weight and have supportive garments if their natural breasts are large.

REFERENCES

1. Persoff MM. Vertical mastopexy with expansion augmentation. Aesthetic Plast Surg 2003;27(1):13–9.
2. Hedén P, Jernbeck J, Hober M, et al. Breast augmentation with anatomical cohesive gel implants: the world's largest current experience. Clin Plast Surg 2001;28(3):531–52.

3. Hedén P, Nava MB, van Tetering JP, et al. Prevalence of rupture in Inamed silicone breast implants. Plast Reconstr Surg 2006;118(2):303–8 [discussion: 309–12].

4. Hedén P, Bone B, Murphy DK, et al. Style 410 cohesive silicone breast implants: safety and effectiveness at 5 to 9 years after implantation. Plast Reconstr Surg 2006;118(6):1281–7.

5. Hedén P. Breast augmentation with anatomical, high-cohesive silicon gel implant. In: Spear SL, editor. Surgery of the breast: principles and art. 2nd edition. Philadelphia: Lippincott Williams and Wilkins; 2006. p. 1344–67.

6. Hedén P. Implant selection and preoperative planning in breast augmentation with form stable cohesive gel filled anatomical implants. In: Szemerey, Bajusz, Hedén, editors. 2008.

7. Hedén P, et al. Breast augmentation. In: Eriksson G, Chung P, Gosain D, editors. Plastic surgery. Burlington (MA): Elsevier Publ.; 2008 [In publication].

8. Hedén P. Form stable anatomical high cohesive silicone gel implants—European experience. In: Hall-Findlay E, Evans G, editors. Aesthetic and reconstructive surgery of the breast. Burlington (MA): Elsevier Publ.; 2008 [In publication].

9. Tebbetts JB. Use of anatomic breast implants: ten essentials. Aesthetic Surg J 1998;18(5):377–84.

10. Tebbetts JB. Patient evaluation, operative planning, and surgical techniques to increase control and reduce morbidity and reoperations in breast augmentation. Clin Plast Surg 2001;28(3):501–21.

11. Cardenas-Camarena L, Ramirez-Macias R. Augmentation/mastopexy: how to select and perform the proper technique. Aesthetic Plast Surg 2006; 30(1):21–33.

12. Arace A, Gavantes G, Araco F, et al. Infections of breast implants in aesthetic breast augmentations: a single-center review of 3,002 patients. Aesthetic Plast Surg 2007;31(4):325–9.

13. Tebbetts JB. Dual plane breast augmentation: optimizing implant-soft-tissue relationships in a wide range of breast types. Plast Reconstr Surg 2001; 107(5):1255–72.

14. Danino AM, Basmacioglu P, Saito S, et al. Comparison of the capsular response to the Biocell RTV and Mentor 1600 Siltex breast implant surface texturing: a scanning electron microscopic study. Plast Reconstr Surg 2001;108(7):2047–52.

15. Heden P, Adams W, Maxwell P, et al. Aesthetic breast surgery; consulting for the future. Plast Reconstr Surg (submitted for publication).

16. Handel N. Health risks of failed silicone gel breast implants. Plast Reconstr Surg 1995;95(6):1129–31.

17. Handel N. Secondary mastopexy in the augmented patient: a recipe for disaster. Plast Reconstr Surg 2006;118(7 Suppl):152S–63S [discussion: 164S–5S, 166S–7S].

18. Spear SL, Boehmler JH 4th, Clemens MV, et al. Augmentation/mastopexy: a 3-year review of a single surgeon's practice. Plast Reconstr Surg 2006; 118(7 Suppl):136S–47S [discussion: 148S–9S, 150S–1S].

19. Spear SL, Pelletiere CV, Menon N, et al. One-stage augmentation combined with mastopexy: aesthetic results and patient satisfaction. Aesthetic Plast Surg 2004;28(5):259–67.

20. Stevens WG, Freeman ME, Stoker DA, et al. One-stage mastopexy with breast augmentation: a review of 321 patients. Plast Reconstr Surg 2007;120(6): 1674–9.

21. Stevens WG, Cohen R, Vath SD, et al. Is it safe to combine abdominoplasty with elective breast surgery? A review of 151 consecutive cases. Plast Reconstr Surg 2006;118(1):207–12 [discussion: 213–4].

Augmentation Mastopexy

Scott L. Spear, MD*, Joseph H. Dayan, MD, Mark W. Clemens, MD

KEYWORDS

- Breast lift • Augmentation mastoplexy • Mammoplasty

Augmentation/mastopexy when performed in a single stage presents more significant challenges than either augmentation or mastopexy alone. The combination of breast augmentation and mastopexy in one stage exponentially increases the risk of complications than either surgery carries alone.[1-3] Its reputation within plastic surgery as a significant source of litigation is well established.[4] The complexity of a one-stage augmentation/mastopexy is a result of combining the expansion of breast volume while at the same time reducing the skin envelope, effectively two opposing goals.[5] As a one-stage procedure, augmentation/mastopexy is associated with all of the risks of breast augmentation and mastopexy, including nipple malposition, inadequate ptosis correction, misshapened areolas, poor scarring, capsular contracture, and implant malposition. Theoretically, increased risks and uncertainties also include wound healing problems, skin necrosis, implant extrusion, infection, and misalignment of the nipple, gland, and implant. Although loss of the nipple is not a risk typically associated with either mastopexy or augmentation alone, it is a risk of augmentation/mastopexy when the two operations are combined.

The inherent risks of this procedure have not affected its popularity among patients. Between 1997 and 2007, there was a 395% increase in the frequency of breast augmentation and an equal increase in breast lift procedures.[6] The number of combined augmentation/mastopexy procedures has similarly increased in frequency because of the convenience of a single-stage operation. The authors have previously written

extensively on the subject of augmentation/mastopexy.[7-14] A review from 2003 to 2006 comparing our experience with breast augmentation, primary augmentation/mastopexy, and secondary/augmentation mastopexy revealed complication rates of 1.7%, 17%, and 23%, respectively.[14]

To better understand why approximately 20% of the combined procedures have revisions or complications, we reviewed the most common complications and causes for revision in a separate publication.[11] This separate series of 34 consecutive revisions after previous augmentation and mastopexy from 1993 to 2001 demonstrated that the most common features of patients having revisions were recurrent ptosis (55%), capsular contracture (55%), implant malposition (35%), size change (30%), poor scars (25%), and nipple malposition (10%). These percentages represent those patients having revision and are not the percent of revisions of the group of augmentation/mastopexies seen as a whole. These revisions were performed after an average interval of 7 years from the previous surgery.

Although a single-stage procedure remains attractive to the surgeon and patient, its successful execution is contingent upon careful preoperative planning and attentive implementation to reduce the severity and frequency of complications. The following discussion is a detailed description of our approach to augmentation/mastopexy, which is focused around several principles as follows:

In most cases, placing the implants first and then tailoring the skin envelope to accommodate the larger breast volume

Dr. Spear is a paid consultant to Lifecell, Ethicon, and Allergan corporations. This study was conducted without any funding. Drs. Clemens and Dayan have no disclosures.
Department of Plastic Surgery, Georgetown University Medical Center, 1st Floor PHC Building, 3800 Reservoir Road NW, Washington, DC 20007, USA
* Corresponding author.
E-mail address: spears@gunet.georgetown.edu (S.L. Spear).

Clin Plastic Surg 36 (2009) 105–115
doi:10.1016/j.cps.2008.08.006
0094-1298/08/$ – see front matter © 2008 Elsevier Inc. All rights reserved.

Addressing breast asymmetries by employing different mastopexy patterns when appropriate

Tailor-tacking the skin with the patient in the upright position in the operating room before finally committing to the planned mastopexy pattern

Conservative superficial undermining of the skin to preserve perfusion to the nipple-areola complex (NAC) and skin flaps to reduce the risk of necrosis and wound healing complications

PATIENT SELECTION AND EVALUATION

A broad spectrum of patients who are candidates for augmentation/mastopexy exists who present with very different challenges. A young patient with a tuberous breast deformity and a short nipple to inframammary fold distance with a tight skin envelope presents with an entirely different problem than a postpartum woman with deflated breasts and loose skin. These factors influence the size and dimensions of the implant and the mastopexy pattern. The decision of whether to perform a mastopexy and with what type of skin excision pattern is dependent upon the size of the breast and the surface area of the skin envelope. Critical to this decision is the relationship among the nipple position, breast parenchyma, and inframammary fold.

The preoperative evaluation begins with a systematic evaluation of the patient's ptosis. Using the Regnault classification, breast ptosis is rated as grade I, nipple lying at the fold; grade II, nipple below the fold but still on the anterior portion of the breast; or grade III, nipple at the most inferior portion of the breast (**Fig. 1**).[15] Breast ptosis can be a complex entity that involves more elements than the relationship between the nipple position and the inframammary fold as designated by the Regnault classification. Several other factors should also be taken into consideration before surgery, including the patient's primary motivation. If breast augmentation is the primary goal, some ptosis may be camouflaged by placing an implant alone, provided that the size of the implant is sufficient to fill out the patient's skin envelope. In the authors' experience, a mastopexy may not be required if there is less than 2 cm of breast overhanging the fold and the nipple is positioned on the anterior surface of the breast, with nonpigmented skin visible between the areola and the inferior border of the breast and a nipple to inframammary fold distance that is not excessively long (<9 cm). If the primary goal is to correct

significant asymmetries, particularly if this involves a significant amount of reduction on one side, the safest plan may be to perform the mastopexies first followed by breast augmentation at a second stage. Accounting for too many variables in one setting may lead to unpredictable and often disappointing results.

The preoperative evaluation also includes an assessment of the size and surface area of the breast, the elasticity of the skin and the quality of the breast parenchyma, as well as the relationship among the nipple, breast gland, and inframammary fold (**Figs. 2–4**). The assessment begins with two key elements: (1) the nipple position in relation to the inframammary fold, as classified by Regnault, and (2) the vertical distance that the breast overhangs the fold. Next, the distance from the nipple to the inframammary fold is measured with the skin placed on tension to simulate the stretch that will be caused when the implant is placed. The more the skin and glandular tissue overhangs the inframammary fold, the less likely that a reasonable size implant alone will be able to successfully fill out the breast.[16] Similarly, the lower the nipple on the surface of the breast, the less likely a prosthesis will elevate the nipple adequately onto the surface of the breast.

When planning the mastopexy pattern, a circumareolar pattern may be more desirable with respect to limiting the amount of scars placed on the breast, but this comes at the cost of placing more tension on the closure and may lead to a flattened appearance, poor scarring, or a distorted NAC.[17] In the vast majority of cases, a circumareolar or, more commonly, a vertical or circumvertical technique is sufficient, leaving a formal "Wise" pattern for only the most severe cases. A circumareolar mastopexy alone works well only for the patient in whom the nipple lies near or just below the fold with the inferior border of the areola no lower than the inferior curve of the breast on frontal view, and when there is less than 4 cm of breast overhanging the fold, leaving an initial nipple-to-fold distance of no more than 8 to 9 cm. In planning a circumareolar mastopexy, as a guideline, the ratio of the outer to the inner diameter of the circumareolar markings should ideally be no greater than 2:1 and certainly no greater than 3:1.

The circumvertical or vertical technique offers the greatest versatility and is most helpful when there is a greater degree of ptosis.[18] This technique is most appropriate when the nipple is more than 2 cm below the inframammary fold, a portion of the areola lies on the inferior curve of the breast, the nipple-to-fold distance is greater than 8 or 9 cm, or the breast overhangs the fold by 4 or more cm. Adding a vertical component to

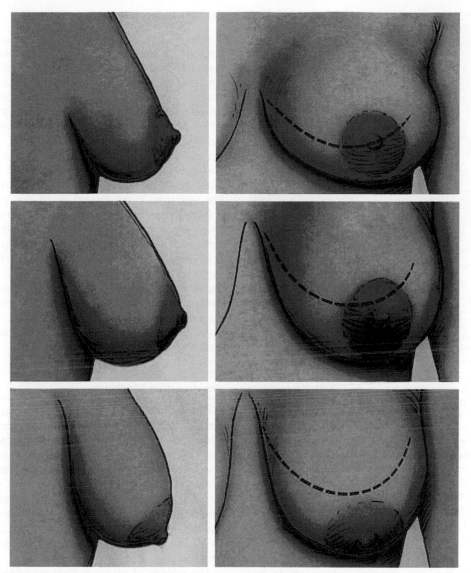

Fig. 1. Evaluation of the position of the nipple in relation to the inframammary fold and its location on the breast mound, the amount of breast tissue below the inframammary fold, and the length of the nipple to inframammary fold is critical in determining the optimal procedure. (*From* Spear SL, Boehmler JH, Clemens MW. Augmentation/mastopexy: a 3-year review of a single surgeon's practice. Plast Reconstr Surg 2006;118:136S–47S; with permission.)

the excision pattern effectively reduces the diameter of the circumareolar closure by approximately one third the distance of the width of the vertical excision (circumference = π D) A circumvertical excision pattern not only places less tension on the circumareolar closure but also increases projection by narrowing and coning the breast. For these reasons, a circumvertical pattern provides the most control in terms of shaping the breast. Even in situations in which an acceptable result using a circumareolar pattern might be

achieved, we will often add a conservative vertical excision to improve the overall shape of the breast.

As a general principle, the final extent and pattern of the excision should not be determined until the implants are placed. The skin envelope and nipple position are then tailor-tacked with the patient sitting upright and then finally adjusted to the dimensions of the newly augmented breast. A transverse scar may be added to keep the nipple to inframammary fold distance from getting too long. The addition of a transverse scar does not

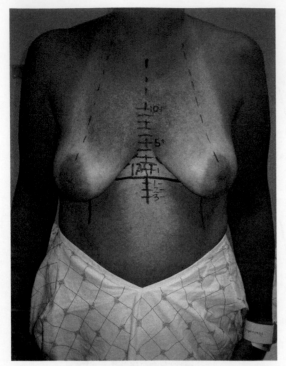

Fig. 2. Preoperative evaluation includes an assessment of the size and surface area of the breast, the elasticity of the skin, and the quality of breast parenchyma. With the patient standing upright, markings begin by noting the chest midline with 1 cm tangent hash marks, the breast meridians, and the inframammary folds. Note the tangent line drawn across the front of the chest for use as a reference for the inframammary lines; in this patient, the nipple falls at the level of the fold. Careful attention is paid to marking the breast meridians because there are often lateral asymmetries of the NAC that should be corrected as much as possible by adjusting the planned excision.

invalidate the circumvertical approach to the procedure.

PREOPERATIVE HISTORY AND CONSIDERATIONS

Several variables may increase the risks of performing a single-stage augmentation/mastopexy, including smoking or a previously performed breast augmentation or breast reduction. Smokers are counseled as to the increased risk and are cautioned to stop smoking. Because the blood supply to the NAC is impaired to some extent in all of these patients, the procedure is performed carefully with minimal undermining. Previously augmented patients have some degree of thinning of the tissues from the implant, and, for the same reasons, a cautious and conservative approach is necessary.

CHOOSING THE IMPLANT

The decision-making process in selecting the appropriate sized implant is more complex in augmentation/mastopexy than in augmentation alone. Because the skin envelope will be reduced, one should measure not only the base width of the breast in its native state but also the base width while pinching the skin to simulate the breast dimensions after the mastopexy (**Fig. 5**). This maneuver will effectively narrow the base width and provides a closer approximation of what the outer limits of the implant diameter should be. For example, if the breast is 13 cm wide with a 2-cm pinch thickness and has a width of 12 cm when simulating the mastopexy, an implant diameter of 10 to 11 cm would probably be more appropriate than one with a diameter of 11 to 12 cm. In terms of implant projection, for deflated breasts, the higher profile models are often preferable in filling out the loose skin envelope. Once these parameters are defined, a discussion with the patient regarding her ideal breast size refines the final choice of implant.

Preoperative Markings

With the patient standing upright, markings begin with the midline, breast meridians, and inframammary folds (see **Fig. 2**). A line is drawn tangent to the inframammary folds across the front of the chest for use as a reference. The midline is marked from the sternal notch to the xiphoid process. Careful attention is paid to marking the breast meridians, because there are often lateral asymmetries of the NAC that should be corrected as much as possible by adjusting the planned excision (**Fig. 3**).

The degree of ptosis is then evaluated, noting the relationship of the nipple to the inframammary fold as well as the nipple-to-fold distance and the amount or volume of breast that overhangs the fold. The sternal notch-to-nipple distance is variable among patients with different heights; therefore, the absolute numerical measurement is not as helpful as the previously mentioned measurements. Nevertheless, it can be used as a guide to assess symmetry of the NAC in each patient. Based on these measurements, a preliminary decision is made in regards to whether to proceed with a mastopexy and, if so, which type to use. If there is significant asymmetry between the two breasts, logic follows that planned skin excisions may be different, and it is made clear to the patient that although the intent is to achieve a more symmetric result, perfect symmetry virtually never happens.

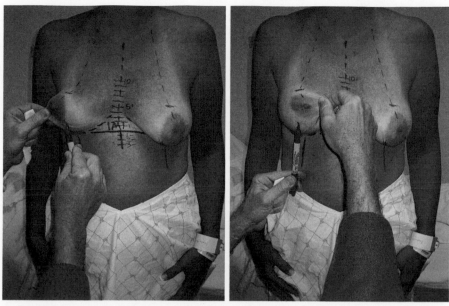

Fig. 3. The distance from the nipple to the inframammary fold is measured with the skin placed on tension to simulate the stretch that will be caused when the implant is placed. The medial and lateral pillars of the vertical mastopexy component are marked while displacing the breast medially and laterally, respectively.

After evaluating the degree of breast and nipple ptosis and forming an initial operative plan, measurements for the implant are made. The base width of the breast is measured at rest and while simulating the mastopexy with a vertical pinch between the surgeon's thumb and fingers (see **Fig. 5**). The upper pole pinch thickness is also measured with calipers. The difference between these values is a guide to the upper limit for the diameter of the implant. Using the implant

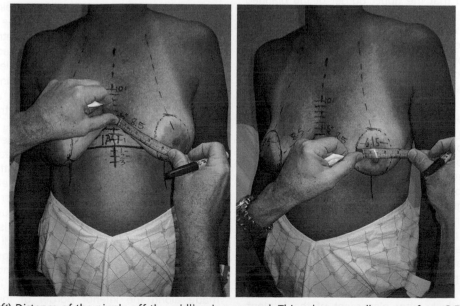

Fig. 4. (*Left*) Distance of the nipple off the midline is measured. This value generally ranges from 8.5 to 10 cm. (*Right*) Nipple width distance is then evened out. Note asymmetric areolar windows of this patient, 7.5 cm versus 6.5 cm, to correct breast asymmetries.

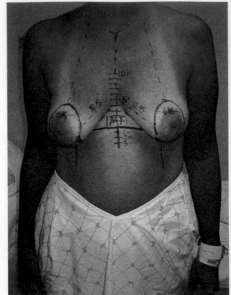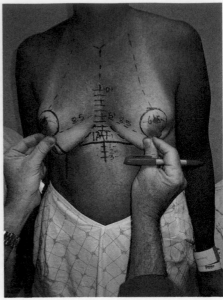

Fig. 5. (*Left*) Because the skin envelope will be reduced, it is important to measure not only the base width of the breast in its native state, (*Right*) but also the base width while tailor-tacking the skin to simulate the breast dimensions after the mastopexy. The base width is narrowed and will require a smaller diameter implant based on the new width. Note red dot denotes new nipple position.

diameter measurement, the height of anticipated breast is marked from the inframammary fold. Markings are made to visualize the implant position on the chest wall and predict appropriate nipple placement.

As part of the initial skin marking in the examination room, the NAC is manually pinched and tailor-tacked so that the upper border of the planned new areola position can be marked on the chest with the nipple at or slightly below the center of the projected dimensions of the breast mound. Gentle downward traction is placed on the superior pole breast skin to simulate the tension that will be created by the mastopexy. Unlike in breast reduction procedures, the NAC is invariably finally marked to lie somewhere above the inframammary fold in augmentation/mastopexy once the implant is in. Although the most serious error is to place the nipple too high, the most common error is inadequate elevation of the nipple. It is important to note the presence of tan lines, because these are another guide to areas that may be exposed in swimwear or some clothing. It is also useful to have the patient wear a bra and mark the upper boundaries of where the bra crosses the breast. These maneuvers can serve as important guides to avoid placing the nipple too high. Ultimately, the final nipple position is still best decided intraoperatively after placement of the implant, tailor-tacking the planned excision, and sitting the patient upright.

Circumareolar Technique

Starting from the planned new upper areolar border and skirting the edges of the NAC, an ellipse is drawn around the lower half of the areola. A total of 5 to 7 cm of skin should be left between the bottom of this ellipse and the fold. Measurements are taken from the midline to the medial edge of the markings on both sides to help provide reasonably symmetric placement of the NAC on the vertical axis. If significant asymmetry exists, the side with the relatively malpositioned NAC is addressed by adjusting the medial or, less often, the lateral extent of the ellipse. Finally, the nipple-to-fold distance is measured again to ensure symmetry of the NAC in the transverse plane (**Fig. 6**).

The procedure begins with the patient in the supine position with the arms tucked or abducted 90 degrees or less. Careful attention is made to padding at the hands and elbows. A 42-mm cookie cutter or other diameter circle is centered over each nipple without undue tension on the skin. In patients in whom it is unclear whether any mastopexy procedure will be necessary, the procedure begins with a periareolar incision for placement of the implant without any de-epithelialization.[19] The incision is usually made along the inferior border of the areola, and dissection is carried down to the pectoralis major muscle.

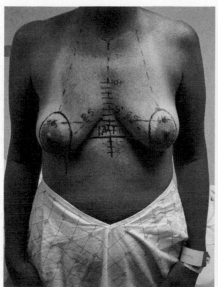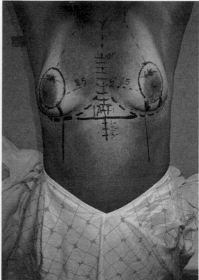

Fig. 6. Patient with all preliminary markings in repose (*left*) and with arms raised (*right*) to demonstrate planned areolar windows, vertical excisions, and inframammary folds. Note planned nipple placement (*red dot*) at approximately +3 cm superior to inframammary folds.

At the authors' center, we prefer a dual-plane approach placing the implant partially retropectorally.[20] The inferior third of the pocket is dissected in the subglandular plane while the upper two thirds or so of the pocket lies in the subpectoral plane. Meticulous hemostasis and irrigation with a triple antibiotic solution are routinely performed to minimize the risk of capsular contracture or infection.[21] After completing the dissection and irrigation, the implant is soaked in antibiotic solution, the field is re-prepped with a Betadine paint stick, and gloves are changed before implant placement. After the insertion of the implant, the incision is stapled closed, and the patient is positioned sitting fully upright. If significant ptosis remains, the previously planned circumareolar pattern is tailor-tacked using a skin stapler. The

nipple position is then reassessed and remeasured and may be fine-tuned as required. The placement of an implant alone will often create the appearance that the nipple has been elevated 2 cm or more. Circumareolar de-epithelialization may then be performed as necessary. This strategy may avoid unnecessary placement of scars on the breast in borderline cases.[22,23]

After de-epithelialization, the outer circumference of the dermis is incised with the Bovie on cutting mode, ensuring that the incision is about 5 to 7 mm away from the skin edge leaving a dermal cuff. Minimal undermining in the subcutaneous plane is performed to redrape the skin. Care is taken not to dissect deep and violate the breast parenchyma to preserve blood supply to the nipple. Usually, only 1 to 2 cm of undermining is

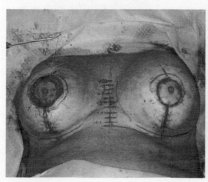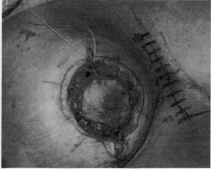

Fig. 7. (*Left*) The interlocking Gore-tex suture technique described by Hammond. Using a CV-3 Gore-tex suture, eight equally spaced bites are placed between the dermal cuff and the dermis of the NAC. Note nipple skin closure after purse-string on contralateral breast. (*Right*) Close-up view of right breast.

required. Classically, a "blocking" technique is used by purse-stringing the dermal cuff with a permanent 3-0 suture.[24] More recently, the authors have adopted the interlocking Gore-Tex suture technique described by Hammond. Using a CV-3 Gore-Tex suture, eight equally spaced bites are placed between the dermal cuff and the dermis of the NAC (**Fig. 7**). The skin is closed with interrupted and running buried Monocryl sutures.

Circumvertical Technique

The circumvertical technique is similar to the periareolar approach but includes a vertical skin excision from the nipple and extends vertically down to or just above the inframammary fold.[25–28] If required, a small transverse skin excision placed in the inframammary fold is performed to eliminate any dog ear and to avoid leaving too much skin inferiorly from the nipple to the fold. This maneuver allows for coning of the breast in cases where greater skin excision is necessary.

The preliminary markings and nipple position are determined as previously described. Superomedial and superolateral traction is applied to the breast, and vertical marks are drawn on the surface of the skin over the projected breast meridian (see **Fig. 3**). These markings extend from the circumareolar marks and join in a "V" or "U" shape down to or just above the fold. These lines are then pinched together to check whether skin closure is possible while anticipating the

effect of the implant (see **Fig. 5**). The length of the vertical limb is directly related to the amount of ptosis but never extends beyond the inframammary fold. If necessary, after tailor-tacking, any residual dog ear can be excised, leaving a small transverse scar in the inframammary fold.

Tailor-tacking is particularly important at this portion of the procedure and should precede any committed excisions of the planned skin design. If the ptosis is severe and the surgeon is confident that a vertical technique is required, the safest way to enter the breast is in a vertical manner within the planned area of de-epithelialization. Theoretically, this dissection would be parallel to the neurovascular supply to the nipple; however, if there is any question regarding the need for a vertical excision, a periareolar approach is used.

The design is tailor-tacked with the patient sitting upright once the implant is in place. The amount of excess skin that can safely be removed is now more accurately determined. These areas are de-epithelialized, and minimal subcutaneous undermining is performed around the areola after incising the dermis, leaving a 5- to 7-mm dermal cuff. The vertical closure is usually 6 to 8 cm in length depending on the implant and final total breast size. Greater vertical lengths are addressed with small transverse triangular excisions based at the inframammary fold. Sometimes, a small excision of excess breast tissue is required in the vertical and transverse components of the design. These maneuvers should be conservative because

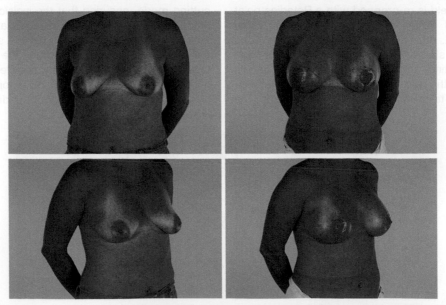

Fig. 8. (*Left*) Preoperative views of the 45-year-old woman seen in previous figures. She had 34B cup breasts and second-degree ptosis with asymmetry. (*Right*) Postoperative view 3 weeks after undergoing bilateral augmentation with Allergan Style 120 textured round silicone gel 400 mL implants with circumvertical mastopexies.

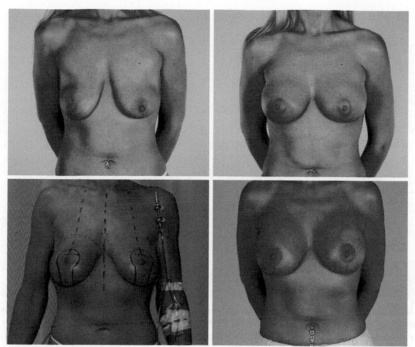

Fig. 9. (*Above, left*) Preoperative view of a 32-year-old woman who lost 100 pounds through exercise and diet. She had 34C cup breasts and second-degree ptosis with asymmetry. (*Above, right*) Postoperative view 6 weeks after under going bilateral augmentation with 280 cc silicone implants with bilateral vertical mastopexies. Despite improvement, the patient desired to be fuller superiorly with more lift. (*Below, left*) Preoperative plan for revision surgery. (*Below, right*) Postoperative view 3 months after undergoing reaugmentation with 500 cc silicone implants and revision vertical mastopexy. (*From* Spear SL, Boehmler JH, Clemens MW. Augmentation/mastopexy: a 3-year review of a single surgeon's practice. Plast Reconstr Surg 2006;118: 136S–47S; with permission.)

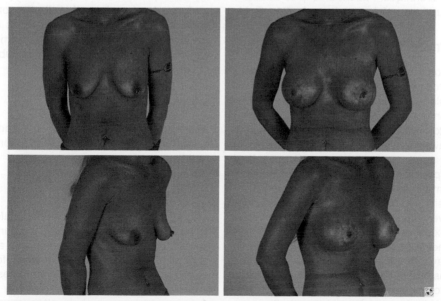

Fig. 10. (*Left*) Preoperative view of a 33-year-old woman who previously had a child and sustained involutional changes in her breasts. She had 32B cup breasts and second-degree ptosis with asymmetry. (*Right*) Postoperative view 4 months after undergoing bilateral augmentation with Allergan right 450 cc and left 425 cc smooth round silicone implants with bilateral circumareolar mastopexies.

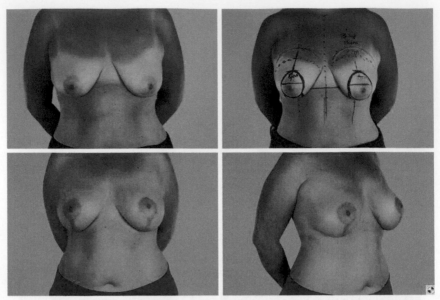

Fig. 11. (*Upper left*) Preoperative view of a 33-year-old woman with 34C cup breasts, second-degree ptosis of both nipples, and breast glands with asymmetry. (*Upper right*) Preoperative markings. (*Bottom*) View of the patient 8 months after undergoing bilateral augmentation with Allergan Style 68 left 250 cc and right 270 cc smooth round saline implants and circumvertical mastopexies.

they increase the risk of implant exposure and vascular compromise. All incisions are then closed using buried interrupted and running Monocryl sutures. If the circumareolar area of excision is significant, the interlocking Gore-tex suture technique may be used for added stability even with the vertical technique. Patient examples at different follow-up time points are shown in **Figs. 8–11**.

COMPLICATIONS AND SIDE EFFECTS

The most common sources of litigation in augmentation/mastopexy include inappropriate use of the circumareolar excision pattern and nipple malposition. When used too aggressively, poor scarring, areolar distortion, and flattening of the breast may occur. To avoid these potential problems, when in doubt, the surgeon should use a circumvertical pattern, especially when the ratio of the outer to inner circumareolar diameter is larger than 3:1.

A malpositioned NAC is usually the result of poor preoperative planning or committing to the planned excision without intraoperative tailor-tacking. These maneuvers are critical because it is not always possible to accurately predict the new dimensions of the breast once the implant is placed. Most commonly, the nipple is inadequately raised, which can be addressed with a simple revision. A NAC that is too high is a more difficult problem because surgical correction is difficult and may leave the patient with a visible

scar in the superior pole of the breast that may be visible in a swimsuit or low-cut dress.

Perhaps the most dreaded complication is nipple necrosis. In patients who have previously undergone breast reduction, mastopexy, or augmentation, the risks may be significant. In secondary cases, when in doubt, the mastopexy may be performed using de-epithelialization only without undermining the skin. If redraping is necessary, undermining should always be performed conservatively (1 to 2 cm) in a superficial subcutaneous plane.

POSTOPERATIVE CARE

Patients are placed in a soft bra and observed closely in the first few days to monitor the nipple and flaps.

SUMMARY

Augmentation/mastopexy can be a safe and gratifying procedure for the patient and surgeon when performed with thoughtful planning and careful execution. Patients should be well informed preoperatively that breast asymmetries may be improved but are never completely corrected. A symmetric approach is often appropriate for mild asymmetries, whereas different excision patterns may be required for significant asymmetries. Care must always be taken in the extent of undermining around the areola and ideally should be limited to the minimum required to redrape the skin. The risk of NAC malposition may be reduced by careful intraoperative tailor-tacking but is ultimately dependent on several unpredictable variables.

REFERENCES

1. Karnes J, Morrison W, Salisbury M, et al. Simultaneous breast augmentation and lift. Aesthetic Plast Surg 2000;24:148–54.
2. Owsley JQ Jr. Simultaneous mastopexy and augmentation for correction of the small, ptotic breast. Ann Plast Surg 1979;2:195–200.
3. Snow JW. Crescent mastopexy and augmentation. Plast Reconstr Surg 1986;77:161–2.
4. Hoffman S. Some thoughts on augmentation/mastopexy and medical malpractice. Plast Reconstr Surg 2004;113:1892–3.
5. Gonzales-Ulloa M. Correction of hypotrophy of the breast by exogenous material. Plast Reconstr Surg 1960;25:15–26.
6. American Society for Aesthetic Plastic Surgery. Available at: www.surgery.org Accessed June 28, 08.
7. Spear SL, Venturi ML. Augmentation with periareolar mastopexy. In: Spear SL, editor. Surgery of the breast: principles and art, Vol. 2. 2nd edition. Philadelphia: Lippincott Williams & Wilkins; 2006. p. 1393–402.
8. Spear SL, Pelletiere CV, Menon N. One-stage augmentation combined with mastopexy: aesthetic results and patient satisfaction. Aesthetic Plast Surg 2004;28:259–67.
9. Spear SL, Giese SY. Simultaneous breast augmentation and mastopexy. Journal of Aesthetic Surgery 2000;20:155–65.
10. Spear SL, Davison SP. Breast augmentation with periareolar mastopexy. Operative Techniques in Plastic and Reconstructive Surgery 2000;7:131–6.
11. Spear SL, Low M, Ducic I. Revision augmentation mastopexy: indications, operations, and outcomes. Ann Plast Surg 2003;51:540–6.
12. Davison SP, Spear SL. Simultaneous breast augmentation with periareolar mastopexy. Seminars in Plastic Surgery 2004;18:189–202.
13. Spear SL. Augmentation/mastopexy: surgeon, beware. Plast Reconstr Surg 2003;112:905–6.
14. Spear SL, Boehmler JH, Clemens MW. Augmentation/mastopexy: a 3-year review of a single surgeon's practice. Plast Reconstr Surg 2006;118: 136S–47S [discussion: 148S–51S].
15. Regnault P. The hypoplastic and ptotic breast: a combined operation with prosthetic augmentation. Plast Reconstr Surg 1966;37:31–7.
16. Brink RR. Evaluating breast parenchymal maldistribution with regard to mastopexy and augmentation mammaplasty. Plast Reconstr Surg 2000;106:491–6.
17. Baran CN, Peker F, Ortak T, et al. Unsatisfactory results of periareolar mastopexy with or without augmentation and reduction mammoplasty: enlarged areola with flattened nipple. Aesthetic Plast Surg 2001;25:286–9.
18. Cardenas-Camarena L, Ramirez-Macias R. Augmentation/mastopexy: how to select and perform the proper technique. Aesthetic Plast Surg 2006; 30:21–33.
19. de la Fuente A, Martin del Yerro JL. Periareolar mastopexy with mammary implants. Aesthetic Plast Surg 1992;16:337–41.
20. Tebbets JB. Dual plane breast augmentation: optimizing implant-soft-tissue relationships in a wide range of breast types. Plast Reconstr Surg 2001; 107(5):1255–72.
21. Adams WP Jr, Rios JL, Smith SJ. Enhancing patient outcomes in aesthetic and reconstructive breast surgery using triple antibiotic breast irrigation: six-year prospective clinical study. Plast Reconstr Surg 2006;118(7 Suppl):46S–52S.
22. Elliott LF. Circumareolar mastopexy with augmentation. Clin Plast Surg 2002;29:337–47.
23. Gasperoni C, Salgarello M, Gargani G. Experience and technical refinements in the "donut" mastopexy with augmentation mammaplasty. Aesthetic Plast Surg 1988;12:111–4.
24. Benelli L. A new periareolar mammaplasty: the "round block" technique. Aesthetic Plast Surg 1990;14:93–100.
25. Ceydeli A, Freund RM. "Tear-drop augmentation mastopexy": a technique to augment superior pole hollow. Aesthetic Plast Surg 2003;27:425–32 [discussion: 433].
26. Gruber R, Denkler K, Hvistendahl Y. Extended crescent mastopexy with augmentation. Aesthetic Plast Surg 2006;30:269–74 [discussion: 275–6].
27. Nigro DM. Crescent mastopexy and augmentation. Plast Reconstr Surg 1985;76:802–3.
28. Persoff MM. Vertical mastopexy with expansion augmentation. Aesthetic Plast Surg 2003;27:13–9.

Commentary

This article nicely summarizes all the approaches to one of the most demanding operations in breast surgery. The authors emphasize that mastopexy may be more challenging or unpredictable when performed simultaneously with breast augmentation. However, the combination of both techniques can be an effective way of producing an aesthetic breast form, as seen in Dr. Spear's postoperative results.

As the breast mound descends on the chest wall, patients display variability in breast shape, tissue laxity, symmetry, parenchymal distribution, and nipple position. Although numerous options exist for restoring a youthful-appearing breast, the common goals are to raise the nipple-areola complex, decrease the skin envelope, achieve symmetry, and improve the breast shape, while maintaining or increasing volume.

Because mastopexy patients are highly concerned with an aesthetically pleasing outcome, we have started performing internal lifts concurrent with an augmentation in a select group of patients who meet distinct criteria. Besides recreating a youthful, firm breast, reducing the extent of scarring is one of the major concerns. Because ptosis includes an enormous spectrum of different shapes and volumes, it is not practical to correct all the different aspects with a single approach. To be able to offer an optimal solution for all augmentation mastopexy candidates, the plastic surgeon has to master more than one technique and will find this article useful and practical.

Allen Gabriel, MD
11175 Campus Street, Suite 21126
Loma Linda, CA 92354

G. Patrick Maxwell, MD
11175 Campus Street, Suite 21126
Loma Linda, CA 92354

E-mail addresses:
agabriel@llu.edu (A. Gabriel)
gpm@maxwellaesthetics.com (G.P. Maxwell)

Clin Plastic Surg 36 (2009) 117
doi:10.1016/j.cps.2008.10.001

Capsular Contracture: What is It? What Causes It? How Can It Be Prevented and Managed?

William P. Adams Jr, MD

KEYWORDS
- Capsular contracture • Breast implants
- Breast augmentation • Breast augmentation outcomes

For more than 40 years, capsular contracture has remained the most common complication in aesthetic and reconstructive breast surgery. This pathologic process occurs in response to the implantation of breast prostheses and is one of the most common causes of reoperation following implantation.[1–3] Despite theories and anecdotal reports, the etiology of capsular contracture and its treatment remain unresolved.

The economic impact of capsular contracture in aesthetic and reconstructive breast surgery is not insignificant considering the data from the Mentor and Allergan pre-market approval studies (PMAs) that cite capsular contracture rates for both saline and gel implants at 15% for augmentation and for reconstruction patients between 15% and 30%. With these current statistics, approximately 45,000 individuals are affected with capsular contracture in the United States alone on an annual basis merely for primary breast augmentation.[4–6]

The etiology of capsular contracture has been considered for many years. Potential etiologies include the hypertrophic scar hypothesis, myofibroblasts, silicone gel bleed, hematoma theory, age, and the infectious theory. Most of these theories do not have sound data to support their relevance; however, the infectious theory has accumulated a plethora of supporting data and remains the leading theory for this condition. Nevertheless, most experts feel that capsular contracture is a multifactorial problem. What we know is at the cellular level capsular contracture is most likely caused by any factor producing inflammation within the periprosthetic pocket and near the developing capsule.

Data have also suggested that capsular contracture and its relation to the infectious theory is a polymicrobial issue with multiple bacteria implicated in the formation of capsular contracture (**Box 1**). Recent work on biofilms and the propensity for these to attach to the silicone elastomer has further supported the infectious theory for capsular contracture, and it is now evident that multiple bacterial strains, both biofilm and nonbiofilm, may cause this condition.[7]

Current understanding of capsular contracture can be viewed as a balance of multiple related factors that affect peri-prosthetic inflammation. There are potentiators of capsular contracture including bacteria, tissue trauma, and blood, and there are suppressors of inflammation including antibiotic irrigations, sound surgical technique, implant type, and, to a lesser extent, other modalities such as massage and vitamins (**Fig. 1**). It is the net sum of the potentiators and suppressors that ultimately result in the pathologic state of capsular contracture.

Financial Disclosures: Investigator for Allergan and Mentor cohesive gel IDE trials. Medical director of Mentor Corporation cohesive gel implant (CPG) trial 2001-2007. Consultant to Ethicon, Allergan. Scientific Advisor - TyRx, Axis-3.

Department of Plastic Surgery, University of Texas Southwestern Medical Center, 6901 Snider Plaza, Suite 120, Dallas, TX 75205, USA
E-mail address: dr@dr-adams.com

Clin Plastic Surg 36 (2009) 119–126
doi:10.1016/j.cps.2008.08.007
0094-1298/08/$ – see front matter © 2008 Published by Elsevier Inc.

Box 1
Established polymicrobial factors in formation of capsular contracture

Staphylococcus epidermidis

Diptheroids

Propionobacter acnes

Enterobacter cloacae

Camphoctophaga

Group D Enterococcus

Propionibacter granulosum

Staphylococcus aureus

Peptococcus

Streptococcus gamma

Propionibacterium avidum

Micrococcus

Clostridium clostridia

Bacillus cereus

Clostridium cadav

Enterobacter agglo

Escherichia coli

Proteus mirabilis

Pseudomonas

Potentiation of capsular contracture is thought to be a result of either bacterial contamination of the pocket or another factor that stimulates inflammation and fibroblast growth, which leads to collagen deposition and contracture.[8,9]

PREVENTION OF CAPSULAR CONTRACTURE

The best defense against capsular contracture is a good offense of techniques that have resulted in a reduced capsular contracture based on sound data. Optimal outcomes for the breast augmentation patient have been reported using the process of breast augmentation, which includes surgical techniques that minimize capsular contracture.[10]

A refined surgical technique has been shown to produce improved outcomes and recovery for breast augmentation patients. Bacteria, including *Staphylococcus epidermidis*, have been cultured from capsules taken from open capsulotomies[11] and the association of capsular contracture has been confirmed.[7,12–15] Multiple other bacterial strains have been cultured around breast implants and implicated in capsular contracture.[16] Data also suggest that some of these bacterial strains live in an armored biofilm that can attach to the silicone elastomer, making eradication of this colonization difficult. Antimicrobial agents/irrigations have been shown to be effective in reducing capsular contracture following breast augmentation and reconstruction.[1,11]

Breast pocket irrigation has been universally practiced and recommended for many years; however, the specifics of this technique have been ill defined. Since multiple bacteria have been implicated in the subclinical infectious theory producing capsular contracture, many of the irrigations used by surgeons have been inadequate to give broad-spectrum coverage against these bacteria. In fact, the first scientific investigation to assess in vitro efficacy of commonly used breast pocket irrigations, including tea-color betadine, double antibiotic solution (polymyxin B and gentamicin), cefazolin (Ancef) irrigation, bacitracin

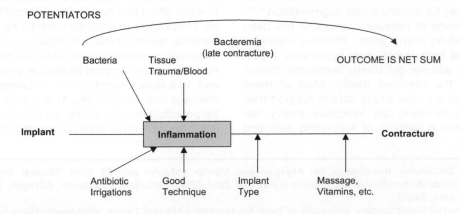

POTENTIATORS

Bacteremia (late contracture)

Bacteria   Tissue Trauma/Blood

OUTCOME IS NET SUM

Implant ——————— Inflammation ——————— Contracture

Antibiotic Irrigations   Good Technique   Implant Type   Massage, Vitamins, etc.

SUPPRESSORS

Fig. 1. Etiology of capsular contracture. The early inflammatory response on the cellular level is the key to understanding the etiology of contracture.

irrigation, determined that all of these irrigation provided inadequate broad-spectrum coverage against the desired bacteria.[17] In a series of investigations, Adams and colleagues[17] considered many of the commonly used breast pocket irrigations and concluded that the most optimal broad-spectrum coverage was provided with a combination of 50 mL of stock betadine solution, 1 g of cefazolin, 80 mg of gentamicin, and 500 mL of normal saline. This combination of irrigation provided excellent broad-spectrum coverage while minimizing the concentration of betadine, which has been shown to be cytotoxic to fibroblast and wound healing. Following this publication, during the saline implant PMA hearings and subsequent approval of saline implants, the Food and Drug Administration (FDA) provided saline implant labeling that included the recommendation for a contraindication to any contact with the implant with betadine. The logic of this restriction has been previously detailed; however, it is important to understand that this concern stemmed from a series of saline implant deflations reported to Mentor Corporation primarily from a single surgeon who was placing betadine irrigation intraluminally in the saline device.[18] Mentor Corporation performed a host of excellent implant-betadine bench testings, all of which indicated no effect of shell integrity with any extraluminal betadine; however, there was a negative effect on shell integrity when betadine was placed within the device intraluminally. In a similar time frame, there were also some data to suggest some elastomer fill tube weakening in Spectrum and Becker port tubings when coming in contact with betadine solution. Interestingly, these fill tubes were vulcanized using a peroxide catalyst that is not used in the room temperature vulcanization (RTV) vulcanization of saline implant shells; however, the peroxide catalyst is used for one portion of the saline implant valve, which is located on the intraluminal portion of the valve. This information further elucidated a coherent and logical explanation for all of the observations and again confirmed that extraluminal betadine would have no effect on shells of implants. Furthermore, at the time of the FDA evaluation and recommendations, there was a host of clinical information particularly randomized clinical trails using betadine and nonbetadine solutions in the same patient, which demonstrated no difference in deflation rates between the betadine and nonbetadine sides.[19] Despite what appeared to be quite definitive data on this issue, the FDA still elected to give their recommendation for a contraindication for contact of betadine with implant shell.

Due to this recommendation, further testings for optimal broad-spectrum nonbetadine-containing solutions were performed.[18] The conclusion of these in vitro studies resulted in the recommendation of a triple antibiotic solution of 50,000 units of bacitracin, 1 g of cefazolin, 80 mg gentamicin, and 500 mL of normal saline. Subsequently, the same group performed a clinical trial using the aforementioned irrigating solutions in a 6-year prospective clinical study with the results finding 1.8% capsular contracture in the augmentation group compared with 9.0% in the saline prospective trials and 9.5% in breast reconstruction patients compared with 27.5% in the saline prospective trials.[1] The clinical trial confirmed the original in vitro findings resulting with a four to five times reduction in the capsular contraction rate in breast augmentation and a threefold reduction in capsular contracture in the reconstruction group.

Furthermore, the study concluded that in addition to the triple antibiotic solution, additional technique recommendations include:

- atraumatic pocket dissection under direct vision avoiding blunt instrumentation
- soaking of implants in irrigation solution during pocket dissection,
- irrigation of pocket with 120 to 150 mL of irrigation without any active evacuation,
- cleansing of skin surrounding incisions with irrigation solution,
- glove change before implant handling,
- aseptic implant insertion
- minimize implant manipulation after insertion (gloves washed with antibiotic solution if further implant handling was required)

Breast irrigation alternatives for the antibiotic-allergic patient are detailed in **Table 1**.

Additional relevant data includes a study by Wiener in 2007, which demonstrated that betadine irrigation 50% was associated with a significantly lower capsular contraction rate than irrigating the pockets with saline alone.[20] Incidentally, there was also no increase in deflation rates in the betadine group. Mechanical properties of explants previously irrigated with betadine were also evaluated and found to have no evidence of mechanical weakening of shell properties.[21]

Given the plethora of data and the science of breast implant irrigation, it is clear that there are ample signs to support a reduction in capsular contraction rates with the use of proper antibiotic irrigations and sound surgical technique. As previously mentioned, tissue trauma and bleeding are also known entities that can increase the inflammatory process at the cellular level, and precise surgical techniques that minimize these factors contribute to low contracture rates, and this is a consensus recommendation in the literature.

Table 1
Recommended alternative solutions for breast irrigation for substitution of the bacitracin-cefazolin-gentamicin triple antibiotic solution components[1]

Allergen	Recommended Alternative Irrigation Solution
Cephalosporin or penicillin	Gentamicin (80 mg), povidone-iodine solution (250 mL), normal saline (250 mL)
Bacitracin	Cefazolin (1 g), gentamicin (80 mg), povidone-iodine solution (50 mL), normal saline (50 mL)
Gentamicin/aminoglycoside	Povidone-iodine (250 mL) and normal saline (250 mL)
Iodine	Bacitracin (50,000 units), cefazolin (1 g), gentamicin (80 mg), normal saline (500 mL)

Data from Adams WP Jr, Rios JL, Smith SJ. Enhancing patient outcomes in aesthetic and reconstructive breast irrigation: six-year prospective clinical study. Plast Reconstr Surg 2006;117:30–6.

Ample data also exist to prove that extraluminal betadine does not have detrimental effects on the silicone elastomer. Finally, many surgeons are strong advocates in the use of antibiotic irrigation; yet, there remain some skeptics. It is cogent to keep in mind that this practice is an inexpensive technique with good scientific proof with minimal to no tradeoffs, and in the end, it is difficult to develop a reason not to use these proven irrigations in any aesthetic or reconstructive breast procedure using implants.

Despite the science, the FDA restriction has created surgeon confusion on which antibiotic irrigations are permitted. It is important to understand that the FDA labeling is a recommendation and ultimately the patient and surgeon will determine the direction of care they feel is optimal. For this reason, the use of off-label betadine-containing irrigations is permissible; however, should be accompanied by a written consent or addition of this off-label use of betadine in the standard operative disclosure.

The next horizon in the arena of breast pocket preparation and irrigation will be techniques and products that help standardize this process. Due to continued surgeon confusion about what irrigations are optimal as well as other factors including pharmacists and nurses preparing irrigations with incorrect concentrations and ratios, products are currently being investigated that would obviate and bypass these confounding variables providing a fully standardized method for pocket preparation available for every procedure in every operating room providing optimal coverage. Furthermore, with the development of biofilms and more resistant bacteria, particularly methicillin-resistant *Staphylococcus aureus* (MRSA), current irrigations do not provide local coverage against MRSA, methicillin-resistant *Staphylococcus epidermidis* (MRSE), and vancomycin-resistant *Enterococcus*

(VRE), all which have become more prevalent in the past 5 years in the community. With the development of novel dug-eluting biodegradable systems, a standardized system providing sound coverage against these bacteria appears to be possible and will hopefully be available to clinical use by 2009 in clinical trials.[22]

ADDITIONAL CONSIDERATIONS IN CAPSULAR CONTRACTURE
Systemic Antibiotics

Although systemic antibiotics have been recommended for preventing initial infection at the wound site following surgery, they are not recommended for a primary mode of preventing capsular contracture. One randomized study in two groups of 23 women undergoing breast augmentation showed that the numbers of culturable bacteria from the breast pocket are reduced initially by administration of prophylactic antibiotics (benzylpenicillin and dicloxacillin) 1 hour before surgery, but they had no effect on capsular contracture.[23] After 1 year, the rate of capsular contracture was similar in the groups that both did and did not receive antibiotics before surgery. Furthermore, from the microbiologic perspective, the routine/ accepted perioperative antibiotics do not provide broad-spectrum coverage for the host of polymicrobes that are known to cause capsular contracture.

Implant Texture

The characteristics of the implant can influence the development of capsular contracture. Since the late 1960s, there have been five generations of silicone gel implants,[24] each of which has represented a change in the manufacturing process and the design. The fourth generation represents the post-1992 moratorium devices, similar to the third-generation devices but produced under stricter manufacturing standards. The fifth-generation devices (Allergan 410 and Mentor Contour Profile gel [CPG]) contain an even more highly cohesive silicone gel fill and a textured anatomic shape.[25,26] The progressing generations have correlated with a decreasing incidence of capsular contracture, although it is not clear if this is entirely because of implant design.[25–27] Surface textures were initially developed to mimic surface of polyurethane implants, which were felt to provide reduction in capsular contracture. Nevertheless, what is currently known now is that any capsular contracture benefit of polyurethane devices was related to biochemical effects on the capsule and not the surface texture.

Studies to determine whether texturing the surface of the implant reduces the risk of capsular contracture have yielded mixed results. The impact of texturing on the risk of capsular contracture appears to be affected by the surgical technique. Texturing of the implant surface has been associated with reduced capsular contracture following subglandular placement of saline and gel-filled implants.[28,29] In contrast, texturing of implants did not have a beneficial effect when other techniques of implant placement were used, including submuscular placement,[29,30] even after 10 years.[31] Currently, there is still a lack of definitive data to support a benefit of texture with regard to capsular contracture.

Historically, the type of fill was thought to influence the development of capsular contracture. Older-generation silicone gel devices were characterized by higher gel bleed than current-generation implants and exhibited much higher rupture rates.[32] Capsular contracture rates were sixfold higher with these devices than with devices containing low-bleed silicone gel fillings ($P < .007$).[33] Women receiving implants with fifth-generation form-stable cohesive silicone gel fillings also had lower rates of capsular contracture.[25,26,34–38]

Implant size, projection, and shape may also affect capsular contracture. Large implant size (>350 mL) is associated with the development of capsular contracture and other complications requiring surgical correction, including hematoma, infection, extrusion, skin wrinkling, and palpation of implant folds.[39] The reasons underlying the correlation between large size and increased complications require further study; however, this association has been borne out in the clinical setting as well. The advent of tissue-based planning to match the implant to the breast dimensions and tissue has reduced complications including capsular contracture and reoperation rates to less than 3% with up to 7 years follow-up.[40]

Although capsular contracture most often occurs and is readily evident during the first year after implantation,[3,41–45] it can occur as much as 10 years later.[31] As logic would suggest, in both augmentation and reconstruction, the longer an implant remains in the body, the greater the cumulative risk of capsular contracture.[46,47] The reasons for delayed development of capsular contracture not totally clear; however, systemic bacteremia (other infections or dental procedures) with concurrent micro-fractures in the existing capsule resulting in an intra-capsular inoculum may be implicated.[46,47]

Postoperative Drains

Postoperative drains were thought to have a role in reducing the risk of capsular contracture. In a 1978 study, use of these drains with low intermittent suction significantly reduced capsular contracture ($P < .05$) and the need for capsulotomy ($P < .02$) as compared with surgeries that did not use drains. If suction was not employed, however, there was no difference in the incidence of capsular contracture.[48] Nevertheless, this study is felt to be outdated because of the many variables present 30 years ago.

Conversely, the use of drains was associated with a fivefold increased risk of infection.[49] Although definitive data do not exist, there is a large body of clinical data showing low capsular contracture rates when a drain is not used.[1,25,26,33,35]

Augmentation Incisions and Capsular Contracture

Two recent studies assessed the association of incision types with Baker grade III/IV capsular contracture. The prospective study, using a Danish registry of 2277 women, found that surgical routes other than inframammary incisions were associated with a relative risk of capsular contracture of 5.8 (95% CI, 1.9–13.0).[39] In addition, a retrospective study of 430 women showed that periareolar incisions were 16.1 times more likely to result in capsular contracture than were inframammary incisions ($P < .0001$).[50] This was a follow-up to a previous study demonstrating that betadine was effective in preventing capsular contracture following breast augmentation. Patients treated with betadine-soaked gauze placed on the nipple-areola complex in addition to irrigation with betadine had the lowest incidence of capsular contracture (0.5% of 211 patients), as well as having no deflation of implants after 10 months.[20] Types of incisions that minimize the exposure of the implant to contaminants can reduce the risk of capsular contracture. Periareolar incisions are more disruptive to the ductal system harboring the bacteria, possibly accounting for the increased risk of capsular contracture.[50]

These data may reshape how certain cosmetic breast procedures are performed, particularly procedures such as augmentation mastopexy where the implant may be placed through a periareolar incision or a separate inframammary incision. A separate incision may be more prudent for reduction of capsular contracture.

Treatment of Capsular Contracture

Treatment of an established capsular contracture typically involves the gold standard of a total capsulectomy removing the entire affected capsule and implant. The majority of capsular contractures occur in the first year postimplantation. The timing of treatment for an early capsular contracture should allow enough time for the process to reach a homeostasis where there is not an ongoing progression in the contracture. Generally 6 to 9 months from the time of diagnosis is adequate for an early capsular contracture.

Due to known issues with biofilms, which are extremely hard to eradicate from the silicone elastomer of the implant, it is advisable to use a new implant in the affected breast when treating the capsular contracture. Other adjuncts to the surgical treatment of contracture include considering a site change and, particularly if the implant is in the subglandular position, a site change to a subpectoral or dual-plane position may be considered or, in extreme cases, sometimes exchanging the implant to a fresh pocket: even subpectoral to a subglandular position may be considered. In the author's experience, a subpectoral or dual-plane pocket plan is optimal, and it is my preference to place implants in the dual-plane pocket position regardless of whether they were previously in that position.

There have also been consistent reports that a total capsulectomy is the gold standard for the treatment of contracture. There has been anecdotal discussion of using a precapsular dissection leaving the existing capsule in place and inserting the new implant between the anterior capsule and the posterior surface of the muscle for treatment of capsular contracture; however, no good data on this technique are available to make a judgment on its efficacy. Given the basis of the pathology and the relation to an antimicrobial source, the logic of leaving a portion of the capsule remains to be fully elucidated.

There has been much interest in the nonsurgical treatment of capsular contracture. A variety of different modalities have been considered, including mechanical implant displacement, antibiotics, Vitamin E, external ultrasound, steroids, nonsteroidal anti-inflammatory drugs (NSAIDs), chemotherapeutics, and leukotriene inhibitors. No definitive data have been reported with a variety of anecdotal experiences presented.

The latter consideration (Accolate and Singulair) has received the most exposure in the past 2 years. Several studies indicate leukotriene receptor antagonists (LTRAs)—specifically Accolate (zafirlukast) and Singulair (montelukast)—may be a potential treatment for capsular contracture. To date, the data indicating zafirlukast or montelukast for capsular contracture prevention or inhibition is anecdotal. Results of a 2006 preliminary study by Scuderi and colleagues[51] suggest zafirlukast may reduce pain and breast capsule distortion for patients with established contracture. A subsequent study in 2007, also by Scuderi and colleagues,[52] supports these findings.

These drugs used for asthma have their pharmacologic effect along pathways thought to be related to the pathogenesis of capsular contracture. There have been some significant (mostly hepatotoxicity-related) adverse effects with these drugs, and without good scientific basis for their efficacy the off-label use of these medications, particularly Accolate, is not recommended.[53,54] Hopefully there will be some more definitive scientific assessment of this modality in the future.

Postoperative Care

Because most contractures manifest within 12 months, patients should be seen several times during the first year and once per year thereafter. No definitive data exist for the postoperative period; however, certain practices deserve comment. A defined postoperative regimen has been demonstrated to contribute to improved patient outcomes. It is permissible to resume light activities of daily living, but any potential trauma or increase in heart rate to above 100 for the first 2 weeks postoperation should be avoided.

Implant displacement exercises have been advocated for many years, although no good data exist regarding their real impact. Smooth implant displacement likely does not cause any negative effects. Implant displacement in a textured device is not recommended as it may interfere with the implant/soft-tissue interface that develops.

SUMMARY

Capsular contracture has been the nemesis of plastic surgeons for over 45 years, but we are beginning to see the light in prevention and treatment of this malady. Although the true etiology of capsular contracture appears to be multifactorial, its basis/source is at the cellular level with factors that increase inflammation resulting in the expression of capsular contracture. Using known techniques including aseptic techniques with appropriate antibacterial pocket irrigations and atraumatic precise bloodless surgical technique, the incidence of capsular contracture has been significantly minimized compared with typical rates seen before these advancements. No doubt, the coming years will be exciting as we further define this problem and again advance the science for the benefit of our patients.

REFERENCES

1. Adams WP Jr, Rios JL, Smith SJ. Enhancing patient outcomes in aesthetic and reconstructive breast surgery using triple antibiotic breast irrigation: six-year prospective clinical study. Plast Reconstr Surg 2006;117:30.
2. Spear SL, Low M, Ducic I. Revision augmentation mastopexy: indications, operations, and outcomes. Ann Plast Surg 2003;51:540.
3. McLaughlin JK, Lipworth L, Murphy DK, et al. The safety of silicone gel-filled breast implants: a review of the epidemiologic evidence. Ann Plast Surg 2007; 59:569.
4. U.S.Food and Drug Administration. Summary of safety and effectiveness data. Available at: http://www.fda.gov/cdrh/pdf3/p0.30053b.pdf. and http://fda.gov/cdrh/pdf2/p020056b.pdf. Accessed October 19, 2007.
5. Spear SL, Murphy DK, Slicton A, et al. for the Inamed Silicone Breast Implant US Study Group. Inamed silicone breast implant core study results at 6 years. Plast Reconstr Surg 2007;120:8S.
6. Cunningham B. The Mentor core study on silicone MemoryGel breast implants. Plast Reconstr Surg 2007;120:19S.
7. Pajkos A, Deva AK, Vickery K, et al. Detection of subclinical infection in significant breast implant capsules. Plast Reconstr Surg 2003;111:1605.
8. Kamel M, Protzner K, Fornasier V, et al. The peri-implant breast capsule: an immunophenotypic study of capsules taken at explantation surgery. J Biomed Mater Res 2001;58:88.
9. Adams WP Jr, Haydon MS, Raniere J Jr, et al. A rabbit model for capsular contracture: development and clinical implications. Plast Reconstr Surg 2006; 117:1214.
10. Adams WP. The process of breast augmentation: 4 sequential steps to optimizing outcomes for patients. Accepted PRS 2008.
11. Burkhardt BR, Fried M, Schnur PL, et al. Capsules, infection, and intraluminal antibiotics. Plast Reconstr Surg 1981;68:43.
12. Virden CP, Dobke MK, Stein P, et al. Subclinical infection of the silicone breast implant surface as a possible cause of capsular contracture. Aesthetic Plast Surg 1992;16:173.
13. Dobke MK, Svahn JK, Vastine VL, et al. Characterization of microbial presence at the surface of silicone mammary implants. Ann Plast Surg 1995;34:563.
14. Netscher DT, Weizer G, Wigoda P, et al. Clinical relevance of positive breast periprosthetic cultures without overt infection. Plast Reconstr Surg 1995; 96:1125.
15. Macadam SA, Clugston PA, Germann ET. Retrospective case review of capsular contracture after two-stage breast reconstruction: is colonization of the tissue expander pocket associated with subsequent implant capsular contracture? Ann Plast Surg 2004;53:420.
16. Ahn CY, Ko CY, Wagar EA, et al. Microbial evaluation: 139 implants removed from symptomatic patients. Plast Reconstr Surg 1996;98:1225.
17. Adams WP Jr, Conner WC, Barton FE Jr, et al. Optimizing breast pocket irrigation: an in vitro study and clinical implications. Plast Reconstr Surg 2000; 105:334.
18. Adams WP Jr, Conner WC, Barton FE Jr, et al. Optimizing breast-pocket irrigation: the post-Betadine era. Plast Reconstr Surg 2001;107:1596.
19. Burkhardt BR, Eades E. The effect of Biocell texturing and povidone-iodine irrigation on capsular contracture around saline-inflatable breast implants. Plast Reconstr Surg 1995;96:1317.
20. Wiener TC. The role of Betadine irrigation in breast augmentation. Plast Reconstr Surg 2007;119:12.
21. Brandon HJ, Young VL, Jerina KL, et al. Mechanical analysis of explanted saline filled breast implants exposed to betadine pocket irrigation. Aesthetic Surgery Journal 2002;22:438.
22. Adams WP. Optimizing breast implant pocket preparation new horizons prevention of experimental capsular contracture in breast implants by antimicrobial-impregnated biodegradable sleeve. Presented at the American Society of Aesthetic Plastic Surgery Annual Meeting, San Diego; May 3, 2008.
23. Gylbert L, Asplund O, Berggren A, et al. Preoperative antibiotics and capsular contracture in augmentation mammaplasty. Plast Reconstr Surg 1990;86:260.
24. Adams WP Jr, Potter JK. Breast implants: materials and manufacturing past, present and future. In: Spear S, Willey SC, Robb GL, et al, editors. Surgery of the breast: principles and art. 2nd edition. Baltimore (MD): Lippincott Williams & Wilkins; 2005.
25. Bengtson BP, Van Natta BW, Murphy DK, et al. for the Style 410 US Core Clinical Study Group. Style 410 highly cohesive silicone breast implant core study results at 3 years. Plast Reconstr Surg 2007; 120:40S.

26. Cunningham B. The Mentor study on contour profile gel silicone MemoryGel breast implants. Plast Reconstr Surg 2007;120:33S.

27. Danino AM, Basmacioglu P, Saito S, et al. Comparison of the capsular response to the Biocell RTV and Mentor 1600 Siltex breast implant surface texturing: a scanning electron microscopic study. Plast Reconstr Surg 2001;108:2047.

28. Pollock H. Breast capsular contracture: a retrospective study of textured versus smooth silicone implants. Plast Reconstr Surg 1993;91:404.

29. Barnsley GP, Sigurdson LJ, Barnsley SE. Textured surface breast implants in the prevention of capsular contracture among breast augmentation patients: a meta-analysis of randomized controlled trials. Plast Reconstr Surg 2006;117:2182.

30. Collis N, Coleman D, Foo IT, et al. Ten-year review of a prospective randomized controlled trial of textured versus smooth subglandular silicone gel breast implants. Plast Reconstr Surg 2000;106:786.

31. Handel N, Cordray T, Gutierrez J, et al. A long-term study of outcomes, complications, and patient satisfaction with breast implants. Plast Reconstr Surg 2006;117:757.

32. Malata CM, Varma S, Scott M, et al. Silicone breast implant rupture: common/serious complication? Med Prog Technol 1994;20:251.

33. Chang L, Caldwell E, Reading G, et al. A comparison of conventional and low-bleed implants in augmentation mammaplasty. Plast Reconstr Surg 1992;89:79.

34. Bogetti P, Boltri M, Balocco P, et al. Augmentation mammaplasty with a new cohesive gel prosthesis. Aesthetic Plast Surg 2000;24:440.

35. Hedén P, Jernbeck J, Hober M. Breast augmentation with anatomical cohesive gel implants: the world's largest current experience. Clin Plast Surg 2001;28:531.

36. Drever J. Cohesive gel implants for breast augmentation. Aesthetic Surg J 2003;23:405.

37. Brown MH, Shenker R, Silver SA. Cohesive silicone gel breast implants in aesthetic and reconstructive breast surgery. Plast Reconstr Surg 2005;116:768.

38. Henriksen TF, Fryzek JP, Hölmich LR, et al. Reconstructive breast implantation after mastectomy for breast cancer: clinical outcomes in a nationwide prospective cohort study. Arch Surg 2005;140:1152.

39. Henriksen TF, Fryzek JP, Holmich LR, et al. Surgical intervention and capsular contracture after breast augmentation: a prospective study of risk factors. Ann Plast Surg 2005;54:343.

40. Tebbetts JB, Adams WP. Five critical decisions in breast augmentation using five measurements in 5 minutes: the high five decision support process. Plast Reconstr Surg 2005;116:35S.

41. Hakelius L, Ohlsén L. Tendency to capsular contracture around smooth and textured gel-filled silicone mammary implants: a five-year follow-up. Plast Reconstr Surg 1997;100:1566.

42. Kjøller K, Hölmich LR, Jacobsen PH, et al. Epidemiological investigation of local complications after cosmetic breast implant surgery in Denmark. Ann Plast Surg 2002;48:229.

43. Coleman DJ, Foo IT, Sharpe DT. Textured or smooth implants for breast augmentation? A prospective controlled trial. Br J Plast Surg 1991;44:444.

44. Tarpila E, Ghassemifar R, Fagrell D, et al. Capsular contracture with textured versus smooth saline-filled implants for breast augmentation: a prospective clinical study. Plast Reconstr Surg 1997;99:1934.

45. Peters W, Smith D, Fornasier V, et al. An outcome analysis of 100 women after explantation of silicone gel breast implants. Ann Plast Surg 1997;39:9.

46. Ablaza VJ, LaTrenta GS. Late infection of a breast prosthesis with Enterococcus avium. Plast Reconstr Surg 1998;102:227.

47. Adams WP. Silicone gel implants: what data do you and your patients need to know? Presented at the American Society of Plastic Surgeons's 21st Annual Breast Surgery and Body Contouring Symposium, Santa Fe, NM, August 23–26, 2006.

48. Hipps CJ, Raju R, Straith RE. Influence of some operative and postoperative factors on capsular contracture around breast prostheses. Plast Reconstr Surg 1978;61:384.

49. Araco A, Gravante G, Araco F, et al. Infections of breast implants in aesthetic breast augmentations: a single-center review of 3,002 patients. Aesthetic Plast Surg 2007;31:325.

50. Wiener TC. Relationship of incision choice to capsular contracture. Aesthetic Plast Surg 2008;32:303.

51. Scuderi N, Mazzocchi M, Fioramonti P, et al. The effects of zafirlukast on capsular contracture: preliminary report. Aesthetic Plast Surg 2006;30:513.

52. Scuderi N, Mazzocchi M, Rubino C. Effects of zafirlukast on capsular contracture: controlled study measuring the mammary compliance. Int J Immunopathol Pharmacol 2007;20:577.

53. Accolate [package insert]. Wilmington, DE: AstraZeneca Pharmaceuticals LP; 2004.

54. Singulair [package insert]. Whitehouse Station, NJ: Merck & Co., Inc.; 2008.

Management of Common and Uncommon Problems After Primary Breast Augmentation

Maurice Y. Nahabedian, MD, FACS*, Ketan Patel, MD

KEYWORDS
- Breast augmentation
- Common problems after breast augmentation
- Rippling • Breast neoplasms • Breast hematoma
- Implant displacement

Breast augmentation continues to be one of the most sought-after cosmetic procedures for women. Since 1962, this operation has continued to evolve and improve as our understanding of the devices themselves, surgical techniques, and patient selection criteria have increased. Current devices are manufactured with better implant shells and filler materials and are available in a variety of shapes and sizes. Surgical techniques emphasize the importance of absolute sterility, meticulous homeostasis, and proper dissection techniques. Patient selection has focused on ideal proportions, optimizing approach, and ensuring realistic expectations. Thus, our ability to deliver reproducible and predictable outcomes has improved as our scientific understanding of breast augmentation and our artistic abilities have increased. Patient satisfaction continues to remain high and current demographics reveal an increase in the demand and delivery of primary breast augmentation.

As a result of these advancements in primary breast augmentation, clinical outcomes have improved; however, they are not always perfect. Many of these imperfections are related to symmetry based on the contour, position, and volume of the breast or nipple areolar complex. These may be appreciated early in the postoperative period or later. Some are relatively common and others are not. Some may be within the control of the operating surgeon and others may not. In either event, many of these problems can be adequately and appropriately managed.

The purpose of this article is to review some of the common and uncommon problems that can arise following primary breast augmentation. Reviews have demonstrated that the incidence is not as low as one would intuitively think with approximately 20% of women developing some type of problem.[1,2] These problems and morbidities are all-inclusive and do not constitute any one condition. This article evaluates several of these morbidities that are encountered within this subset of patients. These include asymmetry, implant displacement, and rippling and wrinkling. Capsular contracture would also be included in this group but will be covered as a separate article. Less common problems will include late hematomas and benign and malignant tumors following breast augmentation, as well as management of complex deformities or distortions. Solutions will emphasize operative correction and prevention. A brief review of postoperative complications precedes the review on common and uncommon problems.

POSTOPERATIVE COMPLICATIONS

As with all surgical procedures, there are inherent risks of bleeding and infection. Fortunately, these

Department of Plastic Surgery, Georgetown University, 3800 Reservoir Rd, NW, 1st Floor, PHC, WA 20007, USA
* Corresponding author.
E-mail address: drnahabedian@aol.com (M.Y. Nahabedian).

Clin Plastic Surg 36 (2009) 127–138
doi:10.1016/j.cps.2008.07.002

plasticsurgery.theclinics.com

morbidities constitute less than 2% of prosthetic breast augmentation procedures.[3-6] Prevention is for the most part related to proper surgical technique; however, there are situations in which complications occur that are outside of the control of the operating surgeon.

Hematoma

Hematoma formation is an uncommon complication following augmentation mammaplasty with an incidence that ranges from 1% to 2%.[3,4] Its prevention dictates meticulous intraoperative hemostasis and the judgmental use of postoperative drains. Possible bleeding sources include perforating vessels based off of the internal mammary, intercostal, and lateral thoracic vascular systems that may be injured during the pocket dissection phase. My preferred technique is to dissect the implant pocket under direct visualization using a lighted retractor or a nonlighted retractor and a headlamp as well as an electrocautery device. Small vessels are visualized and coagulated before dividing them.

Despite adequate intraoperative hemostasis, postoperative bleeding can sometimes still occur. Reasons for this may include undiagnosed coagulopathies such as von Willebrands disease or platelet dysfunction. Although drains are not routinely used in the authors' practice, their use is considered when there is a generalized oozing that is beyond what is normally seen. Diagnosis of a hematoma may be obvious or subtle depending on the degree of swelling. Ultrasound examination of the affected breast maybe useful for detection.

In the event of an early postoperative hematoma, the patient is immediately returned to the operating room for temporary removal of the implant, evacuation of the hematoma, and to control the source of bleeding. Often times, a discrete bleeding vessel is not found. Following the evacuation and control phase, the pocket is irrigated with a dilute hydrogen peroxide solution followed by antibiotic saline solution. The peroxide serves to dissolve and remove adherent clot. It also has a mild thrombogenic effect. Once hemostasis is ensured, the same device is reinserted as well as a moderate-profile drain. Women are referred to a hematologist for proper evaluation and workup when indicated.

Infection

Infections following breast augmentation are not common with a reported incidence of 1.1%[5] and 1.2%.[6] Postoperative infections typically manifest with erythema, swelling, and pain and may be come evident a few days following the operation and in extreme cases months to years following the operation. Reported organisms have included *Staphylococcus aureus* and *epidermidis*, *Streptococcus*, *Pseudomonas aeruginosa*, and *Mycobacteria*. Treatment must be prompt and aggressive.

The management of a patient with a suspected infection can be perplexing.[7] The first consideration is whether or not the implant can be salvaged. This requires differentiating between a superficial and deep or periprosthetic infection. When a woman initially presents with signs and symptoms of an infection, admission to a hospital for intravenous antibiotics and observation are sometimes recommended. Infectious disease consultation can be useful. Our usual first-line antibiotic is Vancomycin or a broad-spectrum cephalosporin. When outpatient therapy is recommended, a broad-spectrum oral antimicrobial drug is selected. Women are usually assessed at various intervals during the initial 24- to 48-hour period. If the signs and symptoms improve, then the antibiotic therapy is continued usually for a 2-week period based on the recommendation of an infectious disease specialist. If the signs and symptoms do not improve, surgical exploration is considered. In the event of periprosthetic purulence, the prosthetic device is removed, the breast pocket is thoroughly irrigated, and the incision is closed over a closed suction drain. Antibiotic therapy is usually continued for 2 weeks. Reaugmentation is considered no sooner than 6 months following the infection.

COMMON PROBLEMS FOLLOWING BREAST AUGMENTATION

Recognizing that the "common problems" do not commonly occur, there are several that warrant further discussion and will be reviewed in the following sections. Many of the common problems that we as plastic surgeons encounter are ultimately related to asymmetries in volume, contour, and position of the breast or nipple areolar complex. These asymmetries are oftentimes evident preoperatively; however, when they are not recognized preoperatively, they can be exacerbated postoperatively. Another mechanism by which these asymmetries can occur is via surgical technique or device selection. In either case, it is important to recognize the occurrence of a postoperative asymmetry and to have an approach for management. Oftentimes these asymmetries will be self-limiting and improve spontaneously; however, there are situations when secondary procedures may be needed. Before proceeding, the reader should keep in mind that many of the concepts, principles, and management schemes are those adhered to by the primary author and that alternative strategies may be advocated by others.

Asymmetries of Breast Volume and Contour

It is a well-known fact that most women when assessed preoperatively will possess some degree of breast asymmetry.[8] This asymmetry may be because of differences in breast volume, contour, chest wall configuration, or relative positions of the nipple areolar complex. Asymmetries in women with micromastia may be subtle and easily overlooked preoperatively. That said, it is often the case that when performing bilateral breast augmentation, the same technique and the same size prosthetic device is used for both sides. In these cases, the usual outcome will be that these subtle preoperative asymmetries will become exacerbated postoperatively and cause some degree of concern to the patient and surgeon.

To prevent this occurrence, it is best to appreciate the asymmetry preoperatively and take the necessary steps to prevent it postoperatively. This is important because some women are not aware that they are asymmetric. It is extremely important to assess the expectations of all women when considering breast augmentation and especially when there is asymmetry involved. One of the roles of the plastic surgeon is to educate women about the anatomic differences and to review the techniques for correction. Sometimes, the solutions will require additional incisions that some women may not be willing to accept.

Quantitating the degree of asymmetry can be difficult but is assisted by obtaining standardized breast measurements. Topographic analysis can provide useful information regarding the relative proportions of the breast but may be inadequate for subtle volume asymmetries. Adjunct procedures include the use of two- and three-dimensional imaging and analysis. It has been my experience that by viewing a static anterior two-dimensional photograph, volume asymmetries can sometimes be better appreciated. Use of three-dimensional imaging systems have been demonstrated to be quite useful for assessment of breast volumes and quantitating volume differences.[9] It should be remembered, however, that with increasing surgical experience comes a well-trained eye that can further discern some of these asymmetries. When noted preoperatively, modifications in surgical technique or device selection can be applied to correct the asymmetry. When noted postoperatively, the volumetric

information can be useful when planning secondary procedures.

Secondary procedures to correct postoperative asymmetries related to breast volume or contour include exchanging the implant for a different size or modifying the skin envelope. The timing of these secondary procedures is usually no sooner than 6 months following the initial operation for the breast to assume its final state. It has been a personal observation that a small percentage of women can have asymmetry because of protracted unilateral breast edema or because of an implant that is slow to "drop" into its final position. Given enough time, some asymmetries will self-correct. When self-correction does not occur, secondary procedures are usually necessary. This is best accomplished by performing a mastopexy for asymmetries related to the skin envelope and/or an implant exchange for asymmetries related to volume.

When performing a secondary mastopexy, several considerations are important. These include the degree of skin elasticity, the relative positions of the nipple areolar complex, and the relative positions of the breast on the chest wall. It may well be the case that a bilateral mastopexy be recommended because of natural breast ptosis. Options for mastopexy in the setting of a prior augmentation include a crescenteric, periareolar, or circumvertical approach. It is usually a good rule of thumb to select the least invasive procedure to obtain the desired outcome. This is because secondary mastopexy in the previously augmented patient is associated with a higher complication rate because of the altered blood supply to the skin and nipple areolar complex.[10] That said, it has been a personal observation that the circumvertical and periareolar approaches are the most effective when properly designed and outlined in properly selected women. The amount of work required on the part of the plastic surgeon performing a secondary mastopexy is variable and can include revision to the skin envelope, nipple areolar complex, capsule, and implant.[11]

When a mastopexy alone is performed, the ideal location of the nipple areolar complex is determined. If the nipple areolar complex (NAC) requires 1 to 3 cm of elevation, then a periareolar approach is considered; whereas, if greater than 3 cm, a circumvertical approach may be used. Once the cutaneous incisions have been created, the dissection proceeds into the parenchymal tissues to better mobilize the cutaneous envelope and reshape the breast mound. In general, the capsule surrounding the breast implant is not violated unless the implant is to be exchanged as well. In the event that a vertical component of skin is to be excised, the amount is based on pinching the skin between the NAC and inframammary fold along the horizontal axis as well as assessing the medial and lateral excursion of the breast to determine how much can be safely removed. The excision design will taper to a point at the inframammary fold.

Implant Displacement

Implant displacement is an uncommon event but is the most common indication for a secondary procedure following breast augmentation, affecting 1.2% of implants.[12] Displacement can occur in essentially all vectors, including inferior, medial, lateral, and superior. Inferior displacement will result in a discrepancy in the location of the inframammary folds (**Fig. 1**), medial displacement can result in symmastia, and lateral displacement will result in a device that falls into the axillary region when supine. Superior displacement is often the result of capsular contracture or faulty positioning of the device.

The evaluation of a woman with implant displacement requires attention to various factors that include the degree of displacement, quality of the skin, and degree of asymmetry. All four types of displacement have been observed and managed. Lateral displacement results in a device that falls into the axillary region when the patient is in the supine position. This may occur because of an overdissected pocket during the initial augmentation procedure or as a result of excessive contraction of the pectoral major muscle such that occurs with exercises that isolate the function of the pectoralis major muscle. Inferior displacement is defined as a device that sits below the level of the contralateral inframammary fold. The distance from the nipple areolar complex to the inframammary fold is usually lengthened and the breast has an appearance of pseudoptosis with

a "high-riding" nipple areolar complex. This can occur over time or because the inframammary fold was lowered during the primary augmentation to insert a larger device. Following division of the inframammary fold attachments, inferior descent seems to be exacerbated over time. Medial displacement occurs most often when the medial border of the breast pocket has been overdissected with disruption of the sterno-pectoral origin. When bilateral, the deformity may result in a symmastia. Finally, superior displacement is sometimes seen with severe capsular contracture or when a device is placed in the total submuscular position. Release of the inferior origin of the pectoralis major muscle as described with the dual plane technique for implant insertion has been effective in optimizing implant position.[13]

The management of implant displacement can be associated with various degrees of difficulty.[14] Although the repairs seem intuitively simple, these displacements tend to recur, especially the inferior and lateral varieties. The concept dictating the method of repair has included reducing the internal dimensions of the breast pocket by specific placement of nonabsorbable sutures. The technique for this has included either scoring or excising a segment of the breast capsule on the chest wall and the breast parenchyma and then suturing these two layers together. The recurrence is ultimately related to the forces that tend to continue along those vectors.

Traditional techniques for repairing a displaced device based on the different locations are similar in concept but slightly different in practice. When repairing an inferior displaced device, the desired inframammary position is determined. This usually requires that the displaced skin between the inframammary incision and the aberrant inframammary fold be placed back on the chest wall. The capsular tissue between these points is scored or excised to permit tissue adherence. A closed suction drain is always inserted. Traditional repair of a medially displaced device has included scoring the capsular tissue and then placing nonabsorbable sutures along the proposed medial border of the breast. If the pectoral origin has been disrupted and the edge of the muscle is visible, it is reattached to the sternal edge. When repairing a laterally displaced device, it is important to determine the ideal location of the lateral mammary fold. The internal capsule is scored or excised and sutures are used to approximate the lateral breast capsule to the chest wall (**Fig. 2**). Postoperative drain use is essential. In many of these cases, downsizing the implant may be considered to reduce the forces applied to the repair and to minimize the chance of recurrence.

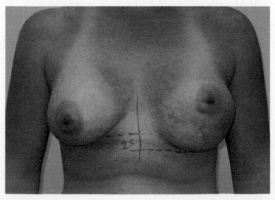

Fig. 1. A woman with 2.5 cm of implant descent following breast augmentation is shown.

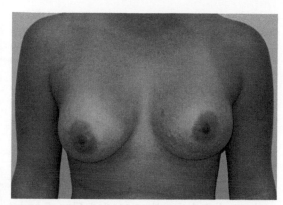

Fig. 2. Postoperative result following excision of inframammary capsule and secondary closure of capsular edges to recreate the inframammary fold. Six-month follow-up.

An alternative technique for repairing the deformity created by a displaced device has included the use of acellular dermal matrices namely Allo-Derm (LifeCell Corporation, Branchburg, NJ).[15] AlloDerm has been used in the authors' practice and found to be very effective in recreating medial, inframammary (**Fig. 3**), and lateral mammary folds. When using AlloDerm in the repair of implant displacement, several caveats should be considered. The AlloDerm should be oriented with the dermal side toward the tissue and away from the device. The use of one or two closed-suction drains is considered important. Finally, there should be no folds in the AlloDerm, in other words, the AlloDerm should be in total contact with the tissue on the

dermal side and the device on the basement membrane side.

The salient technical aspects using AlloDerm include suturing the inferior, lateral, or medial edge of the AlloDerm to the inferior, lateral, or medial chest wall along the fold. The pocket is irrigated with an antibiotic solution. The device is reinserted into the pocket. The opposite edge of the AlloDerm is then sutured to the corresponding site on the breast capsule to prevent the AlloDerm from pleating or drifting. This maneuver will ensure total contact with the AlloDerm and tissue surface. The skin is then closed in the usual manner.

Rippling and Wrinkling

The phenomena of implant rippling and wrinkling (**Fig. 4**) is well known but infrequently reported. Thus, the true incidence is not known. In a recent study of textured saline implants, the incidence of rippling and wrinkling was 37.5%.[16] The occurrence of rippling did not correlate with the fill volume of the device as the difference in rippling between underfilled, recommended filled, and overfilled devices was not significantly different. Personal and reported experience with rippling and wrinkling is that it occurs more frequently following augmentation using saline devices and textured devices; it also occurs when the ratio of implant to parenchyma exceeds 50%.[6,17] It may occur more frequently following subglandular augmentation and when the device is underfilled. The location of the rippling is variable and can occur anywhere on the breast but is usually noticed most inferiorly and superiorly.

The reasons for rippling are variable and depend on the specific factors. When the ratio of device to breast parenchyma exceeds 50%, there is a tendency for the cutaneous skin envelope to atrophy and thin over time leaving the tissues more

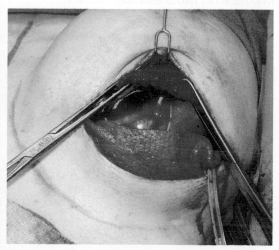

Fig. 3. The use of AlloDerm to set the inframammary fold (IMF) is illustrated. The AlloDerm is sutured to the IMF and to the upper breast capsule to prevent pleats or folds.

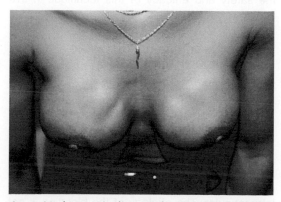

Fig. 4. Moderate rippling and wrinkling following breast augmentation with a round, textured surface, and subglandular implant.

susceptible to rippling. Fill volume is important because if the device is underfilled, there will be folds in the device and the overlying skin will reflect the folding. When the device is overfilled, there may be pleats that form along the perimeter of the device that may be palpable along its course. Textured devices seem to result in more rippling because of the tissue adherence. Thus, any contour issues with the device will translate into a contour irregularity or ripple on the skin surface. Subglandular augmentation may result in increased rippling because there is usually less tissue between the device and the skin surface.

Management of rippling and wrinkling can be complicated, especially if the augmented breast is associated with cutaneous and parenchymal atrophy. First-line treatment would depend on the type, surface characteristics, and location of the device. If it is a saline implant, then exchanging that for a silicone gel implant is considered. If the device is textured, then a smooth device would be considered. If the device is subglandular, then a pocket conversion to the subpectoral space would be considered. Other options would include using the capsule and adjacent layer of fat to add to the thickness of the soft tissues.[18] If the rippling was along the inferior pole, then the upper pole capsule and layer of fat could be incised and rotated inferiorly on a hinge. Another controversial option would be to inject fat into the layer between the skin and capsule of the breast. This would require fat harvesting using standard techniques and injection of the processed fat using fine cannulas into the subcutaneous layer. Temporary removal of the device is recommended during the injection phase. One caveat to fat grafting the noncancerous breast is that fat necrosis and microcalcifications may mimic precancerous changes on mammography and subject the patient to biopsy. Thus, further investigation is needed to determine the safety and efficacy of this technique in this setting.

UNCOMMON PROBLEMS FOLLOWING BREAST AUGMENTATION
Late Hematoma

The occurrence of a late hematoma many years after initial breast augmentation has been reported.[19,20] This will usually manifest as a relatively rapid, unilateral swelling of the breast without signs of infection. The affected breast will be firm and usually not affected with ecchymosis (**Fig. 5**). This is because the hematoma is usually intracapsular. The etiology of the bleeding is not always obvious but is often because of capsular erosion into the surrounding tissues. The bleeding

continues until it tamponades as a result of the increased pressure. Imaging studies such as ultrasound and MRI can be useful in confirming the diagnosis. The management of late hematoma is operative and includes removal of the device and total removal of the capsule. The capsule is usually associated with dense calcifications (**Fig. 6**). The decision regarding reaugmentation is ultimately that of the patients because a new device can be safely inserted. When the interval from initial occurrence to operation has been several months, the skin of the breast has been auto-expanded and will sometimes require partial excision. A postoperative drain will be needed. **Figs. 5** and **6** show patients with late hematoma.

Breast Neoplasms

There is a wide spectrum of neoplasms of the breast that includes benign nonproliferative lesions such as fibroadenomas and fibrocytic and papillary apocrine changes, as well as malignant proliferative lesions such as ductal and lobular carcinomas. Another subset of benign tumors that are locally aggressive but are not considered malignant includes phyloides tumors and desmoid tumors. Despite the benign nature of these tumors, both require aggressive management to minimize the risk of recurrence.

The relationship of breast neoplasms to prosthetic devices has always been a concern. Over the years, there have been several epidemiologic studies conducted that have essentially demonstrated no association between the two.[21] The incidence of breast neoplasms following breast augmentation generally parallels that of women who have not had breast augmentation.

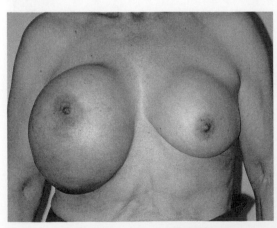

Fig. 5. A woman with a late intracapsular hematoma following breast augmentation many years following the initial operation. There is no ecchymosis and the breast is very firm.

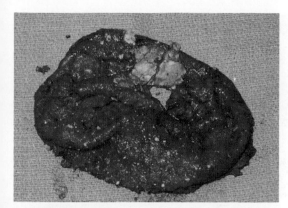

Fig. 6. A typical appearance of the inner aspect of the breast implant capsule following long-standing implantation with late hematoma demonstrating severe calcifications.

Most of these tumors will generally involve the parenchymal tissues of the breast; however, some can involve the chest wall or capsular tissues. Diagnosis of these tumors can be complicated in the presence of breast implants; however, there are a variety of specialized techniques that can facilitate diagnosis. These include displacement techniques during mammography and MRI scans.[22] Studies have demonstrated that breast imaging can be obscured in approximately 30% of women with breast implants.[23,24]

The management of women with breast neoplasms can be complicated in the presence of breast implants. Biopsy is almost always required to rule out malignancy. Superficial lesions that may be palpable can be easily excised using standard biopsy techniques. Deep lesions or microscopic lesions may require temporary removal of the implant to access the breast tissue. Thus, the specific location of the tumor will affect how the breast is managed. Neoplasms involving the chest wall are managed differently than tumors involving the breast parenchyma. The ensuing sections will focus on two different types of tumors. The first will represent that of a desmoid tumor involving the chest wall and the second will represent that of a ductal carcinoma involving the breast parenchyma.

Desmoid tumors following breast augmentation are exceedingly rare with less than a dozen reported cases.[25–29] Although they can occur sporadically in the breast, 30% are associated with antecedent trauma or previous surgery. These benign tumors are characterized by spindle-shaped cells surrounded by abundant layers of collagen with very little cell-to-cell contact. The tumors most likely originate from the capsule surrounding the breast implant and will invade adjacent

structures; however, they can also arise from muscle. The exact etiology is uncertain and may involve a fibroblastic reaction to the capsule of the breast implant. Often they are indistinguishable from scar tissue. The peripheral aspects of the tumor are often observed invading adjacent muscle structures. Recurrence following simple excision is high; therefore, aggressive resection is recommended.

The management of a patient with a desmoid tumor following breast augmentation is depicted in **Fig. 7**. Radiologic imaging with MRI or CT is essential to define the extent of these lesions. Lesions invading the breast parenchyma will require radical resection consisting of a partial or total mastectomy. Lesions invading the pectoralis major and intercostal muscles will require a chest wall resection. The benefit of postoperative radiation therapy or systemic chemotherapy is questionable and is not usually performed; however, they are considered when total excision of the lesion is compromised. Reconstruction of the secondary deformity may be indicated and depends on the extent of the resection. Chest wall resections will often require a reconstruction using methylmethacrylate or another biosynthetic material. Soft tissue reconstruction is best achieved using autologous tissues. Flaps based off the posterior thorax are considered for partial breast defects and abdominal flaps are considered for total breast defects. Insertion of another prosthetic device is sometimes considered following the resection and reconstruction.

Malignant neoplasms following breast augmentation represent a different spectrum of disease and require careful attention.[21,30] Diagnosis is usually made by breast imaging that is usually mammography, although ultrasound and MRI are also used. Some women will present with a palpable abnormality that will prompt additional work-up and biopsy. When mammographic imaging is performed, displacement techniques are used to better visualize the parenchyma.[22] Despite the usefulness of this technique, adequate visualization can be obscured and will depend on the degree of capsular contracture.[23] Detected abnormalities require biopsy that is best accomplished via open biopsy technique rather than fine-needle aspiration or core biopsy because of the presence of the implant. Common breast cancers include ductal carcinoma in situ (DCIS), infiltrating ductal, and infiltrating lobular carcinoma.

The management of a malignant neoplasm following breast augmentation is somewhat controversial. The debate stems over the issue of breast conservation versus mastectomy. Advocates of breast conservation cite the psychologic

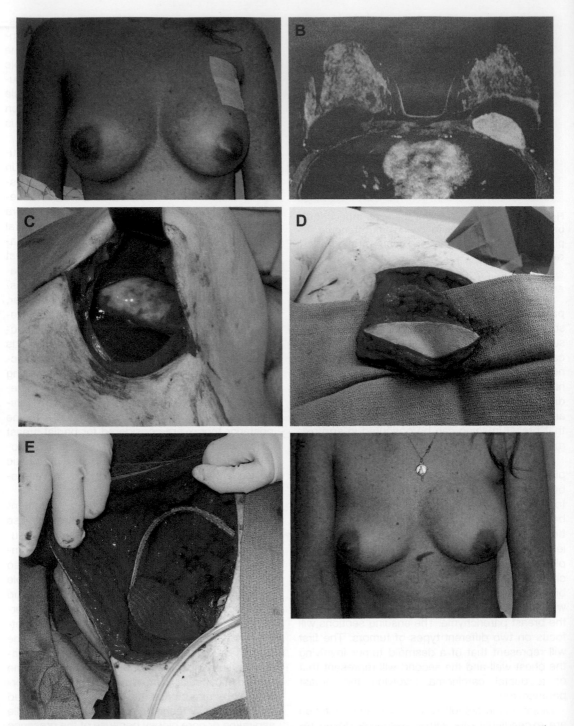

Fig. 7. (A) A woman 3 years following bilateral breast augmentation using saline devices in the subpectoral position. A palpable mass is appreciated in the left breast. (B) MRI demonstrating a large mass in the subcapsular
position of the left breast. (C) Intraoperative photograph demonstrating a large desmoid tumor involving the
capsule of the implant and the underlying chest wall. The resection included the third, fourth, and fifth ribs.
(D) A latissimus dorsi musculocutaneous flap is harvest for reconstruction of the chest defect. (E) The latissimus
dorsi flap is positioned over the methylmethacrylate construct of the chest wall. The skin paddle is deepithelial-
ized and buried. (F) Postoperative view at 1 month. The right and left implants were removed.

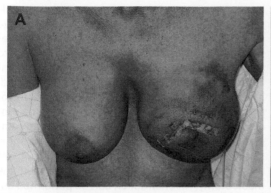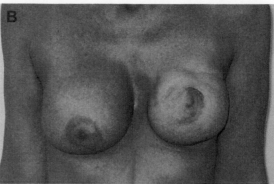

Fig. 8. (*A*) The photograph depicts a woman with left breast cancer following biopsy. The plan is for breast conservation therapy (BCT) and postoperative radiation therapy. (*B*) Two years following BCT, there is moderate distortion and asymmetry with thinning of the subcutaneous tissues.

advantage of preserving the natural breast mound and nipple areolar complex as well as the overall survival rates that are similar to mastectomy.[31] Others will cite the effects of radiation therapy and its high incidence of capsular contracture (60% at 2 years) and the high revision rate of 25%.[32] Advocates of mastectomy and immediate

reconstruction will cite improved cosmesis and the occasional ability to obviate the need for postoperative radiotherapy.[33] Both approaches will be reviewed.

The challenge with breast conservation in a previously augmented breast is to preserve natural breast contours in the face of limited parenchyma.

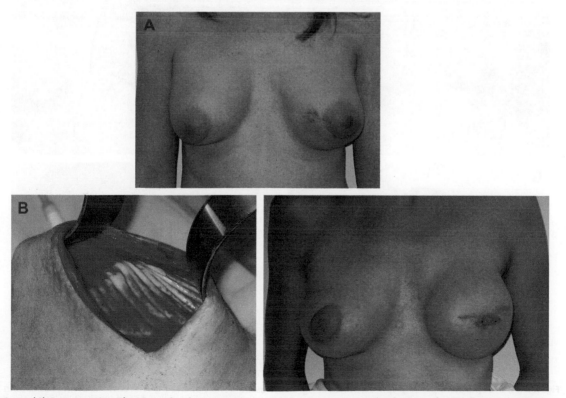

Fig. 9. (*A*) Preoperative photograph of a woman with left breast cancer in the setting of prior breast augmentation. The plan is for mastectomy with two-stage reconstruction using AlloDerm. (*B*) Intraoperative photograph of the AlloDerm demonstrating adherence and viability. (*C*) Postoperative image at 1 year demonstrating good symmetry following left implant exchange and nipple reconstruction and right mastopexy.

Assessing patient expectations is critical in these cases because of potential morbidity related to contour and the postoperative radiation therapy. Often, these women have had implants for several years and the volume of parenchyma relative to the implant is usually less than 50%. The original implant may be removed, retained, or exchanged for a new one depending on the nature and location of the tumor. The excision will usually include both the parenchyma and underlying capsule. Resection of the overlying skin is sometimes necessary. If an implant is reinserted, then the capsular repair is considered. Options include reapproximation when small and leaving the capsular defect as is when large. The skin is closed and adjuvant treatments are planned. **Fig. 8** shows a patient following the initial biopsy and 2 years following breast conservation, implant retention, and postoperative radiation.

Mastectomy following breast augmentation is less controversial than breast conservation and

is often associated with good to excellent outcomes. This is because the breast tissues have in essence been preexpanded with the original device. The approach is much like that of a standard mastectomy in a woman without breast augmentation. A skin-sparing pattern is usually outlined. If the implant is located above the pectoral major muscle, then the mastectomy specimen can include the parenchymal tissue as well as the implant and its associated capsule. If the implant is located under the pectoralis muscle, then there will be two separate specimens. Following the mastectomy, reconstruction can be performed using autologous tissue or prosthetic devices. Oftentimes, women will choose to continue with prosthetic reconstruction based on factors related to speed of recovery, simplicity, potential for excellent outcomes, and because she has already had a device.

Prosthetic reconstruction following mastectomy in a previously augmented patient can be

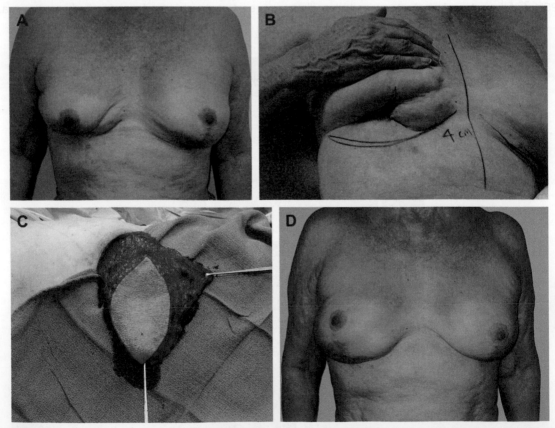

Fig. 10. (A) Preoperative photograph demonstrating a soft tissue deficit of the right breast following subcutaneous infection and debridement after breast augmentation. (B) The extent of the deformity is illustrated in detail. (C) A latissimus dorsi musculocutaneous flap is harvested to replace the tissue deficit and reestablish contour. (D) Postoperative image demonstrating correction of the deformity with reestablishment of the inframammary fold and good symmetry.

accomplished using tissue expanders or implants. If the previous device was subglandular, then a subpectoral pocket is created. If the previous device was subpectoral, then that same pocket can be used. If a nipple or skin-sparing mastectomy was performed, then a permanent saline or silicone gel implant can be inserted. If there was a moderate degree of skin excision, then a tissue expander is considered. Personal preference is to use a tissue expander because the postmastectomy scar and capsule formation will often distort the contour of the first device. During a second stage, this scarring and capsule can be modified to obtain ideal volume, contour, and position.

Another significant advancement in these cases where the reconstruction is performed using prosthetic devices is the use of acellular dermal matrix as a pectoralis major extender and as a means to optimally compartmentalize the tissue expander or implant.[34] Personal experience with AlloDerm has resulted in excellent outcomes and high patient satisfaction. **Fig. 9** illustrates a patient who had breast augmentation who developed breast cancer and had a mastectomy and two-stage reconstruction using a tissue expander and implant.

The use of autologous tissue to reconstruct the breast following mastectomy in the setting of a prior breast augmentation is also a powerful method. With many of the advancements in autologous reconstruction such as deep inferior epigastric perforator (DIEP), superior gluteal artery perforator (SGAP), and other muscle-sparing procedures, outcomes have been maximized while minimizing donor site deformities or problems.[35]

Contour Deformities

Contour deformities of the breast that are outside the realm of expectations may be a result of soft tissue infections, implant removal, and tissue loss for other reasons such as biopsy or excision. These may result in significant breast asymmetry and be very troublesome to the patient. The deformities can involve any area of the breast and management must take into consideration the quality of the tissues, the ratio of breast implant to breast tissue, breast volume, and patient expectations. Correction of these deformities often falls into the category of breast reconstruction because simpler solutions may not always be adequate.

Fig. 10 shows a patient who developed a superficial soft tissue infection of the breast following breast augmentation. This resulted in a significant lower pole deformity following debridement, loss of the inframammary fold, and significant asymmetry. Previous attempts at repair had included revision augmentation, capsular release, and

autologous fat grafting. At the time of my evaluation, the tissues were soft and subtle, the devices were in place, and the patient desired correction of the soft tissue deformity. Options that are typically considered in cases such as this include scar revision, adjacent tissue rearrangement, autologous tissue reconstruction, implant exchange, or implant removal. In this particular case, a latissimus dorsi musculocutaneous flap was selected and served to reestablish lower pole contour, redefine the inframammary fold, and achieve symmetry (**Fig. 10**C).

SUMMARY

The management of common and uncommon problems following breast augmentation can pose a challenge in some situations. The diversity of these problems is remarkable and different principles and concepts should be adhered to for optimal management. This article has reviewed some of these problems and has hopefully provided solutions for prevention and management.

REFERENCES

1. Kjøller K, Hölmich LR, Jacobsen PH, et al. Epidemiological investigation of local complications after cosmetic breast implant surgery in Denmark. Ann Plast Surg 2002;48(3):229–37.
2. Codner MA, Cohen AT, Hester TR. Complications in breast augmentation: prevention and correction. Clin Plast Surg 2001;28:587–95.
3. Rheingold LM, Yoo RP, Courtiss EH. Experience with 326 inflatable breast implants. Plast Reconstr Surg 1994;93(1):118–22.
4. Mladick RA. No-touch submuscular saline breast augmentation technique. Aesthetic Plast Surg 1993;17:183–92.
5. Araco A, Gravante G, Araco F, et al. Infections of breast implants in aesthetic breast augmentations: a single-center review of 3,002 patients. Aesthetic Plast Surg 2007;31(4):325–9.
6. Handel N, Cordray T, Gutierrez J, et al. A long-term study of outcomes, complications, and patient satisfaction with breast implants. Plast Reconstr Surg 2006;117:757–67.
7. Spear SL, Howard MA, Boehmler JH, et al. The infected or exposed breast implant: management and treatment strategies. Plast Reconstr Surg 2004;113:1634–44.
8. Rohrich RJ, Hartley W, Brown S. Incidence of breast and chest wall asymmetry in breast augmentation: a retrospective analysis of 100 patients. Plast Reconstr Surg 2006;118(Suppl 7):7S–13S.
9. Galdino GM, Nahabedian MY, Chiaramonte M, et al. Clinical applications of three-dimensional

photography in breast surgery. Plast Reconstr Surg 2002;110:58–70.

10. Handel N. Secondary mastopexy in the augmented patient: a recipe for disaster. Plast Reconstr Surg 2006;118(7 Suppl):152S–63S.

11. Handel N. Mastopexy in the previously augmented breast. In: Spear SL, editor. Surgery of the breast: principles and art. Philadelphia: Lippincott-Williams-Wilkins; 2006. p. 1457–72.

12. Henriksen TF, Fryzek JP, Hölmich LR, et al. Surgical intervention and capsular contracture after breast augmentation: a prospective study of risk factors. Ann Plast Surg 2005;54:343–51.

13. Tebbetts JB. Dual plane breast augmentation: optimizing implant-soft-tissue relationships in a wide range of breast types. Plast Reconstr Surg 2001; 107(5):1255–72.

14. Clarendon CC. Implant descent: a complication of augmentation mammaplasty and its correction. Ann Plast Surg 1988;21:452–7.

15. Baxter RA. Intracapsular allogenic dermal grafts for breast implant related problems. Plast Reconstr Surg 2003;112:1692–6.

16. Al-Sabounchi S, De Mey AM, Eder H. Textured saline-filled breast implants for augmentation mammaplasty: does overfilling prevent deflation? A long-term follow-up. Plast Reconstr Surg 2006; 118(1):215–22.

17. Brown MH, Shenker R, Silver SA. Cohesive silicone gel breast implants in aesthetic and reconstructive breast surgery. Plast Reconstr Surg 2005;116(3): 768–79.

18. Massiha H. Scar tissue flaps for the correction of postimplant breast rippling. Ann Plast Surg 2002; 48(5):505–7.

19. Nahabedian MY. Explantation of 41 year old implants following primary breast augmentation. Ann Plast Surg 2007;58:91–4.

20. Veiga DF, Filho JV, Schnaider CS, et al. Late hematoma after aesthetic breast augmentation with textured silicone prosthesis: a case report. Aesthetic Plast Surg 2005;29:431–3.

21. Deapen D. Breast implants and breast cancer: a review of incidence, detection, mortality, and survival. Plast Reconstr Surg 2007;120(7 Suppl 1):70S–80S.

22. Ecklund GW, Busby RC, Miller SH, et al. Improved imaging of the augmented breast. Am J Roentgenol 1988;151:469–73.

23. Handel N, Silverstein MJ. Breast cancer diagnosis and prognosis in augmented women. Plast Reconstr Surg 2006;118(3):587–93.

24. Miglioretti DL, Rutter CM, Geller BM, et al. Effect of breast augmentation on the accuracy of mammography and cancer statistics. JAMA 2004;291: 442–50.

25. Schuh ME, Radford DM. Desmoid tumor of the breast following augmentation mammaplasty. Plast Reconstr Surg 1994;93(3):603–5.

26. Schiller V, Arndt R, Brenner R. Aggressive fibromatosis of the chest associated with a silicone breast implant. Chest 1995;108(5):1466–8.

27. Aaron AD, O'Mara JW, Montgomery EA, et al. Chest wall fibromatosis associated with silicone breast implants. Surg Oncol 1996;5(2):93–9.

28. Jandali AR, Wedler V, Meyer VE, et al. Breast implant and desmoid tumor: is there an etiological relation? Handchir Mikrochir Plast Chir 2004;36(6):343–7.

29. Gandolfo L, Guglielmino S, Bosco V, et al. Chest wall fibromatosis after mammary prosthesis implantation. A case report and review of the literature. Chir Ital 2006;58(5):655–60.

30. McIntosh SA, Horgan K. Breast cancer following augmentation mammoplasty: a review of its impact on prognosis and management. J Plast Reconstr Aesthet Surg 2007;60(10):1127–35.

31. Hölmich LR, Mellemkjaer L, Gunnarsdottir KA, et al. Stage of breast cancer at diagnosis among women with cosmetic breast implants. Br J Cancer 2003; 88:832a8.

32. Handel N, Lewinsky B, Silverstein MJ, et al. Conservation therapy for breast cancer following augmentation mammaplasty. Plast Reconstr Surg 1991;87: 873A8.

33. Spear SL, Slack C, Howard MA. Postmastectomy reconstruction of the previously augmented breast: diagnosis, staging, methodology, and outcome. Plast Reconstr Surg 2001;107:1167a76.

34. Willey SC, Robb GC, Hammond DC, et al. Immediate breast reconstruction with tissue expanders and alloderm. In: Spear SL, editor. Surgery of the breast: principles and art. Philadelphia: Lippincott-Williams-Wilkins; 2006. p. 484–8.

35. Nahabedian MY, Momen B, Galdino G, et al. Breast reconstruction with the free TRAM or DIEP flap: patient selection, choice of flap, and outcome. Plast Reconstr Surg 2002;110:466–75.

Complications, Reoperations, and Revisions in Breast Augmentation

Bradley P. Bengtson, MD

KEYWORDS

- Defining complications
- Most common complications in breast augmentation
- Reoperations and revisions
- Classification systems
- Outcomes and evidence based data in augmentation
- Track and document patient data
- Process of breast augmentation
- Capsular contracture, malposition, recurrent ptosis, and coverage problems
- Current literature and solutions

What is your personal complication rate in breast augmentation surgery? How many of your patient complications undergo surgical revisions and over what time period?

Quite frankly, I believe as plastic surgeons, we do not specifically follow or track our own patients closely enough to know these answers. We should each know where we have been to know where we are heading, and know where we are to know where we are going. Complications and their tracking are very dynamic events. Our postoperative patient's breasts are always changing. However we should each have an idea, for a snapshot in time, an average 3- to 5-year follow-up, what our overall complication rate and surgical revision rates are, and etiology of the revision if known. Anecdotal medicine, at least in the United States, ended during the American Civil War, or the War of Northern Aggression if you grew up below the Mason-Dixon Line.[1,2] The statement that war changes and advances medicine, particular the field of surgery, has to be one of the greatest understatements of all time. At least in the United States, it was during these dramatic

times of war that true outcomes-based and evidence-based medicine was born. Every interaction between a surgeon and a sick or injured soldier was meticulously documented and recorded, and the foundation for outcomes-based medicine was born.[3] Somewhere between 1861 and now, particularly in the field of plastic surgery, some of our critical appraisal of science and data, its application to how we practice plastic surgery—the procedures we perform and devices we use, has been partially lost.

This moment of enlightenment came for me when I enrolled in the McGhan Style 410 Form Stable Cohesive Gel Silicone implant study. This was my first experience with an FDA-based, premarket approval protocol where multiple reviewers and organizations were tracking my patients and data. It forced me to look more critically at my own patient outcomes and complications. The results surprised me! I believe most surgeons will tend to overestimate the number of procedures we perform, and underestimate our complications unless we specifically track and record them. Hopefully, this article will encourage you to begin

Department of Plastic Surgery, Medical Education and Research Center & Plastic Surgery Associates, 220 Lyon NW, Suite 700, Grand Rapids, MI 49503, USA
E-mail address: plastb@aol.com

Clin Plastic Surg 36 (2009) 139–156
doi:10.1016/j.cps.2008.08.002

an increased introspective interest and sensitivity to begin this process on your own. If so, then it will have accomplished the most important take-home point. Data collection options include tracking patients with your own individual database, enrolling in one of the patient follow-up studies supported by the breast implant manufacturers (but since not every patient will enroll, additional mechanisms and tracking may be required for complete accuracy), use an implant inventory and tracking software modified for tracking patient complications and revisions, and/or finally, there is an early initiative to reduce complications in breast augmentation by one of the implant companies that may provide a Web- or inventory-based structure to assist with patient data tracking.

The first step is to personally commit to look critically at our own results and begin to follow our patients long term with a method of follow-up that we can integrate into our practices. Then take the next step: for the benefit of all of our patients and colleagues, openly, honestly, and transparently report and present our individual data. Subsequently, to be open to look at other surgeons' methods and data, other ways to do things, and then if they show fewer complications or benefits with acceptable trade-offs, be bold enough to modify or change the way we practice. Because plastic surgery is so dynamic, we should each continue to reevaluate where we are over time. Change is hard and there are many potential obstacles, but even if one of our own patients has an improved outcome or is saved a complication or surgical revision, wouldn't it be worth it? Finally, I believe this is not about globally trying to standardize how things are done or even about establishing "Best Practice" guidelines. It is about looking individually to ourselves and our own practices and to committing to do better. There is a reason why in karate there are no 10th-degree black belts, only 9th. No one can ever be perfect, we can only strive for it. Plastic surgery is no different.

> "I am careful not to confuse excellence with perfection. Excellence, I can reach for; perfection is God's business."
> —Michael J. Fox

Plastic surgery of the breast is unique in that we are not just looking at patency rates following an anastomosis or patient survival rates with one chemotherapy regime over another. It was interesting that in last month's *Clinics in Plastic Surgery*, Sheila Sprague and Paula McKay defined outcome- and evidence-based plastic surgery as, "…the integration of the best research evidence with clinical expertise and patient values into clinical decision making. It can be defined as the conscientious, explicit, and judicious use of the current best evidence in making decisions about the care of individual patients." And they go on to state, "…emphasizing the need to properly evaluate the efficacy of plastic surgical interventions before accepting them as standard surgical practice. It involves the process of systematically finding, appraising, and using research findings as the basis for clinical decisions."[4] Accordingly, there are very few things in medicine and plastic surgery that are "Absolutes," and there remains a great deal of room for individual approaches.[5] Plus we are not giving away our artistry. Plastic surgery is *both* an art *and* a science, not *either/or*. DaVinci was an incredible artist but used scientific and data-driven mathematical "Divine Principles" to analyze, paint, and sculpt the human body, right?

In reviewing these next few pages, my hope is that you will not disconnect the outcomes from the patients, or think, "Oh great, another classification system." No method of documenting or reporting is perfect. Presented will be both tabular and algorithmic methods. However, the main goal is for you to take an individual challenge. Not take the complication personally, but to personalize the process, and if you have not already done so, begin to accurately document and record your patient breast augmentation experiences. Not one method will work for each surgeon or practice, but the first step is to truly make the commitment and begin to look individually at our own results. If you are completely honest and transparent, the results may also surprise you.

COMPLICATIONS, REOPERATIONS AND REVISIONS

com·pli·ca·tion (kŏm'plĭ-kā'shən) when pertaining to medicine is defined by the online Free Dictionary as:

"A secondary disease, an accident, or a negative reaction occurring during the course of an illness and usually aggravating the illness."

Or, a complication may be a problem that arises following a procedure, treatment, or illness. Complications are more of a global, all-encompassing term and they may range in severity from minor to severe, and may or may not result in additional surgery. Why complications are so difficult to categorize is that they include many factors that are preventable and some that are not. They include factors with known causes and many with unknown or just suspected causality. To further "complicate" things, in plastic surgery, there is an elective component to what we do and certain subjectiveness. For instance, what one surgeon may deem a significant capsular contracture, another surgeon may not. Also, most of the procedures we perform including breast augmentation, are elective to begin with. No description or evaluation method is perfect, but regardless of the "grey zones," many complications are definable and many require a medical or surgical intervention. These are the most important, because they are the ones we can potentially impact and change, and they will be the focus of this article. In the past, I have defined "major" complications as those that require a surgical intervention to enhance or correct, and "minor" as one that resolves on its own or without surgical intervention.[6] This also is not perfect, a pulmonary embolus is obviously a major complication in severity, but may not be operable. However, concerning complications we can potentially prevent or treat, this is a helpful classification.

Next, the term "reoperation" has been thrust upon us and is a commonly used term. It has been described in detail,[7] but understanding some basics are important. The Food and Drug Administration (FDA), in order to capture as many complications as possible, includes "reoperations" as any additional surgery a patient may have during her involvement in a study. For instance, a scheduled second-stage reconstruction and expander/implant exchange or a nipple reconstruction is considered a *reoperation*. We are all well aware of how we alter our vocabulary to accommodate an insurance, legal, or governmental organization. We do it every day when we do our CPT coding, but we should understand the distinction in the terminology. The term, "revision," is a more accurate and better term to describe a major complication, or a patient who we are reoperating on who has had the exact or similar prior procedure and had a complication or adverse event that we are enhancing or correcting. A breast augmentation revision patient assumes that she has had a prior breast augmentation. A mastopexy should not be considered a *reoperation* or *revision* unless the patient has had a prior mastopexy, however the FDA and some others would define this as a *re-operation*. It will take some time to work through these semantics, but these terms are important when we discuss or report complications, and I believe "surgical revision" is a more accurate term.

THE PROCESS OF BREAST AUGMENTATION

There are two, and probably more, ways to generally evaluate complications. The most common is to evaluate each complication specifically and work backward to try to determine if anything could have been done differently to have prevented the problem. Another way is to be more proactive and try to determine if there was a breach in the process of breast augmentation that caused the complication, and then to address or change the *Process* to prevent the problem from occurring in the future. In the past I viewed breast augmentation as an event in time, a surgical procedure. I now look at it as a "process." This *process* has been defined and may be separated into four segments: (1) patient education and informed consent, (2) tissue-based operative planning, (3) precise surgical technique, and (4) defined postoperative care (**Fig. 1**).[8]

Many postoperative complications may be traced back to a breach in one or more of these specific *process* areas. For instance, a high implant exchange rate for size may be a failure of adequate informed consent and patient education. A high revision rate for malposition of the inframammary fold may be a technical error or too large of an implant base width, and so forth. When going through these complications and your personal complications, it may be very helpful to try to determine if there was a violation in one or more areas of the breast augmentation *process*.

Fig. 2 depicts the most common postoperative complications following breast augmentation in algorithmic format. It has been modified and expanded since its original publication.[9] In the premarket approval (PMA) studies and recent studies released by the implant manufactures and further studies reported for saline, silicone gel–filled, and silicone-form stable devices list the most common complications and reasons for revision as capsular contracture, implant malposition, ptosis or sagging of the breast, hematoma, and size change request.

The *Process* of Breast Augmentation

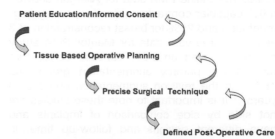

4 Key Steps to Success in Breast Augmentation

Patient Education/Informed Consent

Tissue Based Operative Planning

Precise Surgical Technique

Defined Post-Operative Care

Fig. 1. Breast augmentation is best defined as a series of four main parts or subprocesses verses a specific event or operative procedure. (*From* Adams W, S8 Course ASAPS, 2005; with permission.)

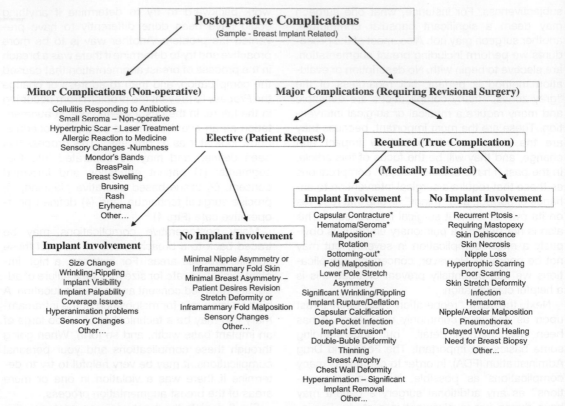

Fig. 2. Algorithmic method of listing breast augmentation complications. The complications are separated into "major" complications that require an operative revision and minor, those that do not. They are further broken down into who is driving the revision, the patient for more of a minimal deformity or the surgeon for a medically indicated problem, and finally whether the complication is implant related or not. (*Modified and expanded from* Bengtson B. Standardizing revision and reoperation reporting. Plast Reconstr Surg 2008;121:1871–2; with permission)

Table 1 shows complications data from the Inamed core data for both augmentation, revision and reconstruction patients.[10] **Tables 2** and **3** show the most common reasons for revisions from the Mentor core data for augmentation and reconstruction cohorts respectively.[11]

In the Allergan Silicone Primary Augmentation PMA study, capsular contracture rates were 13.2%, and 17.0% in the Revision cohort at 4 years. The Saline PMA data for Allergan showed a 9% capsular contracture rates for primary augmentation and 25% for breast reconstruction at 3 years.[10] Three-year data for Mentor PMA study groups revealed an 8.0% capsular contracture rate in the primary augmentation group and 18.9% in the revision augmentation group at 3 years.[11] It is important to note these studies are not side by side comparison of implants and have different designs and follow-up time. In both manufacturers' data, capsular contracture was the number one complication following breast augmentation and the most common reason for surgical revision.

We will review these common complications following breast augmentation and subsequent need for revision. We will also focus on some techniques, methods, or procedures that may be performed to minimize, reduce, or eliminate these complications, or to change our current *process* of breast augmentation to maximally impact these complications. **Table 4** lists complications following breast augmentation in tabular format beginning with common patient complaints, symptoms, or clinical descriptions and some current methods for treatment.

SPECIFIC COMPLICATIONS FOLLOWING BREAST AUGMENTATION
Capsular Contracture

Capsular contracture (**Fig. 3**) remains the number one complication and primary reason for revision in breast implant studies ranging from 15% to 30% with up to 50,000 patients treated yearly.[10–16] The etiology remains somewhat of a mystery but the main implicated factors range from silicone

Table 1
Most common reasons for revisions

Primary Reason	Primary Augmentation (%)	Revision Augmentation (%)	Primary Reconstruction (%)
For reoperation occurring in >8% of reoperations			
Capsular contracture	27.5	18.1	14.5
Implant malposition	14.4	11.7	20.3
Ptosis	12.0	9.6	4.3
Need for biopsy	10.2	8.5	10.1
Hematoma/seroma	6.6	13.8	8.7
Asymmetry	4.2	3.2	17.4
For implant removal (with or without replacement) occurring in >8% of explanations			
Capsular contracture	33.0	22.6	21.2
Patient request for style/size change	20.6	18.9	12.1
Implant malposition	10.3	18.9	27.3
Asymmetry	9.3	1.9	21.2
Suspected rupture	9.3	9.4	6.1

From Spear S, Murphy D, Slicton A. Inamed silicone breast implant core study results at 6 years. Plast Reconstr Surg 2007;120:8S–16S.

Table 2
Most common reasons for revision for the augmentation cohort

Reasons for Reoperation	Primary (%)	Revision (%)
Capsular contracture Baker grade II/III/IV	36.7	39.7
Patient request for style/size change	14.7	12.1
Hematoma/seroma	11.0	8.6
Scarring/hypertrophic scarring	11.0	5.2
Biopsy	5.5	10.3
Asymmetry	4.6	1.7
Ptosis	3.7	1.7
Infection	2.8	1.7
Delayed wound healing	1.8	8.6
Implant malposition	1.8	3.4
Wrinkling	1.8	1.7
Breast pain	0.9	1.7
Implant extrusion	0.9	3.4
Necrosis	0.9	
Suspected rupture	0.9[a]	
Tear in capsule	0.9	
Total	109	105

[a] The device was removed and found to be intact.
From Cunningham B. The mentor core study on silicone memorygel breast implants. Plast Reconstr Surg 2007;120:19S–29S.

Table 3
Most common reasons for revisions for the reconstruction cohort

Reasons for Reoperation	Primary (%)	Revision (%)
Asymmetry	20.3	4.2
Biopsy	13.9	29.2
Capsular contracture Baker grade II/III/IV	12.7	12.5
Implant malposition	11.4	8.3
Patient request for style/size change	11.4	4.2
Infection	5.1	
Scarring/hypertrophic scarring	3.8	
Ptosis	3.8	4.2
Hematoma/seroma	3.8	4.2
Breast cancer	3.8	4.2
Implant extrusion	2.5	4.2
Nipple complications (unplanned)	2.5	4.2
Delayed wound healing	1.3	
Breast pain	1.3	
Implant palpability/visibility	1.3	4.2
Muscle spasm	1.3	12.5
Total	79	24

From Cunnigham B. The mentor core study on silicone memorygel breast implants. Plast Reconstr Surg 2007;120:19S–29S.

gel bleed, lack of compressive forces, pocket position, surface characteristics, and external factors such as radiation to the most common factors of bacterial contamination and hematoma/seroma. Methods that have been tried in attempt to minimize capsular formation include intraluminal or pocket steroids, introduction of low-bleed shells and gels, systemic antibiotics, saline-filled or double-lumen implants, underfilling of implants, creating a larger or "mega pocket," talc-free gloves, implant displacement exercises, avoiding agents that may increase bleeding, submuscular placement, increase heavy surface texturing, and atraumatic techniques that decrease blood and seroma formation. Although many of these factors may influence the occurrence and degree of capsule formation, today most plastic surgeons and researchers would agree that there are two main causal theories of adverse capsule formation resulting in contraction: Bacterial Theory and Hypertrophic Scar Theory.

The Infectious Theory has been championed by many investigators including Burkhardt and colleagues,[17] Adams and colleagues,[18] Weiner,[19] and Pajkos and colleagues.[20] *Staphylococcus epidermidis*, *Propionbacter*, *Enterobacter*, *Bacillus*, and other species have been implicated. The theory involves a low-level contamination of a skin bacteria or seeding of an implant following a transient bacteremia in the implant space, and may involve a biofilm that forms around the implant when present. This has led to the development of various solutions to prevent bacterial contamination in the form of pocket irrigation. The FDA has regulated against the use of Betadine for pocket irrigation based on what appears to have been an anecdotal report in 1998 that Betadine could break down or harm a silicone shell when used intraluminally. This has made its way into the implant product labeling, and in 2000, without specific controlled experimental or clinical data to show that it is truly detrimental, Betadine warnings were put in place including extraluminal use for pocket irrigation. This original isolated report has been refuted by multiple studies and investigators,[19,21] without any policy changes. There have been attempts to have the FDA review and revisit the science of Betadine and silicone shells, but until that reversal, surgeons will need to continue to use other agents or obtain off-label consent. In the interim, varying antibiotic and antibacterial agents are being used including Vancomycin, Hebiclens, Bacitracin, Cephalosporins particularly Ancef, Gentamicin, and others alone or in isolation are being used. One of the more popular pocket irrigation solutions is the "Adams Solution," which includes: Bacitracin 50,000 units, Cefazolin 1 gram, and Gentamicin 80 mg in 500 mL of normal saline for at least a 5-minute contact time without active evacuation, glove changes, and no touch techniques.[18]

The Hypertrophic Scar Theory entails a noninfectious material such as blood or seroma collects around an implant and initiates a capsular contracture.[21–23] Some have identified and implicated a myofibroblastlike cell as being involved.[24] In experimental studies as far back as 1975, Cholmondeley and colleagues[25] noted that hematoma around an implant increased capsular contraction rates. Clinically, Hipps and colleagues,[26] Williams,[27] Freeman,[28] Handel and colleagues,[22] and others have reported an increase in capsular contracture in patients who had seroma or hematomas postoperatively that were not drained. Clinical experience has shown the vast majority of undrained hematomas develop Baker III-IV capsular contractures requiring revision, resulting in a very low threshold to return to operating room for drainage. Concurrently, there are a large number of delayed hematoma reports resulting in capsular contractures. Although less commonly used in primary augmentation, small short-term drains have been advocated by Jewell and others with low reported capsular contracture results.

An extremely interesting and intriguing finding surrounds use of the new Soft Tissue Matrix, or Acellular Dermis, such as Alloderm and Strattice, and its influence on capsular contraction and applications to breast revision cases. For significant contracture to occur, the encapsulation of the implant must be circumferential. Both histologically and clinically there is no attachment of an implant or expander, even heavily textured, to Alloderm or Strattice and also there is no capsule that forms beneath the material (**Fig. 4**). So the question is: Can a clinically significant Baker III-IV capsular contracture form with this material present? How much material is required to prevent the bridging of the capsule across the material? Although only with short-term 6-month follow-up, even for recalcitrant cases, there has been no recurrence when using this tissue. The early results are certainly exciting!

The take-home messages concerning capsular contracture are that because of its unknown etiology, many techniques should be instituted: minimizing bacterial contamination or seeding in the pocket including triple antibiotic irrigation, or meticulous atraumatic cautery dissection with prospective hemostasis under direct vision to minimize blood and fluid formation around an implant. The science would support surgical techniques and methods to decrease hematoma and fluid collection as well as bacterial contamination as ways to effectively reduce capsular contracture rates.

We also tend to be an "either-or" society, when in fact it is more likely that in most cases it may be "both-and." There are likely multiple factors at play in capsular contracture formation, and these may be different in their degree of involvement from patient to patient. There is minimal downside to practice these techniques except for a slight increase in cost. Specific research into the effects of surface texturing, form-stable devices, antibiotic irrigation, and pocket position as well as problems such as double capsule formation continues; we will also drill down into prior published data looking at these factors, and carry on new research into the etiology of capsular contracture. Until these areas are further defined, we should consider doing all we can to minimize its occurrence or recurrence.

Malposition

Implant malposition (**Fig. 5**) is the second most common complication in most studies and is actually a very broad category that encompasses a wide range of complications including lateral malposition; inframammary fold malposition or lower pole stretch (bottoming out) or a combination of both; and synmastia, which is an extreme form of medial malposition, and may also encompass shaped implant rotation and varying degrees of asymmetry. Most implant malpositions are preventable. The importance and significance of the inframammary fold is gaining a great deal more attention and will be covered in more detail later in this article. Lateral and medial malposition most often result from an overdissection of the lateral breast pocket or over-release of the pectoralis muscle off their sternal attachments. For partial submuscular or dual-plane pocket dissection, the muscle may be released off of the rib attachments but the sternal attachments should be preserved. Patients must understand that cleavage will need to be created with external forces, ie, bras, not surgically. Synmastia can be difficult to correct although it can be successfully done in one stage with a capsular flap, Neopocket techniques with further support using a soft-tissue dermal matrix. Care should be taken not to overdissect the lateral pocket, with fine tuning done under direct vision with cautery dissection incrementally if needed after the implant is in position. Tissue-based planning is also critical to avoid malposition. If an implant size is selected that outweighs the soft tissue support of the breast or if the base width of the implant greatly exceeds the base width of the breast, malpositions and stretch deformities are more likely to occur.

Table 4
Classification of breast augmentation complications and secondary breast deformities

Patient Concern/Complaint	Underlying Etiology	Anatomic Deformity/Diagnosis	Treatment Options*
Malposition problems			
Breasts are different	Present preoperatively? Underestimated	Asymmetry	Multiple various approaches including explanation
Too far out/arm rubs against	Over dissection of pocket, implant size	Lateral malposition	Capsulaorraphy, capsular flap, soft tissue matrix
Too far in/breasts touching	Release of pectoralis of sternum	Medical malposition/synmastia	Capsular flap, neopocket/soft tissue matrix, staged
Double bubble/breast coming off implant	Mismatch implant and breast, IMF malposition	Unrecognized constricted breast/double bubble	Plane position change, breast scoring, smaller implant, mastopexy
One breast too low/bottomed-out	Technical error, unrecognized asymmetery preop	Fold malposition	IMF reconstruction, soft tissue matrix
	Implant too large		
Skin stretched out, nipple too high	Lower pole skin stretch	Lower pole stretch deformity/bottoming out	IMF reconstruction, crescent skin resection
Implant spinning/moving/wrong shape	Rotation of shaped implant	Shaped implant rotation/pocket stretch	Exchange to round device, capsular flap-neopocket
Capsular contraction			
Breast too tight	? Etiology unknown	Significant capsular contraction	Capsulotomy
Breast too high	Bacterial theory	Baker III-IV capsule	Capsulectomy
Breast too hard	Hypertrophic scar blood-fluid theory		Antibiotic irrigation
Painful			Implant explanation or exchange
			Change planes
Visible wrinkling/rippling	Thin/poor coverage		Exchange to textural implant
I feel my implants too much	Implant visibility/ palpability		Soft tissue matrix/Acellular Dermis
Soft tissue coverage issues			
Visible wrinkling/rippling	Poor-thin coverage	Wrinkling/rippling	Multiple surgical options
I feel my implants too much	Implant visibility/ palpability	Implant palpability	Pocket change capsular flap, soft tissue matrix

Complaint	Cause	Finding	Treatment
My skin is too thin	Thin tissues/ soft tissue coverage	Breast glandular atrophy	
	Glandular atrophy	Overall thinning	Fat grafting, autogenous flap latissimus flap
	Oversized implant	Soft tissue coverage issues	Capsular/autogenous flap
	Implant style-saline		Implant exchange for gel
	Implant factors - underfill - or low fill volume devices		Implant exchange higher fill volume device
	Capsular contracture		Silicone for saline
Breasts are sagging	High-textured implant		Form-stable device
Bad stretchy skin	Poor skin elasticity	Visible wrinkling	Deeper pocket, soft tissue matrix
Recurrent ptosis			
Breasts are sagging	High-textured implant/concurrent capsular contracture	Waterfall/Snoopy deformity	Mastopexy, capsulotomy, capsulectomy smooth round implant, soft tissue matrix
Bad stretchy skin	Poor skin elasticity	Lower pole stretch	IMF or lower pole skin resection
Breasts falling off implants	Implant too large	Recurrent ptosis	Smaller implant if present
	Residual breasts too large	May be form of double-bubble	Mastopexy, breast plication
Hematoma/seroma			
My breasts are swollen/ painful	Hematoma	Hematoma	Surgical drainage
Breasts are hard	Seroma	Seroma	Surgical drainage/ Postoperative drain placement
Hyperanimation issues			
Moves too much/ looks weird with motion	Submuscular placement	Hyperanimation with submuscular device	Convert to subglandular
"Great at rest but how about when I do this?"	Inadequate pectoralis release	Intermammary widening	Divide muscle further, soft tissue matrix?

(continued on next page)

Table 4
(continued)

Patient Concern/Complaint	Underlying Etiology	Anatomic Deformity/Diagnosis	Treatment Options*
Extrusion			
My implant is coming out! What's this 'blue' color?	Thin tissue coverage, capsular contracture	"Holy $%#@ !!!"	Simple excision and revision? explantation/delayed revision
My skin is too thin	Pressure phenomenon/infection?	Pending extrusion/exposure	Capsular flap/consider acellular dermis
Infection			Local muscle flap
			Capsulectomy-antibiotic irrigation
			Explantation +/− delayed reaugmentation
Infection	Contamination	Infection	Attempted salvage
	Systemic bacteremia		Explantation +/− delayed reaugmentation
Size change			
My breasts are too small/I'm unhappy	Misread of patient expectations	Elective size change	Improved informed consent/patient selection
Too big	Disconnect in patient evaluation/informed consent	Breasts truly disproportionate?	Recommend size change a minimum of 100 mL–150 mL different
Non-implant–related complications			
Hypertrophic scarring			
Thick, ugly, red painful scars	Genetic component/unknown?	Hypertrophic scarring	Vascular laser/dilute steroid injection/silicone sheeting
Bad scars	Poor scarring/infection	Skin dehiscence	
	Black, Asian skin types	Sterile suture abscess?	
Nipple malposition			
My nipples are in the wrong spot	Implant malposition	Nipple malposition/lower pole stretch or bottoming out or fold malposition	IMF skin resection
Sticks out of bra/bathing suit	Poor surgical planning		Nipple repositioning
Pneumothorax			
No symptoms	Puncture through pleura only	Air in pleural space	Evacuate air in pleural space intraoperatively

Short of breath / Sensory changes	Puncture of lung	Pneumothorax	Chest tube
Nipple or breast is numb	Intercostal/lower pole nerve stretch or division	Sensory changes	Avoid division
Skin cellulitis			Tincture of time
Skin is red and hot	Erythema	Cellulitis	Appropriate antibiotics
Mondors bands			
Weird band/string beneath my breast	Occluded veins, superior epigastric vein	Mondors bands	Tincture of time/ reassurance
Prolonged bruising			
Black and blue	Blood	Bruising	Tincture of time
Bruising	Hematoma	Hematoma with textured device	Consider evacuation if with form-stable device

* Explanation without implant replacement is always an outpoint and should be considered for recurrent capsular contracture, recurrent malposition, extrusion, or infection.

Inframammary Fold Malposition

The inframammary fold (IMF) is a very unique structure that deserves a great deal of respect. The surgeon must specifically look for fold asymmetry preoperatively, and if present postoperatively determine if it is attributable to lower pole stretch, a lowering of the inframammary fold, or both, because surgical treatment is different. Acland's group in Louisville has done some very interesting histological work looking at the anatomy of the IMF (**Fig. 6**).[29]

Clinically, this correlates to what I term the resting versus the true fold (**Fig. 7**). Each of us performing a Wise pattern reduction, has initially placed an incision directly in the resting IMF with the patient in a sitting or standing position only to see the incision ride up on the breast postoperatively. This is because of the varying position of the fascial slips and where they insert into the skin. These fascial slips originate from a lower position (true fold) on the chest below and insert at a higher position exerting forces onto the skin (resting fold) deeper fascial layers that insert in a lower position on the chest wall.

Tissue-based principles of implant selection have been refined and can very accurately determine the IMF position based on the style, type, and size of the implant selected and the patient's breast characteristics and measurements.[31–35] Based on these principles, the new ideal fold position may be determined and set or the original true fold maintained. For instance, the implant size or style may be chosen as a priority to minimize or eliminate the need for fold position change. Accordingly, in a constricted breast deformity, it is important to know where the fold should actually sit, based on the implant selected.

The internal position of the resting and true fold may vary from patient to patient up to 2 cm. The IMF may be set or resecured with sutures, such as a 2-0 Vicryl. Although there are multiple methods for correction, one variation has recently been described for repositioning a low IMF.[36]

In your own patients who have had a prior IMF incision, it should be easy to discriminate between stretch of the lower pole of the breast, or bottoming out, and a fold malposition. If the incision remains symmetrical to the contralateral side and there is no additional skin or implant below the incision line, then there is lower pole stretch. If the incision is riding up on the breast then there is a fold malposition. Documenting nipple to fold distances over time is also very helpful. If the lower pole is stretched, then the focus is to reduce the skin envelope. As a generalization, the worst stretch deformities seen for revision are implants

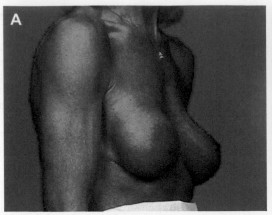
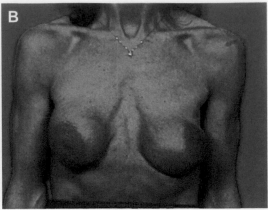

Fig. 3. Lateral (*A*) and frontal (*B*) views of a patient with Baker IV capsular contracture. She has 300 cc round silicone devices 26 years ago placed in the subglandular position.

disproportionate to the patients' soft tissues, saline implants more commonly than silicone, and smooth surface implants in the subglandular position. So a larger, greater than 450-mL implant, smooth saline implant in a subglandular pocket is more likely to present with a stretch deformity. The least likely patient for stretch is a highly form stable, heavily textured implant in the partial submuscular or dual plane position with these patients having less than 1 cm stretch at rest and less than 2 cm on stretch with an average 4-year follow-up. If any stretch deformity is present, along with a crescent skin resection in the IMF, exchange for a silicone device, exchange for a smaller device, changing pocket position to submuscular, and/or adding a soft tissue dermal matrix for further support should all be considered.

Double-Bubble Deformity

This malposition variant may result from a mismatch between the implant diameter and the

base width of the breast. Alternatively, it may occur with a submuscular implant and IMF malposition, or more rarely with a subglandular augmentation of a constricted breast. Prevention of this complication is key in avoiding an IMF malposition and choosing an implant that is the same diameter or slightly smaller than the breast diameter. A real set-up for developing this problem is a constricted type breast with a small breast diameter and a high fold. For a constricted breast, scoring is required to allow the breast to unfold and open up over the device, with the patient also requiring a concurrent mastopexy (**Fig. 8**).

Recurrent Breast Ptosis

Recurrent ptosis has been the most common cause for reoperation in my last 500 primary breast augmentation patients using heavily textured devices. Particularly when using full-height implants, they may remain too high on the breast with the breast becoming recurrently ptotic off the device.

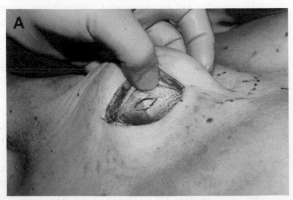
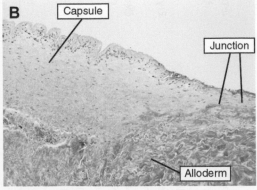

Fig. 4. Both clinically (*A*) and histologically (*B*), the junction of the acellular dermis and implant capsule is depicted. Alloderm and Strattice are both nonadherent to an underlying implant with no extension of the capsular layer beneath the matrix material. The impact of this on the development of capsular contracture will be interesting to follow. Is a 0% capsular contraction rate possible?

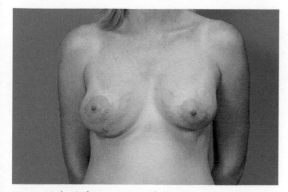

Fig. 5. Right inframammary fold malposition in a patient with a dual plane augmentation.

This may also be termed as a "Waterfall" or "Snoopy deformity" with the breast cascading off of the implant. After switching to smooth implants when raising the nipple more than 4 cm, and performing a simultaneous vertical to full mastopexy, this problem has not recurred. For patients either with an extremely deflated breast and minimal parenchyma or borderline on whether they will require an implant, staging these patients should also be considered.

Wrinkling and Rippling

Soft tissue coverage remains a top priority in breast augmentation. Until devices have no visible wrinkling, or clinical edge palpability, I typically accept the trade-offs with a dual-plane placement for the added coverage. When using the subglandular position, patients should have a minimum of 2-cm pinch thickness. However, even with adequate soft tissue coverage, the gland may atrophy over time and lower pole stretch occur. Saline devices, underfilled gel devices, and heavy surface texturing may all increase the occurrence of wrinkling further prioritizing a partial submuscular position. Visible wrinkling is also a common complication following treated capsular contraction and thinning can be extremely difficult to correct. Exchange to a silicone-filled device, changing planes to retropectoral position, and consideration again for a soft tissue matrix may be beneficial. It is a bit early to advocate soft tissue coverage universally with an acellular dermis; however, early experience with this material is very promising. Both a tenting effect on stretch and a thicker material are advantageous. Clinically, prominent wrinkling above the point where a soft issue matrix stops, but not directly beneath the material, has been evident. The verdict is still out, but this does hold out additional hope and options in treating these very difficult patient problems.

Hyperanimation Deformities

Presentations surrounding distortion with implants in the submuscular position are being increasingly discussed. Actual data on this were recently presented by Spear at the 2008 American Society for Aesthetic Plastic Surgery in San Diego, in which he found approximately 10% of patients had a significant amount of distortion enough to seek surgical solution. He noted that thin, very active

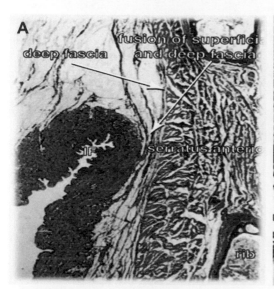
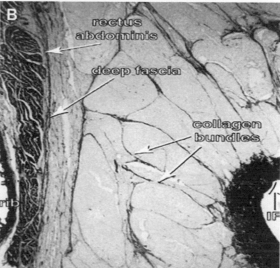

Fig. 6. Histology of the inframammary fold, *A* and *B*, show exceptionally well the dynamics of the fascia in this region where the fascial slips extend from the deeper tissues at an upward angle allowing for an implant to potentially rest in a lower position on the chest than the resting fold where the superficial fiber attach to the skin.

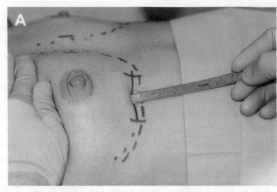
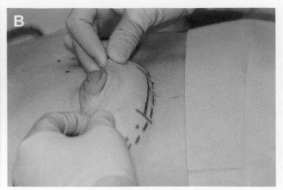

Fig. 7. (*A*) Clinical view of the marked fold at rest in the standing or sitting position where the superficial fiber creates the fold at rest versus (*B*) the internal attachment of the fascia slips that attach at a lower position down the chest wall, up to 2 cm lower in some patients.

muscular patients or body builder types were the most common to present with this problem. He also noted that this is also the exact population that benefits from more coverage and placement of an implant in the submuscular position. Absent from these discussions advocating the subglandular position is any patient follow-up, data, or science concerning the trade-offs of increased glandular atrophy, capsular contracture, visible wrinkling and rippling, and increase in distance of the nipple to fold over time with concomitant lower pole stretch and implant malposition and their frequency in subglandular augmentation. Presentations should also include the reporting of data demonstrating the trade-offs of placing these devices in the subglandular position, particularly

implants greater than 400 mL, with nipple to IMF measurements over time. Hyperanimation may also be more of a significant problem in breast revision patients than primary augmentation, and again may be an indication for a soft tissue matrix as a pectoral extension. In primary augmentation with adequate pectoralis release off of the ribs to the sternal margin and a dual plane, the vector is changed from more of an oblique upper pull to a more direct lateral vector with an increase in cleavage and intermammary distance unconcerning to most patients (**Fig. 9**).

Until more actual science is introduced into this discussion, I am afraid that we will continue to see separate subglandular and submuscular camps showing complications and problems from each

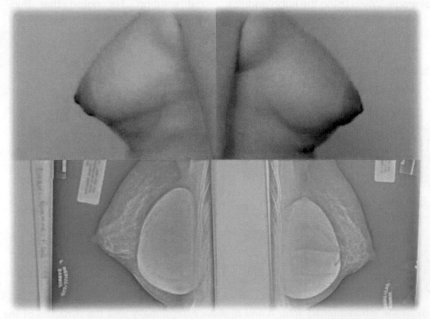

Fig. 8. Double-bubble deformity beautifully depicted on a Xero-mammogram following augmentation of a patient with a constricted breast deformity.

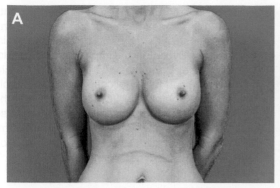
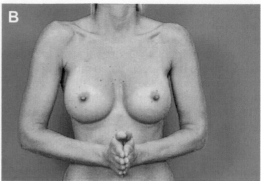

Fig. 9. (*A* and *B*) Form-stable implants have been placed in a partial retro-pectoral position with release off the rib insertions and dual-plane release but preservation of the sternal attachments. The vector of pull is changed from oblique to transverse with additional resistance of the animation from the stability of the device resulting in minimal widening of the cleavage and intermammary distance.

approach, with the surgeons left to decide for themselves which trade-offs they believe are most significant. Subfascial breast augmentation and soft tissue matrices have yet to fully weigh in here as well.

Hematoma and Seroma

Hematoma rates have been reported and range from 0.5% to 2.0%. Although some would advocate more of a conservative approach, I believe the risk of capsular contracture and not treating a hematoma far outweigh the risks if left untreated. Conversely, if treated and drained when diagnosed, healing typically proceeds normally. This is a definite instance where a surgical drain should be placed postoperatively. An additional topic that needs addressed is the use of nonsteroidal medications such as Celebrex preoperatively and ibuprofen postoperatively. Motrin is commonly used as the main or only postoperative medication without an increase in hematoma rates. In the *Physicians Desk Reference*, bleeding is not a listed side effect of this nonsteroidal, although associations have been made. One last point, as heavily textured form-stable devices are increasingly used, surgeons should recognize that a hematoma may not appear as an expanding fluid collection, but may expand directly into the tissues going down the flank or back because of the tight pocket. If significant ecchymosis occurs with a heavily textured device, this should be considered and treated like a hematoma.

Size Change

Elective implant size change remains one of the top reasons for breast augmentation revision surgery and makes up 1.5%, or half of my personal

primary breast revisions over the past 7 years. This complication may create a significant and costly revision for the surgeon and the patient, and often represents a failure of the first *process* of patient education and informed consent. There is a subset of patients who get caught up in the specifics of numbers and sizes of devices. Because of this, it is best to present a range of implants, of approximately 100 ml, to patients based on their specific tissue-based planning assessment that optimizes the fill of her breast. It is also important to emphasize that it will take 100 to 150 mL for her to see a visual difference in her breast and overemphasize that the next breast implant size up or down will have minimal to no visible change! "Even though 300 mL sounds like a lot more than 270 mL, it is 2 tablespoons!" Concurrently, if a patient comes in demanding a specific size or projection, this is a real "red flag." Showing multiple before and after photographs of patients with similar breasts, potentially trying on sizers, bra stuffing, may be used, but regardless of the method this remains as one of the most difficult aspect of the preoperative process. Truly educating a patient in this area takes time and it is very important that patients understand, are involved in, and sign off on the implants that are selected.

Over the past few years there has been an increased use of photographic imaging, particularly 3-D imaging. This is a very exciting area, but just as in rhinoplasty, until we can deliver what we are simulating, surgeons must do everything in their power not to imply a warranty and use the systems as an educational tool.

Finally, understanding the physical differences between silicone and saline are important. Briefly, silicone weighs less, and is less dense than saline. Try placing a saline implant next to a silicone device in a saline- or water-filled basin. Silicone floats. Saline implants hover and are isodense. Next, saline implants, because of their increased density and contribution of the weight of the shell, are 7% to 15% heavier. So when replacing a 300-mL saline implant filled to 330 mL, it actually weighs 350 to 360 grams. Weigh it on your scale next time. So you will need to use a silicone device approximately 10% larger just to get back to baseline because silicone implants are prefilled and their final weight includes their surrounding shell. Because of this, along with silicone implants typically being less projecting, and revision patients wanting to be larger, this information is helpful to know what implant sizes to order. This is even more significant in reconstruction with tissue expanders adding up to 80 grams or up to 20% of the overall weight of the final expander. For example, you should be prepared to replace a tissue expander filled with 350 mL with a 420- to 450-mL silicone implant.[37]

Device-Related Complications

Device-related complications are mainly a manufactural issue; however, there are a few critical pieces to discuss. Implant rupture and shell failure is implant-style dependent[10,11,30] with the new form-stable devices having by far and away the lowest shell-failure rates of less than 1%.[31–34] As surgeons, we likely remain the number one reason for implant failure—iatrogenic. The implant may be impacted with the front or back of a needle, grabbed with a forceps, or scraped with a lighted retractor or other instrument, which may initiate the problem. Attempting to place an implant through too small of an incision, particularly a silicone gel, and even more so a form-stable device, may generate damage to the shell or internal gel. A minimum of a 4.0-cm incision for a round device and 5.0-5.5-cm incision for a highly form-stable

device should be used, even longer for implants over 400 mL. Lubricants such as sterile xylocaine or protective sleeves may also be useful to assist with insertion. Evolution and improvement of breast implant devices continues and the future is exciting. By the time of this publication, the form-stable devices will hopefully be FDA approved and the next generation of implants entering trials. Also keep your eye on new detection methods for implant failure in situ such as the new high-resolution ultrasound (**Fig. 10**) to detect implant shell failure.[37]

Other Nonimplant–Related Complications

Although more common in revisional breast surgery and less frequent in primary augmentation, it is important to mention a few main principles. Always obtain prior operative notes and review your own before any revision, and at the same time do not completely trust everything you read. Have a very healthy respect (in fact, fear is good) of potential skin and nipple loss in prior augmentation mastopexy patients. Consider other incisions, such as inframammary for revision patients, and either stage the mastopexy or perform minimal nipple repositioning de-epithelialzation only without undermining. Recognize that new complications following a revisional breast operation are much higher, 5- to 10-fold in prior PMA studies, and care should be taken to avoid creating a new complication while addressing another, i.e., creating a malposition when correcting a capsular contracture. Keep your eye on fat grafting and the future of new tissue matrix substitutes, as they have a great deal of applications by providing additional tissue that further supports and stabilizes repairs and helps to prevent additional malpositions and recurrent capsular contracture.

Unfortunately we do not have the space to cover the less common problems of implant exposure,

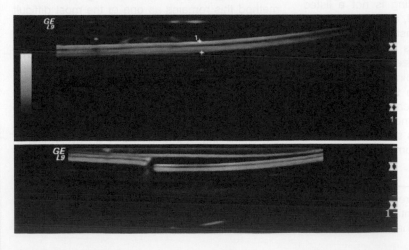

Fig. 10. New high-resolution ultrasound images of an intact and cut "ruptured" smooth silicone Style 15 (Allergan) implant shell visualized with a GE LOGIQ-9 and M12Lprobe.

infection, asymmetry, and others. Even with pocket irrigation, no touch techniques, and parenteral antibiotics, infection may occur. Consideration for placing an Opsite or Tegaderm over the nipple, or using a larger Barrier drape for suspected rupture or to reduce infection should be entertained.[38,39] Pending or frank implant exposure in the absence of a deep space infection may be salvaged. Capsular flaps may also be beneficial in these instances.[40–43]

This article has dealt mainly with the description and classification of complications following breast augmentation, presenting literature on their occurrence and some suggestions for avoiding complications. There are some excellent resources on surgical algorithms and solutions to correct or enhance these complications and revisional breast augmentation surgery listed here along with sources focused on prevention of complications.[35,42–46] Again my hope would be that you will accept the challenge to look back and also move forward to track your personal patient data, openly and honestly share your results and data for the benefit of your colleagues and future breast augmentation patients, and, even though it is difficult, where required, to be open enough to change the way you practice. If only **one patient** is saved a revision or a major complication following breast augmentation, wouldn't it be worth it?

"Clinical Impression is what's left in your chair when you stand."

— Les Hovey

REFERENCES

1. Bengtson B, Kuz J. Photographic atlas of Civil War injuries. Grand Rapids (MI): Medical Staff Press; 1996.
2. Kuz J, Bengtson B. Orthopedic injuries of the Civil War: an atlas of orthopaedic injuries and treatments during the Civil War. Grand Rapids (MI): Medical Staff Press; 1996.
3. Barnes J, Woodward J, Otis G. The medical and surgical history of the war of the rebellion 1861–1865. United States General Printing Office, 1870–1888.
4. Sprague S, McKay P, Thoma A. Study design and hierarchy of evidence for surgical decision making. Clin Plast Surg 2008;35:195–205.
5. Bengtson B. Absolutes, beliefs and preferences. Plast Reconstr Surg 2006;118:798–9.
6. Bengtson B, Schusterman M, Baldwin B, et al. Influence of prior radiotherapy on the development of postoperative complications and success of free tissue transfers in head and neck cancer reconstruction. Am J Surg 1993;166:326–30.
7. Spear S. Reoperations or revisions. Plast Reconstr Surg 2007;119:1943–4.
8. Adams W, Jewell M, Bengtson B. S8 Course—redefining decisions, practice, and outcomes in breast augmentation. New Orleans (LA): American Society for Aesthetic Plastic Surgeons; 2005.
9. Bengtson B. Standardizing revision and reoperation reporting. Plast Reconstr Surg 2008;121:1871–2.
10. Spear S, Murphy D, Slicton A. Inamed silicone breast implant core study results at 6 years. Plast Reconstr Surg 2007;120:8S–16S.
11. Cunningham B. The mentor core study on silicone memorygel breast implants. Plast Reconstr Surg 2007;120:19S–29S.
12. Wong C, Samuel M, Tan B, et al. Capsular contracture in subglandular breast augmentation with textured versus smooth breast implants: a systematic review. Plast Reconstr Surg 2006;118: 1224–36.
13. Handel N, Jensen J, Black Q, et al. The fate of breast implants: a critical analysis of complications and outcomes. Plast Reconstr Surg 1995;96: 1521–30.
14. Pollock H. Breast capsular contracture: a retrospective study of textured versus smooth silicone implants. Plast Reconstr Surg 1993;91:123–30.
15. Henrikson T, Holmlch L, Fryzek J, et al. Incidence and severity of short term complications after breast augmentation: results from a nationwide breast implant registry. Ann Plast Surg 2005;54:343–50.
16. Gylbert L, Asplund O, Jurell G. Capsular contracture after breast reconstruction with silicone-gel and saline-filled implants: a 6-year follow-up. Plast Reconstr Surg 1990;93:118–27.
17. Burkhardt B, Dempsey P, Schnur P, et al. Capsular contracture: a prospective study of the effects of local antibacterial agents. Plast Reconstr Surg 1986;77: 919–28.
18. Adams W, Conner W, Chad H, et al. Optimizing breast pocket irrigation: an in vitro study and clinical implications. Plast Reconstr Surg 2000;105: 334–42.
19. Weiner T. The role of betadine irrigation in breast augmentation. Plast Reconstr Surg 2007;119:12–5.
20. Pajkos A, Deva A, Vickery K, et al. Biofilm detection of subclinical infection in significant breast implant capsules. Plast Reconstr Surg 2003;111:1605–11.
21. Brandon H, Young V, Jerina K, et al. Mechanical analysis of explanted saline-filled breast implants exposed to betadine pocket irrigation. Aesthc Surg 2002;22:438–44.
22. Handel N, Cordray T, Gutierrez J, et al. A long-term study of outcomes, complications, and patient satisfaction with breast implants. Plast Reconstr Surg 2006;117:757–67.
23. Prantl L, Schreml S, Fichtner S, et al. Clinical and morphological conditions in capsular contracture

formed around silicone breast implants. Plast Reconstr Surg 2007;120:275–84.

24. Baker J, Chandler M, LeVier R, et al. Occurrence and activity of myofibroblasts in human capsular tissue surrounding mammary implants. Plast Reconstr Surg 1981;68:913–4.

25. Cholmondeley W, Aston S, Rees T. The effect of hematoma on the thickness of pseudosheaths around silicone implants. Plast Reconst Surg 1975;56:194–8.

26. Hipps C, Raghava R, Straith R. Influence of some operative and postoperative factors on capsular contracture around breast prosthesis. Plast Reconst Surg 1978;61:384–9.

27. Williams J. Experience with a large series of silastic breast implants. Plast Reconst Surg 1972;49:253–8.

28. Freeman B. Successful treatments of some fibrous envelope contractures around breast implants. Plast Reconst Surg 1972;50:107–13.

29. Muntan C, Sundine M, Rink R, Acland R. Inframammary fold: a histological reappraisal. Plast Reconstr Surg 2000;549–56.

30. Heden P, Nava M, Van Tetering J, et al. Prevalence of rupture in inamed silicone breast implants. Plast Reconstr Surg 2006;118:303–8.

31. Heden P, Boné B, Murphy D, et al. Style 410 cohesive silicone breast implants: safety and effectiveness at 5 to 9 years after implantation. Plast Reconstr Surg 2006;118:1281–7.

32. Brown M, Shenker R, Silver S. Cohesive silicone gel breast implants in aesthetic and reconstructive breast surgery. Plast Reconstr Surg 2005;116:768–79.

33. Bengtson B, Van Natta B, Murphy D. Style 410 highly cohesive silicone breast implant core study results at 3 years: silicone breast implants outcomes and safety. Plast Reconstr Surg 2007;120: 40S–8S.

34. Cunningham B. The mentor study on contour profile gel silicone memorygel breast implants. Plast Reconst Surg 2007;120:33S–9S.

35. Tebbetts J, Adams W. Five critical decisions in breast augmentation using five measurements in 5 minutes: the high five decision support process. Plast Reconstr Surg 2005;116:2005–16.

36. Bucky, in press Ch 18.

37. Bengtson B, American Society for Aesthetic Plastic Surgeons, San Diego, 2008.

38. Shestak K, Askari M. A simple barrier drape for breast implant placement. Plast Reconstr Surg 2006;117:1722–3.

39. Bengtson in press PRS.

40. Spear S, Howard M, Boehmier J, et al. The infected or exposed breast implant: management and treatment strategies. Plast Reconstr Surg 2004;113: 1634–40.

41. Chun J, Schulman M. The infected breast prosthesis after mastectomy reconstruction: successful salvage of nine implants in eight consecutive patients. Plast Reconstr Surg 2007; 120:581–9.

42. Adams W, Bengtson B, Tebbetts J, et al. Decision and management algorithms to address patient and Food and Drug Administration concerns regarding breast augmentation and implants. Plast Reconstr Surg 2004;114:1252–7.

43. Handel N. Managing complications in augmentation mammaplasty. In: Spear SL, editor. 2nd edition, Surgery of the breast, vol. 102. Baltimore (MD): Lippincott Williams & Wilkins; 2006. p. 1417–35.

44. Tebbetts J, Tebbetts T. An approach that integrates patient education and informed consent in breast augmentation. Plast Reconstr Surg 2002;110: 979–89.

45. S8 Instructional Course, American Society for Aesthetic Plastic Surgery, New Orleans, 2005.

46. Adams W, S8 Instructional Course, American Society for Aesthetic Plastic Surgery, New Orleans, 2005. Course ASAPS, 2005.

The Anatomy of Revisions After Primary Breast Augmentation: One Surgeon's Perspective

Scott L. Spear, MD*, Joseph H. Dayan, MD, Justin West, MD

KEYWORDS

- Breast augmentation • Revision • Implant • Reoperation

Although breast augmentation is a procedure with a high patient satisfaction rate, at some point in time, some patients will need a revision. While some revisions may be unrelated to the original operation, such as a patient who develops breast ptosis after undergoing a breast augmentation years prior, other revisions may be directly related to the surgery, and in theory, potentially avoidable. Individual reports of revisions by plastic surgeons are consistently more favorable than those reported in peer-reviewed multicenter studies.[1–5] This discrepancy prompted us to quantify our revision rate and closely examine the nature of those revisions. A better understanding of what leads to revisions is desirable to determine whether the frequency of revisions can be reduced. With that in mind, we reviewed all revisions in a consecutive series of primary breast augmentation patients operated over a 3-year period with a minimum follow-up of 2 years. The following is a detailed description of our method of the preoperative evaluation of patients undergoing primary breast augmentation, our surgical technique, a review of the incidence of revisions, and an investigation into whether these revisions could be avoided in the future.

PREOPERATIVE EVALUATION

Before the surgeon visits with the patient, a trained nurse, nurse practitioner, or physician's assistant conducts the initial interview. The initial interviewer answers general questions and provides basic breast augmentation and breast implant information. Realities of the surgery and information about implants of various types are discussed. This helps to set the tone for the consultation and prepares the patient for what her realistic expectations should be. The conversation with the patient is systematic, and begins with identifying the patient's concerns regarding ptosis, symmetry, enlargement, or a combination of these. The discussion goes on to get a sense of the patient's more specific expectations regarding size, naturalness, perkiness, and symmetry. While most patients in the senior author's practice favor a conservative, natural appearance, there are occasional patients who desire a less natural look. This conversation eventually helps guide the surgeon as to what type and size of implant might be most satisfactory. As with any surgery, a relevant medical history is required and not limited to the patient's breast history but should include general illnesses, medications, and knowledge of any family history of breast or other cancers. Documentation of a recent mammogram is strongly recommended for women over the age of 35 or even younger if the patient has a strong family history of breast cancer, similar to the guidelines of the American Cancer Society.[6]

The physician's portion of the interview begins by reviewing with the patient and nurse together

Dr. Scott Spear is a paid consultant to Allergan, Ethicon, and Lifecell.
Department of Plastic Surgery, Georgetown University Hospital, 1st Floor PHC Building, 3800 Reservoir Road NW, Washington, DC, USA
* Corresponding author.
E-mail address: spears@gunet.georgetown.edu (S.L. Spear).

Clin Plastic Surg 36 (2009) 157–165
doi:10.1016/j.cps.2008.07.001

the history and questions generated by the previous interview. The physical examination begins with a first impression, or "blink" response.[7] The breasts are assessed for symmetry and degree of ptosis, if present. The overall build of the patient is noted since there are different challenges associated with either very thin or heavy individuals. There are a number of specific anatomic challenges that should be looked for, including skeletal abnormalities such as pectus excavatum, pectus carinatum, or significant chest wall asymmetry, tuberous breast deformities, a short nipple to inframammary fold distance, a narrow base width, and an unusually wide chest, among others.

The physical examination of the breast and chest should be detailed, systematic, and thoroughly documented. This begins with measurement of the breast base width using calipers, as well as noting the idealized base width if it is different from the existing base width. The intermammary distance and superior pole pinch thickness are also measured with calipers. Using a tape measure, the nipple to inframammary fold distance is assessed with the skin on stretch to simulate the expansion of the skin envelope once an implant is placed. The suprasternal notch to nipple distance may also be measured. This is less critical in decision making, but may be used for documentation regarding nipple symmetry.

Finally, the breasts are evaluated for ptosis using several criteria that ultimately guide the operative plan. The amount of gland that overhangs the fold, the relationship of the nipple to the inframammary fold, the amount of skin available from the nipple to the fold (previously measured as the nipple to inframammary fold distance), and the position of the areola in relationship to the inferior pole of the breast is always assessed.

Once these data are gathered, a general plan is formulated regarding the need for mastopexy, whether asymmetries require correction, and the proposed dimensions and style of the implant. One should consider whether a mastopexy is appropriate if there is any degree of ptosis. In the senior author's experience, in general, if there is mild ptosis with less than 2 cm of gland overhanging the fold, and there is nonpigmented skin visible on frontal view between the lower border of the areola and the inferior pole of the breast, one can usually address this degree of ptosis with an implant alone. More significant ptosis may require some form of mastopexy.[8]

Significant asymmetries also need to be assessed. This may include size, level of the inframammary folds, nipple position, breast width, and differences in the shape and projection of the underlying chest wall on either side. Most of the time, mild asymmetries are acceptable and not addressed. If the asymmetry is significant, and detracts from the overall appearance of the breasts, the easiest way to address it is whenever possible by performing a mastopexy. A more difficult method of managing asymmetry is with different size implants. If there is a large volume discrepancy, a breast reduction with placement of a high profile implant in the smaller breast may be an option. Patients who present with significant asymmetries are told that the asymmetry cannot be corrected but efforts can be made to try to reduce the disparity between the breasts.

Taking all of the above into account, one can narrow down the implant options. The senior author attempts to provide an appropriate range of choices of implant diameters for a given patient. Frequently, the minimal diameter is defined by the base width of the breast minus the upper pole soft tissue pinch thickness. For the normal breast, the upper limits of the implant diameter often approximate the base width of the breast. With the exception of the tuberous breast and other unusual abnormalities, the implant should be compatible with not only the base width but also the available skin and soft tissue cover. In patients who have very tight skin envelopes, low- to moderate-profile implants would probably be the right choice. In patients with a loose skin envelope such as those patients who have had children or have mild ptosis, a moderate- to high-profile implant might be more appropriate. These variables define the outer lower and upper boundaries of the size and dimension of the implant as well as help make a decision whether to place the implants in a subglandular or a subpectoral pocket. In the senior author's practice, greater than 90% of patients having breast augmentation choose to undergo subpectoral breast augmentation. Most of these patients are conservative Washingtonians, which is more representative of the northeastern United States and may not represent patient preferences in cities such as Las Vegas, Los Angeles, Miami, or Dallas. In the senior author's experience, all things considered, subpectoral augmentation is typically favored for the benefits of reduced incidence of capsular contracture, implant visibility, palpability, rippling, and improved visualization of the breast parenchyma on mammography. However, there are some patients who might be better served with a subglandular implant, specifically, those who are committed to weight lifting or frequent exercise, based on a recent study conducted at Georgetown University Hospital.[9]

ELICITING PATIENT FEEDBACK

The nature of implant dimensions and resulting volumes is discussed with the patient using sample implants in the office to demonstrate various choices. The patient is allowed to wear and model the representative implants to help decide on the size and dimensions she feels most comfortable with, within the limits of the surgeon's implant options. This portion of the consultation allows for sufficient time for both the patient and nurse educator to become comfortable with the recommendations and ultimate implant choice. The surgeon should resist allowing the patient to go outside the previous bracketed options without reexamining and reassessing the situation with the patient.

OPERATIVE TECHNIQUE

The most common technique used for breast augmentation in the senior author's practice is a variation on the dual-plane approach.[10] The concept is placement of the implant in a subpectoral pocket, but performing a limited subglandular dissection to allow the breast parenchyma to redrape over the implant and pectoralis major muscle. This is particularly beneficial in patients with some degree of ptosis in the effort to avoid an irregularity between the interior border of the breast tissue and the inferior border of the implant producing a "snoopy" or "double bubble" deformity.

Dissection proceeds down to the level of the pectoralis major muscle and then the subglandular dissection is performed incrementally, as necessary. The greater the amount of ptosis, the more superior the dissection, sometimes as high as the level of the superior border of the areola. Following the subglandular dissection, the pectoralis major muscle is grasped with an Allis clamp and a subpectoral pocket is created using the Bovie and dividing the inferior pectoral attachments, while leaving the sternal attachments intact. We rarely use a sizer in a straightforward primary breast augmentation, but if one is to be used, this is the point at which the sizer is introduced into the subpectoral pocket and the patient is placed in the upright position to evaluate the shape and symmetry of the breasts. Fine-tuning of the pocket dissection is performed as needed and then the pocket is irrigated with Betadine followed by triple-antibiotic solution. The field is re-prepped, gloves are changed, and a final check for hemostasis is performed. The implants are then introduced into the subpectoral pocket followed by closure of the superficial fascia with interrupted 3-0 polydioxanone suture and skin closure with buried interrupted and running subcuticular 3-0 absorbable monofilament suture.

ANALYSIS OF REVISIONS

To better understand the nature of revisions, we reviewed a cohort of consecutive patients undergoing primary breast augmentation by the senior author over a 3-year period from January 2003 to December 2005. The minimum time elapsed from surgery was 2 years with a range of 2 to 4 years. Of note, most cases in the senior author's practice involve secondary surgery, so primary simple breast augmentation represents only a small fraction of the practice.

Based on a careful review of our office records, the revision rate and nature of revisions was recorded. In the series of patients who were reviewed, the overall revision rate with a minimum of 2 years of follow-up was 10%. The primary indications for revision included 2% malposition (bottoming out), 2% capsular contracture, 4% size change, and 2% switch from saline to silicone. During this period there was not a single patient who requested switching from a subpectoral to a subglandular position. Because of the retrospective nature of this study, the number of revisions may underestimate the true incidence, because we can only report those revisions we know of based on our office records. If a patient had a revision elsewhere, and there was no record of it, this fact would be missing from this study. The following cases are those patients who underwent primary breast augmentation by the senior author and subsequently underwent revision surgery. Details of the original preoperative plan, the surgical technique, and operative strategy for the secondary procedure were reviewed in an attempt to identify if anything could be done to reduce the incidence of the revision.

CASE REPORTS

Patient 1 was a 45-year-old woman who desired to have larger, more proportional natural-appearing breasts (**Fig. 1**). She was 5 feet 7 inches tall and weighed 128 pounds with 34AA breasts. The patient's soft tissues were of average laxity. The breast base width was 13.5 cm bilaterally with an intermammary distance of 1.5 cm and an upper pole pinch thickness of 1.8 cm. She had no significant ptosis. There was 6.5 cm of skin available from the nipple to the inframammary fold. The patient had a mild pectus deformity. There was also a 2.5-cm mass in the left breast.

Because of the left breast mass, the patient was referred to a breast surgeon. A mammogram was normal and an ultrasound-guided core needle biopsy revealing benign fibrocystic changes. The breast surgeon recommended excisional biopsy

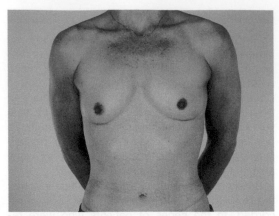

Fig. 1. Preoperative photographs of a 45-year-old woman requesting natural-appearing, larger breasts.

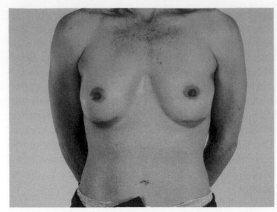

Fig. 2. Patient is shown here 11 months following her primary augmentation with Allergan style 410FM 270-g implants and feels she is "one size too small."

of the mass via a periareolar incision at the time of breast augmentation, given that possible future core needle biopsies would prove to be more difficult with an implant in place.

Based on the patient's preoperative measurements, the original plan was to use an implant with a diameter between 11 and 12 cm introduced via an inframammary incision. A variety of silicone and saline models were considered in volumes that ranged from 200 mL to 270 mL. Low- to moderate-profile styles were chosen based on the patient's conservative goals. After discussing the options, the patient ultimately chose the Allergan (Allergan, Inc., Irvine, CA) style 410FM anatomic textured form-stable 270-g implants (full height, moderate projection) with a diameter of 11.5 cm, which were placed in the subpectoral dual-plane position. The patient reported that she was satisfied overall with the results but that she was "one size too small" and that she had diminished nipple sensation, which did not return on long-term follow-up. Although the patient did not mention it, her implant sat slightly below her incision in the inframammary fold (**Fig. 2**). Thirteen months postoperatively, the patient underwent a revision with a larger implant, an Allergan style #410FF 375-g implant with a diameter of 12.5 cm via the same inframammary incision and same dual-plane pocket. The patient recovered uneventfully with soft breasts when last seen at 2 years after her revision. When last seen, she was still considering increasing the size of her implants even further at some point in the future (**Fig. 3**). Upon review of this case, the patient desired larger implants than those selected during the preoperative consult. Despite another operation to increase the implant size, the patient was still considering an even larger implant. It is hard to criticize the original choice of implant or the decision to enlarge the

implant later. The only way to have avoided a revision here would have been to simply refuse to perform a revision for size change.

Patient 2 was a 42-year-old woman who was interested in larger breasts more proportional to her body (**Fig. 4**). The patient was 5 feet 8 inches tall and weighed 140 pounds with 34A breasts. The breast base width was 13 cm bilaterally with an intermammary distance of 3 cm and an upper pole pinch thickness of 2 cm. The breasts were not ptotic. The right breast was slightly larger than the left.

Based on the preoperative assessment and patient goals, a periareolar dual-plane procedure was planned using implants with a diameter between 11 and 12 cm, which included Allergan style #68 medium- and high-profile implants in the 250- to 300-mL range. Ultimately, style #68 moderate profile 300-mL saline implants with an 11.9-cm diameter filled to 320 mL bilaterally were placed in

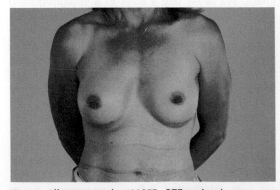

Fig. 3. Allergan style 410FF 375-g implants were placed for greater volume and projection. The patient is shown here at 14 months following her second operation.

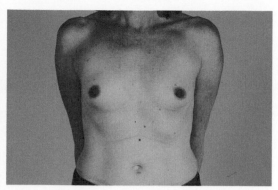

Fig. 4. Preoperative photographs of a 42-year-old woman interested in breast augmentation and wanted to look more proportional.

a subpectoral pocket using the dual plane technique.

The patient was fine at 3 weeks (**Fig. 5**), but by 3 months, she developed Grade III capsular contracture of the left breast (**Fig. 6**). The capsular contracture was tackled 14 weeks following her primary augmentation with a left partial capsulectomy and replacement of her previous implant with a new implant of the same size and style. Clear fluid inside the implant capsule was sent for culture but had no growth.

Five weeks following revision surgery, the patient complained of a mass in her left breast. The patient was referred to a general surgeon and underwent mammography and biopsy with benign findings. At the 6-month follow-up the patient reported that she was satisfied with her overall result. However, by 9 months after her revision for capsular contracture, she began to develop a recurrent capsular contracture on the left breast (**Fig. 7**). Twelve months following the initial revision augmentation, the patient was treated for a recurrent capsular contracture of the left breast with placement of the same implant in a neo-

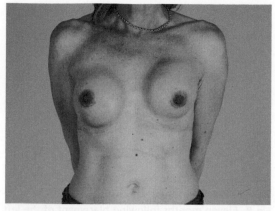

Fig. 6. Three months following breast augmentation with Allergan style 68MP 300-mL smooth round saline implants filled to 320 mL. bilaterally. The patient presented with a Baker grade III capsular contracture on the left breast requiring revision.

subpectoral pocket. This technique involves creating a new space deep to the pectoralis major muscle but superficial to the anterior implant capsule. Both breasts remained soft without recurrence of capsular contracture at 11 months following the neo-subpectoral procedure. However, the patient's left breast implant eventually became inferiorly malpositioned (**Fig. 8**). Consideration has been given for yet a third revision to tack up the inframammary fold, but for the time being nothing is being done.

Patient 3 was a 38-year-old woman who requested larger, fuller "C" cup breasts (**Fig. 9**). The patient had a prior mastopexy and abdominoplasty in 2004. She was 5 feet 5 inches tall and

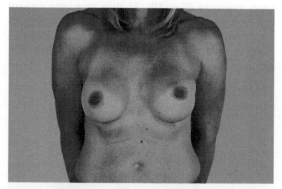

Fig. 7. The patient is shown here at 9 months status post left partial capsulectomy and placement of a new implant using the same style and size. The patient developed a recurrent capsular contracture with the breast parenchyma riding superiorly on the implant. The patient subsequently underwent revision using the same implant with placement in a neo-subpectoral pocket.

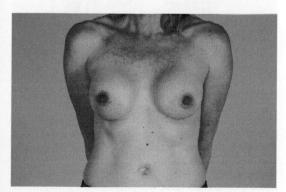

Fig. 5. Result at 7 weeks following primary subpectoral breast augmentation.

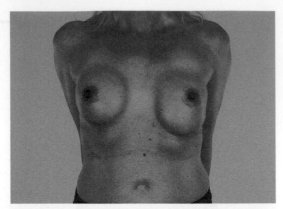

Fig. 8. Eleven months following placement of the left implant into the neo-subpectoral pocket, the patient's breasts remained soft without evidence of capsular contracture. However, the left implant has clearly dropped over time, and consideration is being given for another revision to elevate the left inframammary fold.

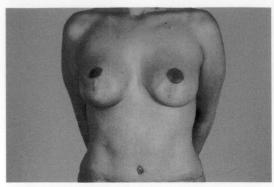

Fig. 10. Three months following subpectoral breast augmentation with Allergan style #68MP 300-mL implants filled to 335 mL bilaterally. The patient developed inferior malposition of both implants. The patient also wanted larger breasts with more projection.

weighed 151 pounds with 34B breasts. The breast base width was 13.5 cm bilaterally with an inter-mammary distance of 1.5 cm and an upper pole pinch thickness of 3 cm. There was no nipple ptosis, and in fact, the nipple was malpositioned superiorly after the previous mastopexy. The gland extended 3 cm below the fold. The nipple to inframammary distance was 9 to 10 cm.

The patient underwent breast augmentation with an Allergan style #68 moderate profile 300-mL implant (diameter 11.9 cm) filled to 335 mL bilaterally placed in a "dual plane" subpectoral pocket.

Three months following surgery the patient presented with the appearance of bottoming out of both implants (**Fig. 10**). At that time, the patient also requested larger implants with more projection. Six months following her initial augmentation procedure, the patient underwent bilateral revision

augmentation/mastopexy. The inframammary folds were raised on both sides by performing an inferior capsulorrhaphy using multiple rows of 3-0 PDS suture. The old implants were replaced with Allergan style 68 high-profile 350-mL implants filled to 420 mL bilaterally (11.4-cm diameter). Things looked fine at her 6-day follow-up appointment, but the patient was subsequently lost to follow-up until a phone interview more than 2 years later with the patient now living in Germany revealed no remaining problems and no further need for revision (**Fig. 11**).

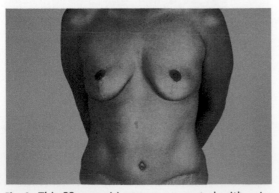

Fig. 9. This 38-year-old woman presented with prior mastopexies and desired fuller "C" cup breasts.

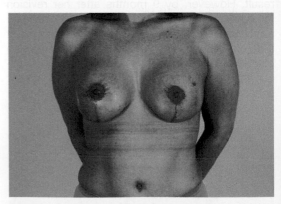

Fig. 11. The patient is shown here at 6 days following revision with elevation of the inframammary folds, revision of her mastopexy with lowering the nipple and shortening the nipple to inframammary distance, and exchange of implants to Allergan style #68 high-profile 350 mL filled to 420 mL. The patient was subsequently lost to follow-up until a phone interview more than 2 years later, the patient now living in Germany, who revealed no remaining problems and no further need for revision.

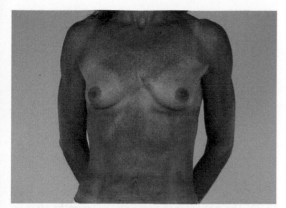

Fig. 12. Preoperative photographs of a 45-year-old woman desiring larger "C" cup breasts.

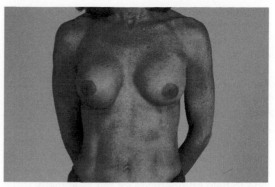

Fig. 14. The patient is shown here at 16 months following revision augmentation. Her saline implants were exchanged for silicone implants with a wider diameter; specifically Allergan style 20, 350-mL implants. An attempt was made to elevate the right inframammary fold via capsulorrhaphy using interrupted and running 3-0 PDS suture.

Patient 4 was a 45-year-old woman who desired larger "C" cup breasts (**Fig. 12**). She specifically requested silicone implants with an inframammary incision. She was very toned at 5 feet 6 inches and weighed 112 pounds with 34A breasts. The breast base width was 10 cm on the right and 11 cm on the left. There was 5.5 cm of skin available from the nipple to the inframammary fold. There was minimal breast asymmetry and no significant ptosis.

Although the patient would have preferred a silicone implant, they were not available at that time. Allergan style #68 medium- and high-profile smooth round saline implants in a volume range of 210 (10.6-cm diameter) to 320 mL (11.1-cm diameter) were considered. Ultimately, 280 mL (10.6-cm diameter) high-profile smooth round saline implants were placed in the subglandular pocket via an inframammary approach.

Three months following her augmentation, the patient complained that her right breast was lower than the left and that she had rippling bilaterally (**Fig. 13**). Nine months following her initial procedure the patient underwent bilateral revision with capsulorrhaphy on the right and exchange for 350-mL (11.4-cm diameter) high-profile, smooth, round silicone implants. She was very happy with her result 16 months after her revision despite some lingering asymmetry in the appearance of the breasts and the inframammary folds (**Fig. 14**).

Patient 5 was a 41-year-old woman who wanted to be a "full C" (**Fig. 15**). She was 5 feet 10 inches tall and weighed 147 pounds with 36A cup breasts. The breast base width was 13.5 cm bilaterally with an intermammary distance of 2.5 cm and an upper pole pinch thickness of 2.2 cm. She did not have any significant ptosis. The nipple to fold distance was 8 cm on the right and 8.5 cm

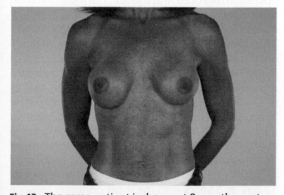

Fig. 13. The same patient is shown at 8 months postoperatively after undergoing breast augmentation using the dual-plane technique with Allergan style #68 high profile 280 mL filled to 270 mL bilaterally. The patient complained of rippling and that her inframammary fold was too low on the right side.

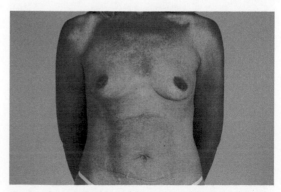

Fig. 15. This is a 41-year-old woman who desired larger full "C" cup breasts.

on the left. There was mild volume asymmetry with the left side slightly larger than the right.

Based on the preoperative evaluation, the initial plan was to use an implant with a diameter between 11.9 and 12.7 cm via a periareolar or inframammary approach. Smooth round saline medium- and high-profile implants were considered in volumes ranging from 350 to 450 mL. Allergan style #68 high profile 425-mL (12.3-cm diameter) implants were placed via a periareolar incision in a "dual-plane" pocket and filled to 425 mL on the right and to 415 mL on the left side to help compensate for the asymmetry.

The patient was initially happy with the results but at her 1-year follow-up appointment expressed interest in switching to larger implants (**Fig. 16**). Nineteen months following her primary augmentation, the patient underwent revision augmentation, ventral hernia repair, and abdominoplasty. Allergan style #68 high profile 650-mL implants (14.0-cm diameter) were used and filled to 700 mL bilaterally. Capsulotomies were performed bilaterally to accommodate the larger implants.

Two months following surgery the patient found a mass on self-examination. Mammogram and MRI revealed intact implants with no evidence of malignancy. The patient is very satisfied with her results and her breasts remain soft at 2 months postoperatively (**Fig. 17**).

DISCUSSION

The value of looking more closely at reoperations or revisions after breast augmentation is to obtain a better understanding of what the term "reoperations" encompasses and to look for opportunities for both surgeons and manufacturers to improve results, reduce complications, and lower the number of revisions.

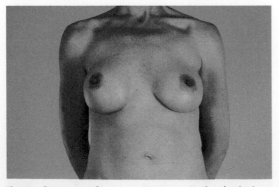

Fig. 16. One year after augmentation in the dual-plane with Allergan style #68 high-profile 425-mL implants with right filled to 425 mL and the left filled to 415 mL.

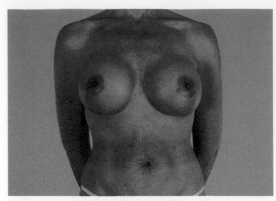

Fig. 17. The patient is shown here at 2 months after revision with exchange to larger volume–filled implants, Allergan style #68 high profile 650 mL (diameter 14.0 cm) filled to 700 mL.

Until recently and even now, the term "reoperations" was poorly defined and not well understood. It is a very broad category designed to capture all events that occur to a woman every breast augmentation. As such, it suffers from being overly broad and includes many events that plastic surgeons would consider irrelevant or unrelated such as breast biopsies, scar revisions, and steroid injections.[4,5]

Unfortunately, several groups have used reoperation rates as a means to discredit plastic surgeons, much as political activists might use rates of the uninsured or unemployed to attract attention or make political points rather than look more closely at the issue to define areas of possible improvement. However, it is still worthwhile to review prospective data with long-term follow-up on reoperation rates to help frame this discussion. The Inamed (now Allergan) silicone breast implant core study published 6-year follow-up results of 455 patients yielding a reoperation rate of 28% at 6 years. The most common reason for reoperation in the study was capsular contracture (14.8%) and style/size change (10%).[1] The Mentor core study on silicone breast implants also published in December 2007 involved a prospective 3-year follow-up of 551 patients undergoing primary breast augmentation. The overall reoperation rate in this group was 15.4% at 3 years. The most common reason for revision was capsular contracture (8.1%) followed by style/size change (2.8%).[2] The Allergan style 410 highly cohesive or "form-stable" silicone implant core study published in 2006 reported an overall reoperation rate of 12.5% at 3 years with the most common reasons for reoperation being change in style/size (4.7%), implant malposition (2.6%), and capsular contracture (1.9%).[3]

After reviewing these data and after close inspection of the case presentations, the relevant question is whether the incidence of these revisions can be reduced. The purpose of this exercise was to take a detailed look at the actual revisions after one series of breast augmentations to flesh out as much as possible what one center's revision rates actually are, what types of revisions are actually done, and whether we have learned any lessons about how we can, or whether we should do something to lower our revision rates.

This retrospective series included 50 consecutive primary breast augmentations without mastopexy for whom at least 2 years had elapsed since their breast augmentation procedure. We excluded revision breast augmentation patients and one-stage augmentation/mastopexy patients because we already know that they are a more diverse group of more complex cases with a higher revision rate. Of our 50 consecutive cases, there were five revisions (10%) that we could find after a careful chart review. The primary driver of revision was size change in two of the five. Thus, 4% of all 50 patients had a revision for size change, and so 40% of the revisions were for size change. One patient had a unilateral capsular contracture representing 2% of patients and 20% of the revisions. One patient, or 2% of the group, had a revision for malposition and finally one patient had revision for visible rippling, which was addressed by switching from saline to silicone.

Clearly, one way to reduce the revision rate in this series would have been not to agree to alter the size of the implants once the size had been appropriately selected and the surgery performed. Similarly, the capsular contracture could have been left unrepaired and that too would have reduced the revision rate; the same is true for visible rippling.

After reviewing this series, our response is mixed. A 10% revision rate after a minimum of 2 years after surgery is disappointingly high, but a 2% revision rate for capsular contracture looks awfully good. After all, is it reasonable to expect the revision rate for capsular contracture to be zero or stay zero?

The issue of size change is a complex one. It is possible there is not just one right size for any given patient, that a woman's perspective can change, her body can change, and the breasts can change after the initial implants. Although every revision comes with risk(s) as great, or greater than the primary procedure, it is possible that the patients who chose to enlarge their implants at a later date were well served by that decision, and that those larger implants would not have been the best decision at the time of the primary procedure. Refusing to offer a patient a re-augmentation would reduce our revision rate, but would not necessarily be in the best interest of the patient.

In summary, it would seem that in this series of patients, the indications for revision such as malposition, capsular contracture, and size change appear to be mostly reasonable and to some extent unavoidable, and although it would improve our data to choose not to operate on these patients, the claim of a lower revision rate should not necessarily drive the surgeon's decision to deny the patient the option of a potentially better result. Overall, the significance of revision rates is probably a matter of perspective. A revision rate approaching zero may not necessarily be the ideal end point; avoiding revisions entirely may reflect the surgeon's preference of strictly limiting the criteria to offer a revision, or may indicate limited follow-up or underreporting. Nevertheless, it remains important to constantly review the specific nature of revisions to better inform our patients and to try to reduce the frequency of revisions to the lowest possible reasonable rate.

REFERENCES

1. Spear SL, Murphy DK, Slicton A, et al. Inamed silicone breast implant core study results at 6 years. Plast Reconstr Surg 2007;120(7 Suppl 1):8S–16S.
2. Cunningham B. The mentor core study on silicone memorygel breast implants. Plast Reconstr Surg 2007;120(7 Suppl 1):19S–29S.
3. Bengtson BP, Van Natta BW, Murphy DK, et al. Style 410 highly cohesive silicone breast implant core study results at 3 years. Plast Reconstr Surg 2007; 120(7 Suppl 1):40S–448S.
4. Spear SL. Reoperations or revisions. Plast Reconstr Surg 2007;119(6):1943–4.
5. Adams WP, Teitelbaum S, Bengtson BP, et al. Breast augmentation roundtable. Plast Reconstr Surg 2006; 118(7S Suppl):175S–87S.
6. Smith RA, Saslow D, Sawyer KA, et al. American Cancer Society guidelines for breast cancer screening: Update 2003. CA Cancer J Clin 2003;53:141.
7. Gladwell M. Blink: the power of thinking without thinking. New York: Little, Brown & Company; 2005.
8. Spear SL, Boehmler JH, Clemens MW. Augmentation/mastopexy: a 3-year review of a single surgeon's practice. Plast Reconstr Surg 2006;118(7S Suppl):136S–47S.
9. Spear SL, Maxwell GP, Eskenazi L, et al. Panel discussion: animation deformities following breast augmentation: should we be concerned? Presented at Annual Meeting of the American Society for Aesthetic Plastic Surgery. San Diego, May 5, 2008.
10. Tebbetts JB. Dual plane breast augmentation: optimizing implant-soft-tissue relationships in a wide range of breast types. Plast Reconstr Surg 2001; 107(5):1255–72.

Possible Future Development of Implants and Breast Augmentation

G. Patrick Maxwell, MD, Allen Gabriel, MD*

KEYWORDS
• Breast • Technology • Augmentation
• Implants • Fat • ADM

Following the introduction of the silicone gel prosthesis in 1962,[1] breast augmentation has become one of the most frequently performed operations in plastic surgery.[2] It is estimated that more than 1% of the adult female population in the United States (between 1 and 2 million) has undergone breast augmentation.[3]

Czerny[4] reported the first augmentation mammaplasty, in which he transferred a lipoma to the breast, in 1895. Longacre[5] attempted autogenous "flap" augmentations in the 1950s, and the use of various injectable substances such as petroleum jelly, beeswax, shellac, and epoxy resin soon followed.[6] Uchida[7] reported the use of injectable silicone in 1961. Solid materials implanted in the 1950s and early 1960s included polyurethane, Teflon, and polyvinyl alcohol formaldehyde (the Ivalon sponge).[6]

On the other hand, in the early twentieth century, Lexer[8] described placing a fat graft as large as two fists into a breast, with an excellent result 3 years later. Others have described transplanting fat to the breast; however, none of the techniques ever became widely used. In the early 1980s, liposuction provided us with a new potential source of autologous tissue for breast augmentation, and surgeons soon described placement of the fatty tissue removed with liposuction into the breast.[9–12]

After Mel Bircoll[9,10] described his fat grafting at the California Society of Plastic Surgeons in 1985, a heated discussion over the safety of fat grafting to the breast ensued at regional and national meetings.

BREAST IMPLANTS

The modern era of breast augmentation began in 1962 with the introduction of silicone gel breast implants.[1] The silicone gel implants commercially available in the United States today are a refined and safer device than their predecessors. The Cronin and Gerow[1] mammary implant of the 1960s, which was manufactured by Dow Corning, was composed of a viscous silicone gel contained within a thick silicone shell in the shape of a teardrop. These early devices had such a high incidence of capsular contracture that a new generation of silicone implants was developed by various manufacturers in the mid to late 1970s in an attempt to produce a more natural result. The third generation of smooth-surfaced silicone implants, developed in the early to mid 1980s, focused on improving the strength and integrity of the silicone shell as well as on minimizing the silicone bleed phenomenon.[13,14] This generation of implants was characterized by two layers of "high-performance" elastomer with a thin fluorosilicone "barrier coat" in between (produced by McGhan Medical, Heyer-Schulte, Dow Corning, and Cox-Uphoff). Third-generation silicone gel implants with the application of a textured surface can be considered fourth-generation devices,

Department of Plastic Surgery, Loma Linda University Medical Center, Loma Linda, CA, USA
* Corresponding author.
E-mail address: gabrielallen@yahoo.com (A. Gabriel).

Clin Plastic Surg 36 (2009) 167–172
doi:10.1016/j.cps.2008.08.005
0094-1298/08/$ – see front matter © 2008 published by Elsevier Inc.

and cohesive silicone gel–filled implants can be considered fifth-generation devices.

TECHNOLOGICALLY ADVANCED BREAST IMPLANTS
Cohesion

All silicone gel implants are cross-linked to maintain a gel consistency, and thus all silicone gel has cohesive properties. As the cross-linking is increased, the consistency or firmness of the "liquid-feeling" gel changes to that of a soft cheese. The enhanced cohesive nature of these implants makes them "form stable." This refers to the implant's maintaining its shape in all positions (shape maintenance). These implants are designed in various anatomic dimensions in addition to round shapes and are collectively referred to as cohesive silicone gel implants. These form-stable implants are currently popular worldwide and are undergoing Food and Drug Administration (FDA)-approved clinical trials in the United States.[15]

Anatomic

The original Cronin and Gerow silicone gel implants had a teardrop shape, as did a number of the early saline- and gel-filled devices. Problems with capsular contracture, however, led manufacturers to design round, smooth-surfaced low-profile implants, which would move within their surgical pockets. These round, smooth designs dominated the market for nearly 20 years. Only when the phenomenon of immobility with softness was appreciated was the creation of anatomic devices clinically appropriate.[16–35] The polyurethane Optimum and Replicon devices (no longer available) were early-generation anatomic-shaped implants popular in the 1980s.[36,37] The adherence of the polyurethane surface, in fact, lent itself to the "stacking" of these implants, one on top of another, to produce an anatomic shape with enhanced projection.[32]

The tissue adherence observed with tissue expanders that had the Biocell surface led McGhan to develop anatomically shaped expanders and subsequently an internally stacked style 153 gel anatomic-shaped implant.[20,32,35] Favorable clinical experience and advanced product design led to a matrix of variable height-to-width ratio anatomic expanders and implants, the Style 133 expanders and Style 410 Matrix cohesive implants. The latter enjoy widespread international use in aesthetic surgery[38] and have completed their initial FDA clinical Investigative Device Exemption study in the United States, awaiting longer follow-up.

Silimed (Brazil) markets polyurethane-covered cohesive silicone gel implants in anatomic shapes.[16] These devices also enjoy international popularity, but to date, no clinical investigative studies have taken place in the United States.

Mentor introduced a midheight Siltex anatomic-shaped tissue expander in 1997 and other height options in 2003. In the fall of 2002, an Investigative Device Exemption study on a midheight anatomic cohesive gel implant was initiated. These "contour"-shaped devices are covered with the Siltex texture. Because tissue adherence does not generally occur, the pocket must be exact and only minimally larger than the footprint of the reduced height device to minimize the possibility of implant rotation.[39,40]

Anatomic-shaped saline inflatable implants are available in the United States manufactured by both Mentor and Allergan (INAMED), and there is debate among plastic surgeons about the merit of each relative to the resultant breast form.[41–46] This debate seems confined to saline-filled implants alone, as virtually all tissue expanders marketed for breast reconstruction in the United States are textured and anatomically shaped. It is predicted that once cohesive gel anatomic implants and other gel implants are available in the United States, the issue will be of less concern as evidenced by surgeons' preferences worldwide.

FAT GRAFTING

As with any surgical procedure, the technique used, the execution of the technique, and the experience of the surgeon affect the outcome. The technique must maximize survival of the fatty tissue, not only by minimizing trauma during harvesting and refinement but also by placing the living fatty tissue in small aliquots rather than large clumps. Minimizing the amount of graft with each pass of the cannula will maximize the surface area of contact between the grafted fat and the recipient tissue. The proximity of the newly grafted fat to a blood supply encourages survival and minimizes the potential for fat necrosis and later calcification.[47]

In contrast, when fat is placed into the recipient site in large clumps, some of the fat cells may be too far from a blood supply, leading to fat necrosis, causing not only lumps and calcifications, but also the formation of liponecrotic cysts in the breasts.[48–51] Therefore, transplanting fat in large clumps should be avoided.

Cytokines

Tissue engineering is the science of generating tissue by using the principles of molecular biology and material engineering. The main elements to be optimized in tissue engineering are the cell and extracellular matrix and critical interaction between these elements.[52]

The cell is the center of all events at the molecular level and is a prerequisite player in the regeneration and maintenance of the tissue. Use of pluripotential mesenchymal stem cells or noncommitted precursor cells are favored because of their high capacity for prospective differentiation and multiplication. The noncommitted precursor cells can be stimulated to differentiate to a specialized cell type, which declares the main constitution for the targeted tissue and acts as the primary cell structurally and functionally. There are specific transcription factors serving for different tissue transformation processes.[52]

Adipose tissue is formed by terminally differentiated adipocytes and their committed precursor cells called preadipocytes. The earlier members of adipocyte lineage include noncommitted stem cells and adipoblasts, which are speculated to exist in various compartments. Multiple steps of adipose cell differentiation involve fatty acid activated receptor, peroxisome proliferator-activated receptor γ, insulin-like growth factor-1 (IGF-1), insulin, retinoids, triiodothyronine, and prostaglandins (I2, D, and J series).[53,54] There are both cyto-inducing and cyto-inhibitory factors that can be involved in this process. Further research will delineate each cytokine and help us understand the differentiation process of preadipocytes.[55] Clearly, in the future we do expect to see chemicals that can be added before or after centrifugation to further refine and enhance graft take and differentiation.

Limitations

Breast augmentation alone using this technique can be a more time-consuming procedure, and the large volume changes commonly attained with implants are not possible using structural fat grafting.

For many years, plastic surgeons have rejected fat grafting to the breast because of speculation that transplanted fat might die and cause lumps or calcifications that would interfere with breast cancer detection. Fat necrosis and calcifications occur in patients with every type of breast surgery: breast biopsy,[56,57] implant procedures,[58–61] radiation therapy,[62] breast reduction,[63,64] breast reconstruction,[65,66] and liposuction of the breast.[67] The incidence of calcifications after all types of breast operations varies but has been reported to be as high as 50% of patients after 2 years. With advances in breast imaging, radiologists are now more adept at distinguishing the calcifications of malignant causes from the benign calcifications resulting from fat necrosis.[47,64–66]

DISCUSSION

The ultimate goal of any breast augmentation is the natural aesthetic appearance and softness, which are mostly influenced by the implant shape. With advances in implant technology involving both enhanced texturing and cohesion, more consistent aesthetic breast forms can be achieved. These implants (Mentor, Allergan, Silimed) are anatomically shaped like a normal aesthetic breast. There is less upper pole fullness compared with the round counterparts since the implant volume is distributed more in the lower poles depending on the projection of the implant. The lower capsular contracture rates can be credited to its textured surface and improved surgical techniques. Owing to the high cohesivity, the anatomic shape is maintained despite the position of the implant. In addition to no gel bleeding, we have also experienced decreased rippling, wrinkling, and bubbling with highly cohesive gel implants. However, since the implant maintains its anatomic shape, proper surgical positioning is of utmost importance, as too large of a pocket may cause an unfavorable rotation of these implants.

Even though currently the fifth-generation implants are being evaluated by the FDA in the United States, the rest of the world has moved on to using the sixth-generation devices with great success. The style 510 implants (Allegan) are an example of how cohesion coefficients can be modified at different levels to accommodate the maintenance of the breast shape. European surgeons have also seen a greater lift of the nipple areolar complex by using these implants.

The future is bright for our aesthetic patients as recently both manufactures (Mentor and Allergan) reported their long-term follow-up data. The results were very strong and supportive. Mentor's Core MemoryGel 10-year study included 1007 women at 3-year follow-up with 8.1% capsular contracture,[68] whereas Allergan's 10-year core study included 940 females at 6-year follow-up with 14.8% capsular contracture for augmentation mammaplasty.[69]

Both manufacturers had less capsular contractures with the highly cohesive gel implants. The Mentor CPG Gel study at 2-year follow-up showed a 0.8% capsular contracture in augmentation mammaplasty.[70] On the other hand, Allergan's style 410 highly cohesive breast implant core study at 3 years showed a 1.9% capsular contracture rate.[71] The data provided by both manufacturers demonstrates safety and efficacy of these medical devices.

As we strive for perfect results, it is important to continue to gather and review data evaluating innovative techniques and devices. Now we even have more options available for breast augmentation, whether we use them in combination or stand alone. While it is not in the scope of this article to discuss acellular dermal matrix (ADM) products, we believe that it is important to keep this option in mind. We have used this product in primary breast augmentations to correct asymmetries. We have used the combinations of acellular dermal matrix products, silicone implants and fat grafting successfully in a variety of primary and secondary breast augmentation cases.[72] By combining all of the available options (ADM, silicone implant, fat grafting), we have been able to create "bioengineered breasts" with high patient and surgeon satisfaction. As always in plastic surgery, our concerns are always safety and as newer technology and products are introduced to us, patient education, consent, and follow-up remain important.

REFERENCES

1. Cronin TD, Gerow FJ. Augmentation mammoplasty; a new "natural feel" prosthesis. Transactions of the third international congress of plastic surgery. October 13–18, 1963. Amsterdam, Excerpta Medica Foundation, 1963;41–9.
2. National Clearing House of Plastic Surgery Statistics, 2001 Data. Arlington Heights (IL), American Society of Plastic Surgeons.
3. Terry MD, Skovron ML, Garbers S, et al. The estimated frequency of cosmetic breast augmentation among US women 1963 through 1988. Am J Public Health 1995;85:11–22.
4. Czerny V. [Plastic replacement of the breast with a lipoma]. Chir Kong Verhandl 1895;2:216–21.
5. Longacre JJ. Correction of the hypoplastic breast with special reference to reconstruction of the "nipple type breast" with local dermofat pedicle flaps. Plast Reconstr Surg 1954;14:431–8.
6. Bondurant S, Ernster V, Herdman R. Safety of silicone breast implants. Washington, DC: National Academy Press; 2000.
7. Uchida J. Clinical application of crosslinked dimethylpolysiloxane, restoration of breast, cheeks, atrophy of infantile paralysis, funnel-shaped chest, etc. Japanese Journal of Plastic and Reconstructive Surgery 1961;4:303–10.
8. Hinderer UT, Del Rio JL. Erich Lexer's mammaplasty. Aesthetic Plast Surg 1992;16:101–9.

9. Bircoll M. Cosmetic breast augmentation utilizing autologous fat and liposuction techniques. Plast Reconstr Surg 1987;79:267–303.
10. Bircoll M, Novack BH. Autologous fat transplantation employing liposuction techniques. Ann Plast Surg 1987;18:327–34.
11. Matsudo PK, Toledo LS. Experience of injected fat grafting. Aesthetic Plast Surg 1998;12:35.
12. Fournier PF. The breast fill. In Liposculpture; The Syringe Technique. Paris: Arnette-Blackwell; 1991. p. 357–64.
13. Price JE Jr, Barker DE. Initial clinical experience with "low bleed" breast implants. Aesthetic Plast Surg 1983;7:255–304.
14. Barker DE, Retsky MI, Searles SL. New low bleed implant—Silastic II. Aesthetic Plast Surg 1985;9:39.
15. Heden P, Jernbeck J, Hober M. Breast augmentation with anatomical cohesive-gel implants. Clin Plast Surg 2001;28:531–52.
16. Hester TR Jr, Tebbetts JB, Maxwell GP. The polyurethane-covered mammary prosthesis: facts and fiction. Clin Plast Surg 2001;28:579–86.
17. Barone FE, Perry L, Maxwell GP, et al. The biomechanical and histopathologic effects of surface texturizing with silicone and polyurethane in tissue implantation and expansion. Plast Reconstr Surg 1992;90:77–87.
18. Maxwell GP, Hammond DC. Breast implants: smooth versus textured. Adv Plast Reconstr Surg 1993;9:209–18.
19. Danino AM, Basmacioglu P, Saito S, et al. Comparison of the capsular response to the Biocell RTV and Mentor 1600 Siltex breast implant surface texturing: a scanning electron microscopic study. Plast Reconstr Surg 2001;108:2047–58.
20. Maxwell GP, Falcone PA. Eighty-four consecutive breast reconstructions using a textured silicone tissue expander. Plast Reconstr Surg 1992;89:1022–30.
21. Hakelius L, Ohlsen L. Tendency to capsule contracture around smooth and textured gel-filled silicone mammary implants: a 5-year followup. Plast Reconstr Surg 1997;100:1566–78.
22. Burkhardt B, Eades E. The effect of biocell texturizing and povidone-iodine irrigation on capsule contracture around saline-inflatable breast implants. Plast Reconstr Surg 1995;96:1317–28.
23. Coleman DJ, Foo IT, Sharpe DT. Textured or smooth implants for breast augmentation? A prospective controlled trial. Br J Plast Surg 1991;44:444–9.
24. Malata CM, Felderg L, Coleman DJ, et al. Textured or smooth implants for breast augmentation? Three year followup of a prospective randomized controlled trial. Br J Plast Surg 1997;50:99–110.
25. Burkhardt BR, Demas CP. The effect of Siltex texturing and povidone-iodine irrigation on capsule

contracture around saline inflatable breast implants. Plast Reconstr Surg 1994;93:123–31.

26. Batra M, Bernard S, Picha G. Histologic comparison of breast implant shells with smooth foam and pillar microstructuring in a rat model. Plast Reconstr Surg 1995;95:354–60.

27. Ersek RA, Salisbury AV. Textured surface, non-silicone-gel breast implants: four years clinical outcome. Plast Reconstr Surg 1997;100:1729–38.

28. Spear SL, Mardini S. Alternative filler materials and new implant designs. Clin Plast Surg 2001;28: 435–42.

29. Choudhary S, Cadier MAM. Local tissue reactions to oil-based breast implant bleed. Br J Plast Surg 2000;53:317–28.

30. Papanastasiou S, Odili J, Newman P, et al. Are tri-glyceride breast implants really biocompatible? Ann Plast Surg 2000;45:172–9.

31. Rohrich RJ, Beran SJ, Ingram AE Jr, et al. Development of alternative breast implant filler material: criteria and horizons. Plast Reconstr Surg 1996;98:455–64.

32. Hester TR, Cukic J. Use of stacked polyurethane-covered mammary implants in aesthetic and reconstructive breast surgery. Plast Reconstr Surg 1990;10:503–9.

33. Hammond DC, Perry LC, Maxwell GP, et al. Morphologic analysis of tissue expander shape using a biomechanical model. Plast Reconstr Surg 1993;92:255–62.

34. Maxwell GP. Breast reconstruction utilizing subcutaneous tissue expansion followed by polyure-thane-covered silicone implants. [discussion]. Plast Reconstr Surg 1991;88:640–8.

35. Maxwell GP, Spear SL. Two-Stage breast reconstruction using biodimensional system. Santa Barbara (CA): McGhan Medical Corporation; 1995.

36. Ashley FL. Further studies on the natural-Y breast prosthesis. Plast Reconstr Surg 1972;49:414–9.

37. Capozzi A, Pennisi VR. Clinical experience with polyurethane-covered gel-filled mammary prosthe-ses. Plast Reconstr Surg 1981;68:512–9.

38. Bronz G. A comparison of naturally shaped and round implants. Aesthetic Surg J 2002;22:238–45.

39. Baeke JL. Breast deformity caused by anatomical or teardrop implant rotation. Plast Reconstr Surg 2002; 109:2555–62.

40. Hamas RS. The postoperative shape of round and teardrop saline-filled breast implants. Aesthetic Surg J 1999;19:369–75.

41. Hamas RS. The comparative dimensions of round and anatomical saline-filled breast implants. Aes-thetic Surg J 2000;20:281–9.

42. Hobar PC, Gutowski K. Experience with anatomic breast implants. Clin Plast Surg 2001;28:553–62.

43. Tebbetts JB. Breast augmentation with full-height anatomic saline implants: the pros and cons. Clin Plast Surg 2001;28:567–73.

44. Tebbetts JB, Tebbetts TB. The best breast: the ultimate discriminating woman's guide to breast augmentation. Dallas (TX): CosmetXpertise; 1999.

45. Kessler DA, Merkatz RB, Schapiro RA. A call for higher standards for breast implants. J Am Med Assoc 1993;270:2607–15.

46. Kessler DA. The basis of the FDA's decision based on breast implants. N Engl J Med 1992;326: 1713–20.

47. Coleman SR, Saboeiro AP. Fat grafting to the breast revisited, safety and efficacy. Plast Reconstr Surg 2007;119:775–83.

48. Castello JR, Barros J, Vazquez R. Giant liponecrotic pseudocyst after breast augmentation by fat injection. Plast Reconstr Surg 1999;103:291–9.

49. Maillard GF. Liponecrotic cysts after augmentation mammaplasty with fat injections. Aesthetic Plast Surg 1994;18:405–9.

50. Montanana VJ, Baena MP, Benito RJ. Complications of autografting fat obtained by liposuction. Plast Re-constr Surg 1990;85:638–45.

51. Kwak JY, Lee SH, Park HL, et al. Sonographic findings in complications of cosmetic breast augmentation with autologous fat obtained by liposuction. J Clin Ultrasound 2004;32:299–308.

52. Shenaq SM, Yuskel E. New research in breast re-construction: adipose tissue engineering. Clin Plast Surg 2002;29:111–20.

53. Hauner H, Petruschke TH, Rohrig K. Effects of epidermal growth factor, platelet growth factor and fibroblastgrowth factor on human adipocyte development and function. Eur J Clin Invest 1995;25: 90–9.

54. Gregorie FM, Smas CM, Sul HS. Understanding adipocyte differentiation. Physiol Rev 1998;78:783–90.

55. Katz AJ, Llull R, Hedrick MH, et al. Emerging approaches to the tissue engineering of fat. Clin Plast Surg 1999;26:587–94.

56. Isaacs G, Rozner L, Tudball C. Breast lumps after reduction mammaplasty. Ann Plast Surg 1985;15: 394–9.

57. Kneeshaw PJ, Lowry M, Manton D, et al. Differentiation of benign from malignant breast disease associated with screening detected microcalcifications using dynamic contrast enhanced magnetic resonance imaging. Breast 2006; 15:29–39.

58. Huch RA, Kunzi W, Debatin JF, et al. MR imaging of the augmented breast. Eur Radiol 1998;8:371–9.

59. Handel N, Jensen JA, Black Q, et al. The fate of breast implants: a critical analysis of complications and outcomes. Plast Reconstr Surg 1995;96:1521–30.

60. Leibman AJ, Kruse BD. Imaging of breast cancer after augmentation mammaplasty. Ann Plast Surg 1993;30:111–9.

61. Fodor J, Udvarhelyi N, Gulyas G, et al. Ossifying calcification of breast implant capsule. Plast Reconstr Surg 2004;113:1880–8.

62. Cyrlak D, Carpenter PM. Breast imaging case of the day: fat necrosis of the breast. Radiographics 1999; 19:S80–9.

63. Netscher D, Meade RA, Friedman JD, et al. Mammography and reduction mammaplasty. Aesthetic Surg J 1999;19:445–51.

64. Mandrekas AD, Assimakopoulos GI, Mastorakos DP, et al. Fat necrosis following breast reduction. Br J Plast Surg 1994;47:560–9.

65. Leibman AJ, Styblo TM, Bostwick J. Mammography of the postreconstruction breast. Plast Reconstr Surg 1997;99:698–775.

66. Mendelson EB. Evaluation of the postoperative breast. Radiol Clin North Am 1992;30:107–15.

67. Abboud M, Vadoud-Seyedi J, De Mey A, et al. Incidence of calcifications in the breast after surgical reduction and liposuction. Plast Reconstr Surg 1995;96:620–8.

68. Cunningham B. The mentor core study on silicone memorygel breast implants. Plast Reconstr Surg 2007;120:19S–29S.

69. Spear SL, Murphy DK, Slicton A, et al. Inamed silicone breast implant core study results at 6 years. Plast Reconstr Surg 2007;120:8S–16S.

70. Cunningham B. The mentor study on contour profile gel silicone memorygel breast implants. Plast Reconstr Surg 2007;120:33S–9S.

71. Bengtson BP, Van Natta BW, Murphy DK, et al. Style 410 highly cohesive silicone breast implant core study results at 3 years. Plast Reconstr Surg 2007;120:40S–8S.

72. Harrington H, Gabriel A, Gupta S, et al. Revisionary breast augmentation and augmentation/mastopexy with acellular dermal matrix. Abstract presented at California Society of Plastic Surgeons Annual Meeting, June 5–8, 2008.

Index

Note: Page numbers of article titles are in **boldface** type.

A

Anatomic shaped implants, 5–6, 168

B

Biocell textured implants, 4–5
Breast, asymmetries of volume and contour of,
    primary breast augmentation in, 129–130
    contour deformities of, following primary breast
      augmentation, 136, 137
    esthetics of, changes in, and long-term
      outcomes, 76
    neoplasms of, following primary breast
      augmentation, 133–137
    nerve supply of, 50
    rippling and wrinkling of, following primary breast
      augmentation, 131–132, 151–152
Breast augmentation, 1988–1992 (crisis), 15–17
    1993–1995 (dark years), 15–17
    1962–1988 (prologue to problems), 15–17
    1996–2000 (quiet years), 18–19
    2006 and beyond (future promise), 19–20
    2000–present (enlightenment), 19
    aesthetic outcome following, assessment of,
      23–24
    and implants, possible future development of,
      167–172
    capsular contracture following, 142–145, 150
    case for doing better in, 77–78
    complications of, classification of, 146–151
      reoperations and revisions in, **139–156**
    device-related complications following, 154–155
    double-bubble deformity following, 151, 152
    form-stable devices in, 77
    hematoma and seroma following, 153
    history of, 1, 15
    hyperanimation deformities following, 152–153
    implant malposition following, 145, 151
    incidence of, 1, 23
    inframammary approach to. See *Inframammary
      approach to augmentation*.
    inframammary fold following, 145–150
    measuring patient outcomes in, BREAST-Q©
      augmentation module, **23–32**
    patient-reported outcome measures (PROMS),
      23–24
    periareolar approach to. See *Periareolar approach
      to augmentation*.
    primary, anatomy of revisions after, **157–165**
      contour deformities following, 136, 137

hematoma following, 128
implant displacement following, 130–131
in asymmetries of breast volume and contour,
    129–130
infection following, 128
late hematoma following, 132
neoplasms of breast following, 132–137
postoperative complications of, 127–128
problems after, management of, **127–138**
revisions after, analysis of, 159
    case reports of, 159–164
    operative technique for, 159
    patient feedback for, 158–159
    preoperative evaluation for, 157–158
rippling and wrinkling following, 131–132,
    151–152
process of, 141–142
recurrent breast ptosis following, 151
revisions of, 143–144
size change revisions following, 153–154
transaxillary approach to. See *Transaxillary
    approach to augmentation*.
transumbilical. See *Transumbilical breast
    augmentation*.
with silicone gel implants, 167–168
Breast implants. See also specific types of implants.
    anatomic shapes of, 5–6, 168
    and breast augmentation, possible future
      development of, **167–172**
    capsular contracture and, 8–10
    cohesion in, 168
    displacement of, following primary breast
      augmentation, 129–130
    evolution of, **1–13**
    history of, and Food and Drug Administration,
      15–21
    malposition of, following breast augmentation,
      145, 151
    safety and regulatory issues concerning, 6–7
    shaped, evolution of, 75
    Siltex-covered, 5
    technologically advanced, 168
    textured-surface, 3–5
    trilucent, 5
Breast pocket irrigation, 120–121
    alternative solutions for, 119–120
BREAST-Q© augmentation module, development of,
    25–27
    cognitive debriefing interviews in, 27
    development of conceptual model, 25–26
    field testing and final scale development in,
      26–27

Clin Plastic Surg 36 (2009) 173–175
doi:10.1016/S0094-1298(08)00115-6

Moving?

Make sure your subscription moves with you!

To notify us of your new address, find your **Clinics Account Number** (located on your mailing label above your name), and contact customer service at:

E-mail: elspcs@elsevier.com

800-654-2452 (subscribers in the U.S. & Canada)
314-453-7041 (subscribers outside of the U.S. & Canada)

Fax number: 314-523-5170

Elsevier Periodicals Customer Service
11830 Westline Industrial Drive
St. Louis, MO 63146

*To ensure uninterrupted delivery of your subscription, please notify us at least 4 weeks in advance of move.

Printed and bound by CPI Group (UK) Ltd, Croydon, CR0 4YY

03/10/2024

01040362-0015